Perspectives on Cancer Care

Perspectives on Cancer Care

Edited by

Josephine (Tonks) N Fawcett

BSc (Hons) RN MSc RNT FHEA

Anne McQueen

BA RGN SCM RCNT NT MSc MPhil FHEA

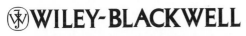

WILEY-BLACKWELL

A John Wiley & Sons, Ltd., Publication

This edition first published 2011
© 2011 Blackwell Publishing Ltd

Blackwell Publishing was acquired by John Wiley & Sons in February 2007. Blackwell's publishing program has been merged with Wiley's global Scientific, Technical and Medical business to form Wiley-Blackwell.

Registered office: John Wiley & Sons Ltd, The Atrium, Southern Gate, Chichester, West Sussex, PO19 8SQ, UK

Editorial offices: 9600 Garsington Road, Oxford, OX4 2DQ, UK
          The Atrium, Southern Gate, Chichester, West Sussex, PO19 8SQ, UK
          2121 State Avenue, Ames, Iowa 50014-8300, USA

For details of our global editorial offices, for customer services and for information about how to apply for permission to reuse the copyright material in this book please see our website at www.wiley.com/wiley-blackwell.

The right of the author to be identified as the author of this work has been asserted in accordance with the UK Copyright, Designs and Patents Act 1988.

Library of Congress Cataloging-in-Publication Data

Perspectives on cancer care / edited by Josephine (Tonks) N. Fawcett and Anne McQueen.
p. ; cm.
Includes bibliographical references and index.
ISBN 978-1-4051-9570-6 (pbk. : alk. paper) 1. Cancer–Nursing. 2. Cancer–Patients–Care. I. Fawcett, Josephine N. II. McQueen, Anne.
[DNLM: 1. Neoplasms. 2. Patient Care. QZ 200 P4671 2011]
RC266.P48 2011
616.99'40231–dc22

                                                                                                    2010020479

A catalogue record for this book is available from the British Library.

This book is published in the following electronic formats: ePDF 9781444329315; ePub 9781444329322

Set in 10/12.5pt Times Roman by Thomson Digital, Noida, India.
Printed and bound in Malaysia by Vivar Printing Sdn Bhd

1 2011

Contents

Colour plate section follows page 50

Contributors

Ashley Brown, MD (London), FRCS (England), is currently Demonstrator of Human Anatomy in the University of Cambridge and teacher in Surgery at the London School of Surgery, Imperial College London, UK.

Patricia B. Campbell, BS, RGN, MS, is Clinical Nurse Specialist, Clinical Trials, Cancer and Palliative Care, Western General Hospital, Edinburgh, UK.

Roseanne Cetnarskyj, PhD, PG cert (education), BSc(SPQ), RGN, is Lecturer in Nursing/ Honorary Genetics Counsellor, School of Nursing, Midwifery and Social Care, Edinburgh Napier University, Edinburgh, UK.

Margaret Colquhoun, MA, RGN, SCM, MN, PG cert (TLHE), is Senior Nurse Lecturer at St Columba's Hospice, Edinburgh, UK.

Antonia Dean, BSc(HONS), Dip onc nurs, PG cert (counselling), is Clinical Nurse Specialist, Breast Cancer Care, London, UK.

Josephine (Tonks) N. Fawcett, BSc (HONS), MSC, RN, RNT, FHEA, is Senior Lecturer, Nursing Studies, School of Health in Social Science, The University of Edinburgh, Edinburgh, UK. Honorary Senior Lecturer, NHS Lothian University Hospitals Division, Edinburgh UK.

Rachel Haigh, RGN, BSC, PGDip, MSc, is Colorectal Cancer Nurse Specialist, Edinburgh Cancer Centre, Western General Hospital, Edinburgh, UK.

Vicky Hill, BA, BSC, RGN, RN (mental health), is Clinical Audit and Effectiveness Facilitator at St Columba's Hospice, Edinburgh, UK.

Gillian Knowles, RGN, BA, MPhil, is Nurse Consultant in Cancer, Edinburgh Cancer Centre, Western General Hospital, Edinburgh, UK.

Rosemary Mander, MSC, PhD, RGN, SCM, MTD, is Emeritus Professor of Midwifery in the School of Health In Social Science The University of Edinburgh, Edinburgh, UK.

Shanne McNamara, RGN, Diploma Cancer Nursing, MSC, is Specialist Nurse for Neuro-oncology, Edinburgh Centre for Neuro-oncology, Western General Hospital, Edinburgh, UK.

Anne McQueen, BA, MSC, Mphil, RGN, SCM, RCNT, NT, FHEA, is Honorary Lecturer, Nursing Studies, School of Health in Social Science, The University of Edinburgh, Edinburgh, UK.

Papiya B. Russell, BMedsci (pharmacology), MB, ChB, MRCP(UK), is Staff Grade Physician in Palliative Medicine, Marie Curie Hospice, Edinburgh, UK.

Lillian Sung, MD, PhD, is Clinician Scientist at The Hospital for Sick Children, as well as an Associate Professor in the Pediatrics and Health Policy Management and Evaluation Departments at the University of Toronto, Toronto, Canada.

Anil Tandon, MB, BS, FRACP, is Consultant Physician, Palliative Care Service, Sir Charles Gairdner Hospital, Perth, Australia.

Deborah Tomlinson, MN, RN, Dip Cancer Nursing, is Clinical Research Nurse Coordinator, Child Health Evaluative Sciences, The Hospital for Sick Children, Toronto, Canada.

Foreword

The original proposal for this book described it as a 'reader' and, in the era of sound-bites delivered by kilobytes, this is very welcome. I am as guilty as anyone of turning to a well-known search engine for every bit of information I need, rarely reaching for the book-shelves. In fact, I pride myself in being able to answer every question posed by my research students within minutes, by the above means; the supervision session usually ending with 'You could have done that!' With information being so readily available – but often only precisely what you needed to know and no more, and not always from a verifiable source – a reader seems the perfect antidote to the relatively recent phenomenon of 'hit and run' learning.

Perspectives on Cancer Care is described by the editors as a book that will inspire, offer insight, enhance knowledge and encourage best practice, and as one that will sit alongside more comprehensive cancer textbooks. As such, the book presents expert views that would have been unlikely to be gathered together under another cover. Had these authors been writing a textbook, they would have been less free to express their expert views, given that textbooks can often constrain writers rather than get the best out of them.

Few of us have not been touched by cancer, either as a matter of personal experience or the experience of a close family member. Despite some of the outer fringes of the 'let's be positive about the cancer experience' movement, it is a fact that more people now live with and through cancer to survival than ever before. Many reflect on the time as life-changing and on having found new resources and inner strength. However, as the first editor, Tonks Fawcett, says in her opening chapter on the cancer experience: 'Once said, in terms of a diagnosis, the word cancer cannot be unsaid.' I am not aware of anybody who has welcomed a diagnosis of cancer, nor has it elicited envy in others as a result. This opening chapter is an excellent essay on cancer and deserves to be read widely as it reflects on the medical, sociological and even the political aspects of cancer, and offers insights into the personal journey. Realistically, the book ends with end-of-life care; cancer continues to kill people who, without expert care, will suffer pain and distress which will instil fear in those close to them and, so much worse, may lead to the loss of hope.

Without some knowledge of molecular biology and the insensible second-by-second homeostatic adjustments that our bodies make – and just how close we live to cancer in our daily existence – few of us know how likely we are to develop some kind of cancer. I write this in my mid 50s, knowing full well that I harbour (as does every man of my age) cellular changes in my prostate that the prospect of longevity only makes more likely to manifest itself as cancer of the prostate. Therefore, for many, survival into old age with the decline in the protective mechanisms which, for lack of a better metaphor, 'fight' cancer at the level of our DNA, makes the development of cancer a strong possibility. For some, however, this prospect is heightened by not choosing their parents carefully and, speaking from personal experience, I am now filmed from a particular angle that few would choose voluntarily, every five years, through my poor choice of parents. The inclusion of a chapter on genetics and cancer is, therefore, entirely appropriate.

It is impossible to mention every author in the book in the space available, and this is not a review, but three other chapters in *Perspectives on Cancer Care* deserve special attention, purely from the perspective of novelty. Rosemary Mander's chapter on the care of the childbearing woman with cancer presents a situation that few would automatically consider when they think of cancer: bringing forth new life in a body that is having its own struggle to survive. While Mander, a midwife, may not agree with me, childbearing seems sufficiently dangerous without the added stress of cancer and there is a great deal more to consider than merely the effect on the woman: what effect does treatment have on the rapidly developing fetus, and is breast-feeding possible while taking chemotherapy? Ashley Brown considers cancer and the surgeon, and even raises the possibility of surgeons becoming redundant with respect to cancer as medical treatments become more successful. Metaphors about turkeys and Christmas come to mind and Brown – a surgeon – describes the changing role of the surgeon and the new possibilities that are developing for different types and levels of surgical intervention as cancer treatment improves. The third chapter worth mentioning in this light is the one on the role of the clinical research nurse in cancer clinical trials, by Patty Campbell. Research nurses are a vital but, arguably, neglected group in clinical research, often going unnoticed. However, this is being addressed in the United Kingdom through proper training and increasing recognition by way of, for example, well-deserved co-authorship. The inclusion of this chapter in this reader is very welcome.

To learn about cancer, its effects and its treatments, this book provides me with much that I need to know, short of experiencing cancer myself. The book is a reader aimed at nurses and others learning in the context of higher education, but it could also provide a useful reader for the person suffering from or being with someone being treated for cancer. As nurses and other clinicians, we often seek insight into conditions so that we may understand them better and provide better care. This book should achieve that and it may also provide, as it did for me, a greater insight into the work of people who care for people with cancer.

Roger Watson FRCN FAAN
The University of Sheffield School of Nursing and Midwifery,
Sheffield, UK

Acknowledgements

First and foremost my sincere thanks go to my good friend and colleague Anne McQueen whose co-editing of this reader was invaluable. Equally sincere thanks must go to all our contributors, clinical and academic, without whose enthusiasm and expertise, the project would not have come to fruition. Thanks also must go to Roger Watson for his lively foreward and, of course, to Wiley–Blackwell for supporting the proposal through to publication. Last, but by no means least, so much appreciation must go to the undergraduate student nurses at the University of Edinburgh who inspired this reader in the first place.

Tonks N Fawcett
August 2010

Introduction

Tonks N. Fawcett and Anne McQueen

The real voyage of discovery consists not in seeking new lands but in seeing with new eyes.
                                                                  Marcel Proust

Nursing care in the 21st century requires not only an understanding of scientific evidence on which to base care decisions, but also the sensitive appreciation of the human response to illness, the primacy of caring and the paramount skills of communication – the heart and art of nursing. The challenge for nurses, and for all heathcare professionals, is to maintain, simultaneously, their mastery of the state of the science and their capacity for the art of patient care.

This book is concerned with caring for individuals with cancer. The authors of the individual chapters write from their own particular expertise and passion on the subject of cancer care; they aim to communicate their enthusiasm for their particular topic and their commitment to the highest quality of care for those diagnosed with cancer. The styles in which the chapters are written also demonstrate the authors' perspectives. Some are writing from the perspective of 'hard' scientific evidence from which best practice emerges. Others look more qualitatively at the experiential aspects of cancer. All the chapters contribute to developing knowledge, understanding and the professional care of those experiencing cancer.

The text is considered to be a 'reader' to support commonly taught undergraduate or postgraduate programmes and courses, or can be seen as a supplementary book providing special insights from clinicians, based on their specific expertise and experience. It is not intended to be a comprehensive text on cancer care but rather (as the title suggests) to offer some perspectives on cancer care that can inspire readers and encourage high-quality care through an enhanced understanding of patients' needs and carers' skills.

In accordance with the title, *Perspectives on Cancer Care*, the text presents a series of chapters highlighting some central issues in the management of patients with cancer. Different circumstances and approaches to the complex reality of cancer care are presented. The text addresses both practical and interpersonal skills and each chapter is based on sound research findings and critical appraisal of the relevant literature. The holistic approach to total care is a prominent feature in cancer care and this is illustrated through the different cancer scenarios represented in the various chapters. The special need

Perspectives on Cancer Care.   Edited by Josephine (Tonks) N. Fawcett and Anne McQueen
© 2011 Blackwell Publishing Ltd

for sensitivity, trust, empathy and support in the care of patients with cancer and their families is illuminated through the book.

Purpose of the text:

- To collate and present perspectives on cancer care that highlight particular issues in cancer care;
- To provide a concise volume with some insights and experience that can be of value to others in the field.

Aims of the text:

- To inspire readers caring for individuals with cancer;
- To give insight into patients' needs and how these can be addressed;
- To enhance knowledge of literature and its relevance to practice;
- To encourage best practice and a high quality of care for individuals facing cancer.

The aim and purpose of the text is achieved by drawing on the expertise of specialist practitioners in the field of cancer care.

Cancer care: an introductory overview

Cancer is common in the United Kingdom (UK) and indeed it is prevalent worldwide. Although causes and risk factors related to our current lifestyle are associated with cancer, it is not a new disease. Around 400 BC, Hippocrates, a Greek physician and the father of medicine, is claimed to have given the name cancer to tumours whose appearance resembled a crab; and he is credited with distinguishing between benign and malignant tumours. However, Hippocrates was not the first to discover the disease since the earliest case to be documented was reported on a papyrus, in Egypt, some time between 3000 and 1500 BC (www.cancerresearchuk.org). It was not until the 19th century that the concept of metastases via the bloodstream was appreciated. However, since Francis Crick and James Watson described the structure of deoxyribonucleic acid (DNA) it has been possible to study cancers at a molecular level, and now to have the possibility of developing new and exciting treatments.

It is recognised that there are more than 200 types of cancer, originating from different causes, presenting with different symptoms and requiring different forms of treatment or management. It is estimated that more than one in three people will develop some form of cancer during their lifetime. In July 2010 Cancer Research UK reported in the region of 298,000 new cases of cancer (excluding non-melanoma skin cancer) being diagnosed each year in the UK; breast, lung, large bowel (colorectal) and prostate cancers accounting for over half (54%) of all new cases (http://info.cancerresearchuk.org/ 2010). Almost 11 million new cases of cancer are diagnosed each year worldwide, 26% of these being in Europe (http://info.cancerresearchuk.org/cancerstats/world/ 2009).

Cameron and Howard (2006: 258) state that 'the key to understanding the clinical behaviour of cancers lies in their biology'. Cancer results from an error or defect in cell division; usually resulting from defects or damage in one or more of the genes involved in cell division. The damaged or mutated genes can start to divide uncontrollably and these defective cells multiply to form a lump of abnormal tissue, the tumour. Four main types of genes are involved in cell division, and defects of these can be seen in cancer:

- Oncogenes
- Tumour suppressor genes
- Suicide genes
- DNA repair genes

When oncogenes are activated, they speed up a cell's growth rate. When one is damaged cell division becomes uncontrolled. *Tumour suppressor genes* inhibit cell division and require to be 'switched off' by other proteins before a cell can grow. Apoptosis, or cell suicide, can occur when something goes wrong with a cell, to prevent damage to neighbouring cells. If the *suicide genes* become damaged, then a faulty cell can keep dividing and become cancerous. *DNA repair genes* enable damaged genes to be repaired. Body cells contain many proteins which are able to repair damaged DNA and the majority of DNA damage is probably repaired quickly, with no ill effects. However, if the DNA damage occurs to a gene which is responsible for making a DNA repair protein, a cell's ability to repair itself will be reduced. This can allow errors to build up in other genes over time and can result in cancer, something now thought of as genome instability.

In malignancy, for whatever reason, 'the homeostatic mechanisms related to cell division fail' (Watson & Fawcett 2003: 78) and the cancerous cells divide uncontrollably usually to form a tumour. Tumorigenesis is a multistep process, the developing tumour seen as clonal expansions. Such tumours may initially be symptomless according to their location but may press on nerves, block the digestive tract, obstruct blood vessels, or release hormones that can interfere with normal body processes. Cancers can spread to other tissues, distant to the primary source. This occurs when a single cancerous cell breaks away from the main tumour and travels via the circulatory or lymphatic system, the cerebrospinal fluid or via serous cavities to other tissues of the body. At the new site, new blood vessels grow to provide it with oxygen and nutrients (angiogenesis). Indeed, Hanahan and Weinberg (2000) identify six capabilities of cancers, acquired directly or indirectly through mutations in specific genes.

1. Self-sufficiency in growth signals, this autonomy modulated by oncogenes;
2. Insensitivity to antigrowth factors that normally regulate cell advance through the G1 phase of the cell cycle);
3. Evasion of apoptosis, programmed cell death, often associated with deactivation of the tumour suppressor gene, p53;
4. Limitless ability to replicate as a result of the above capabilities leading to uncontrolled proliferation;
5. Sustained angiogenesis via an 'angiogenic switch' in the course of cancer progression;
6. Tissue invasion and metastases which depend on all the above capabilities.

If left undetected and untreated the individual will, sometimes sooner, sometimes later, experience the consequences of this 'intimate enemy' (Marieb 2001: 142).

Cancer is recognised as a major fear by the public and this is not surprising since one in four of all deaths in the UK occurs as a result of cancer. However, half of the number of people diagnosed with cancer now survive for more than five years, and the average ten-year cancer survival rate has doubled over the last 30 years. Notably, the overall cancer death rate has fallen by 10% over the last decade (www.cancerresearchuk.org). Much of the improved prognosis is due to advances in knowledge and technology, facilitating earlier diagnosis and more refined treatments.

Although cancer affects individuals, and is not infectious, it is a disease that has effects on the whole family. Those within the family are affected by the changes cancer imposes on the individual; changes to their role within the family, the implications of ongoing treatments and their side effects, emotional upsets on a day-to-day basis, and worries about the future for their loved one and for themselves. Treatment for an individual with cancer therefore requires to include the needs of the family and this forms an important part of the nurse's role.

The prevalence of cancer means that all practising nurses will be involved in the care of individuals with cancer and will require knowledge and skills to cope with their particular needs. However, advances in cancer treatment and care have also provided opportunities for the emergence of nursing specialties such as the clinical nurse specialist in cancer care, the genetic counsellor, the genetic research nurse and the palliative care nurse, to name but a few. These specialists apply their expertise to provide the required sensitive, dedicated care to cancer patients and their families through the different stages of their cancer journey.

Such specialists are among the contributors to this book. This 'reader' is essentially written for student nurses and qualified nurses, not necessarily specialising in oncology, but who will meet patients with cancer in their varying nursing roles. However, it may also be of interest to specialist nurses in cancer care since the specialist practitioners contributing to the book express and share their passion for best practice in cancer care. The virtue of such a text is that it looks to bring together issues in cancer care that are well recognised, and some perhaps less well-recognised areas of expertise. Whilst issues such as pain management and hope are recognised as central in cancer care, they are included here together with genetic issues and the important position of the cancer research nurse. The chapter headings are intentionally selective and diverse in nature, highlighting issues that the authors believe to be significant in cancer care and where there is a need for attention to be focused in a reader. While this adds to the existing literature base, it is a unique text, 'speaking to' the readers and at the same time allowing them to explore critically the knowledge, skills and evidence presented to enhance their professional practice. As already suggested, this is not intended to provide comprehensive coverage of the domains of cancer care; rather as a 'reader' the content seeks to reflect differing perspectives of the chosen contributors, collected into a single volume for publication.

Chapter 1 explores what is meant by cancer as a journey of discovery. The developments affecting cancer care over the last several decades are examined with an appreciation of the tremendous progress that has been made, affecting a patient's cancer career. An analysis is made of the use of metaphors for discussing and understanding cancer, and consideration is given to how their meanings have changed with the social, technological and professional advances. An examination is made of how the notion of cancer and the cancer journey, from presentation to outcome, is different in the 21st century, and the relevance of concepts such as victim, sufferer, survivor, hope, fear, courage and loss through the cancer journey.

Chapter 2 illustrates how cancer genetics is integrated into healthcare, and its value in cancer care. The authors emphasise the importance of having knowledge of cancer family history, and fundamental to this is the current guidance from government and professional bodies. The skills and knowledge required to elicit a family history and construct a three-generation pedigree using universal nomenclature is outlined, and inheritance patterns in relation to cancer predisposition gene changes are explained. An overview is included of currently known gene changes that increase the risk for common cancers and of genetic testing available in the UK. Integral to the chapter is the role of cancer genetic services in the UK. The chapter is supported with case studies to assist understanding.

In Chapter 3, the author considers the care of the childbearing woman with cancer. The prospect of having a baby is generally considered to be a happy event, but when a pregnancy is overshadowed with a diagnosis of cancer it brings with it a range of issues for the childbearing woman, her unborn baby, her family and those who provide care. Some of these issues relate to the woman's survival, as the death of the mother may need to be considered. Other issues relate to the treatment of the woman's cancer, raising questions about maternal and fetal harm and benefit. Thus, decision-making about the timing of treatment becomes significant. In this chapter the traditional role of the midwife, as being 'with woman', will be considered. This role is comparable with that of the palliative care nurse attending a person with cancer. In palliative care the concept of 'being with' assumes special importance, and the role of the midwife in caring for the childbearing woman with cancer may yet need to be addressed more explicitly through research and education.

In Chapter 4 the focus is on the importance of research in addressing the practical realities that patients with cancer are confronted with. Research into the nursing and caring needs of cancer patients is vital to their optimum management and the dissemination of best practice across professional care. In this chapter the authors illustrate the need for a methodical and comprehensive oral assessment tool for use in children with oral mucositis. In order to conduct clinical trials of mucositis prevention and treatment, reliable, valid, sensitive and easy-to-use instruments are required. Considerable effort has resulted in many different mucositis scales being developed, primarily for adults with cancer receiving chemotherapy and radiotherapy. Oral mucositis research in children receiving anticancer therapy has been impeded by the lack of an acceptable, appropriate assessment scale. The authors of this chapter are two of the experts who have been working together to produce an oral mucositis assessment scale that will be appropriate for use in children. This chapter describes the processes involved in the development of the Children's International Mucositis Evaluation Scale (ChIMES) that resulted from this research group.

In Chapter 5 the author outlines the diagnosis, symptoms and treatment of malignant brain tumours. Particular attention is given to the need for a multidisciplinary approach to care. The specific problems experienced by patients, such as physical dysfunction, communication difficulties, cognitive impairment and psychological distress, are explored. The management of seizures is discussed along with the implication of seizures for the patient's quality of life. Additionally radiotherapy, chemotherapy and other therapeutic agents are summarised in relation to survival, and quality of life. Finally there is a discussion on palliative care and end-of-life management for this group of patients.

In Chapter 6 the author looks specifically, and quite distinctly, from the perspective of the surgeon's role in cancer care, arguing that, to date, the surgeon has been pre-eminent in cancer treatment but that the role of the surgeon may be changing. Surgical decisions are now firmly and axiomatically embedded in the multidisciplinary team, in which the key role of the cancer clinical nurse specialist is acknowledged. Along with other advances in cancer care, the author outlines the exciting new surgical developments to consider, including minimally invasive, micro and robotic techniques for achieving an optimal surgical outcome for the patients with cancer.

In Chapter 7 the author addresses cancer pain – a significant cause of fear in cancer patients. Pain in cancer is much more than a physical sensation; it is an open floodgate for fear. Patients in pain may fear that the cancer is worsening, that they will die imminently or in distress, fear losing their composure with those they love, or even the fear that they are being punished for some misdemeanour which bodes badly for their afterlife. Identifying and addressing these fears is a challenging but important step to managing pain, and effectively managing physical pain will in turn help resolve the fear in patients and their families. This chapter explores the different aspects of pain, and demonstrates the use of the World Health Organization analgesic ladder. While the focus is on the use of opioids, the value of adjuvant medication in clinical management is also acknowledged.

Chapter 8 addresses the incidence and experience of fatigue in the cancer patient, which is one of the most commonly reported side effects following treatment. The potential causes are identified and a review of the literature evaluates management strategies. The author discusses whether nurses and allied health professionals can take a more active role in the ongoing care of patients with fatigue, as the 'treatments' that have the highest evidence base appear to be psychosocial support, education and exercise. If it is accepted that patients can expect optimal management of this condition, the National Health Service may have to adapt both existing service provision, and perhaps traditional nursing roles, to accommodate this.

Chapter 9 explores the nature of clinical trials in cancer research and the roles of the clinical research nurse within clinical trials. It discusses the role of the nurse in providing and communicating complex trial and treatment information to patients and families, carefully tailored and paced to meet individual needs. The author explores the role of the nurse as pathfinder – helping patients negotiate the web of information and services available to them – and examines the relationships developed between patients and research nurses in the clinical trial setting. The direct caregiver role and the provision of expert care are also discussed.

Chapter 10 illuminates the emotional nature of work involved in caring for individuals with cancer. Cancer care can provide nurses with much satisfaction but also has the potential to lead to emotional strain. The caring work involved in nursing patients with cancer can facilitate the development of strong professional relationships as nurses and patients communicate and interact with each other in the course of the patients' therapeutic journey. Furthermore, the communication with and support for the patients' families, that is very real in this area of nursing, enhances the nurse's role in the total care for the patients' wellbeing and adds to the emotional and psychological input of nursing work in this context. In this chapter the author presents an understanding of caring and emotional work within a therapeutic relationship in the context of nursing patients with cancer.

In Chapter 11 the authors show how the treatments for gastrointestinal cancer have increased survival, but not without side effects. With a greater emphasis on early diagnosis and treatment of gastrointestinal cancer, there has been a significant increase in the number of survivors. However, multimodal treatment of surgery, chemotherapy and abdominal and pelvic radiation is not without side effects, which can persist into the survival period after therapeutic interventions have been completed. The treatments can have adverse effects on the bowel, the urinary system and sexual function. Inevitably such side effects adversely affect the quality of life and have important implications for body image and self-esteem. This chapter addresses the complications that patients may experience following treatment for bowel cancer, and explores the current research in an attempt to minimise side effects and improve the quality of life.

In Chapter 12, the authors clearly illustrate the value of hope. This is considered important through all stages of the cancer journey; and no less at the time of end of life care. Access to competent and compassionate end-of-life care, where it is needed and when, is a key issue on the national and local agenda. This type of care addresses physical, psychosocial and spiritual issues. Evidence suggests that patients and families may remain hopeful if pain and symptoms are managed, if individuals feel valued, and when caring relationships are maintained. A range of frameworks and models, such as the NHS Gold Standards Framework and integrated care pathways, are being promoted to ensure a cohesive approach to end-of-life care. This closing chapter uses case studies to explore how such models and frameworks may assist healthcare professionals to sustain hope in patients with cancer and their families at the end of life.

References

Cameron DA, Howard GCW (2006) Oncology. In: Boon NA, Colledge NC, Walker BR (eds) *Davidson's Principles and Practice of Medicine*, 20th edn. Edinburgh: Churchill Livingstone.

Cancer Research UK (2009) http://info.cancerresearchuk.org/cancerstats/world/

Cancer Research UK (2010) http://info.cancerresearchuk.org/

Hanahan D, Weinberg RA (2000) The hallmarks of cancer. *Cell* **100**(1): 57–70.

Marieb EN (2001) *Human Anatomy and Physiology*, 5th edn. San Francisco: Addison Wesley Longman.

Watson R, Fawcett TN (2003) *Pathophysiology, Homeostasis and Nursing*. London: Routledge.

Chapter 1

Cancer: a journey of discovery

Tonks N. Fawcett

Life is a journey undertaken on an ocean of experience. All human development, including the experience of illness and health, involves discoveries made on a journey across that ocean of experience.

Barker (2002: 43)

The aim of this opening chapter is to explore what is meant by the cancer journey in its many manifestations. An analysis will be made of the use of metaphors for discussing and understanding cancer, and consideration will be given to how their meanings have changed with social, technological and professional advances. The developments affecting cancer care over the last several decades will be examined, with an appreciation of the tremendous progress that has been made affecting a patient's cancer experience. An examination will be made of how the notion of cancer and the cancer journey, from presentation to outcome, is different in the 21st century and the relevance of concepts such as victim, sufferer, survivor, hope, fear, courage and loss through the cancer journey.

Cancer

Once said, in terms of a diagnosis, the word cancer cannot be unsaid. The word hangs in the air with all its connotations that, in our culture at least, put fear, often abject fear, into the heart of even the most optimistic and knowledgeable individual. After the day of diagnosis, life is never quite the same. Whether, for whatever reason, the diagnosis is realised to be imminent, or whether it comes as some shocking cataclysm, the individual, now suddenly the patient, must seek to make sense of what this means and how it will affect not only the normality of daily life but any possible life aspirations. Questions without answers, or with answers wanted, tumble through the brain as the individual looks for meaning, moving from primeval concerns as to punishment for wrongs committed or to more mundane regrets over such as overexposure to the sun, the curse of nicotine addiction or that casually rejected environmental hazard.

Perspectives on Cancer Care. Edited by Josephine (Tonks) N. Fawcett and Anne McQueen
© 2011 Blackwell Publishing Ltd

Cancer as metaphor

In the search for meaning, humans look to metaphors to liken their reality to something which is perhaps more manageable and examinable. Metaphors, Lakoff and Johnson (1980) argue, allow the understanding of one thing in terms of another, giving illness such as cancer a certain symbolism. For most of the 20th century cancer has mainly been seen as a mortal disease, and a dreadful and dreaded disease to be fought, though not often beaten. The notion of cancer as a battle can give some order to the chaos of the diagnosis, as physicians, oncologists and surgeons share a common purpose and the 'fighting spirit' is encouraged. Reisfield and Wilson (2004) argue that war is an apposite metaphor with the enemy, the commander, the combatant, allies and an armoury of weapons to hand. Such a metaphor also implies vigour, hope and a serious purpose to offset the sense of hopelessness so ready to surface (Hammer et al. 2009).

Such a metaphor is still very potent and embedded in our cancer care language, but it has been much criticised in recent years. Sontag (2001), rejecting any cultural and societal value of such metaphors, argued that the body is not a battlefield and that such metaphors perpetuate stereotypes and stigma. It has to be recognised that Sontag held a particularly jaundiced, and arguably limited, belief that cancer sufferers were seen as victims of suppressed or failed emotions. She asserted that cancer is not a curse or a punishment and certainly not an embarrassment and that, as understanding of cancer causality and treatment advances, metaphors should become irrelevant. Perhaps what Sontag did not wish to acknowledge was that the use of metaphors is deeply embedded culturally, and energy should be focused on the sensitive and positive role that metaphors offer. The illustration of this can be seen in the widespread use of the metaphor of the cancer experience and trajectory as a journey.

Cancer as a journey

The metaphor of the journey is not exclusive to cancer or to illness, but is used in many challenges in life, from sport to intellectual activity. Life is acknowledged to be a journey, despite the abiding difficulty for many of confronting the endpoint. The journey for the cancer sufferer is not just linear, through diagnosis, treatment and the consequences thereof, but also an emotional rollercoaster. Not only that, the biology of cancer is itself seen as the transformation journey of a tumour cell (Kumar & Weaver 2009). The idea of serious illness as a journey has had its own potency. Davis (1963), addressing polio-myelitis, saw it as a form of crisis management from prelude and warning stages to the impact stage of diagnosis and the stage of treatment, and its corollary, which Davis described as the inventory stage. Despite its pervasive applicability, the journey defies a unitary description. As indicated above, it is not merely a linear journey through the stages, however real; each patient will travel in their own way. Reisfield and Wilson (2004: 4026) describe the journey metaphor as 'quieter than the military metaphor' but still having the 'depth, richness and gravitas to be applicable to the cancer experience'. They then use the analogy of the cancer as diverting the individual from the freeway to consider the alternative byways imposed by cancer that bring with it the real concerns of uncertainty, fear, anxiety, guilt, loss and anger. They also suggest, however, that these byways may also bring new meanings to life's journey and new insights as to the nature of the traveller and those who care for and journey alongside the traveller. The journey metaphor, they argue, does not talk in terms of winning or losing, but rather of different roads to travel.

However, this author might part company with Reisfeld and Wilson at this point (to continue the analogy) as the whole notion of fostering hope and positive thinking, at least in the early stages of the cancer journey, is inextricably bound up with optimistic outcomes of winning and even, despite this metaphor, successfully defeating an enemy. Perhaps that is the mistake, and those who support and encourage the traveller on the journey should focus equally on the quality of the journey rather than where it will eventually lead them. While embracing the popularity of the journey metaphor, it must not be forgotten that people create their own metaphors of life and life changes, often reflecting their life worlds, for example, as their most demanding performance, their personal race for life, a labyrinth, or a game of chess. Lerner (1994: xiii) combines many metaphors and likens the cancer experience to 'that of a soldier who is given orders . . . to parachute into a jungle war zone without a map, a compass or training of any kind', and Rachel Clark describes navigating round cancer like 'being dropped in a strange city, without a map or a compass. There are no landmarks and no familiar faces . . . no signs, no-one speaks your language' (Clark et al. 2002: 1). Crane-Okada (2007), also using the metaphor of a compass, looking to helping patients on their journey, likens the features of a compass to the holistic support nurses can provide. Barker (2002) suggests a seafaring, 'tidal' metaphor for life itself, with crises such as cancer as piracy followed by the possibility of shipwreck before sea legs can be regained and the ship sets sail again. For those caring and in the caring professions, listening to patients' narrative metaphors will provide insights into the unique journey and unique meanings for the many byways of their cancer journey (Skott 2002). For some, the cancer journey may remain real, but their search for a meaning is 'not always tidy and neat' (Quinn 2003: 170) and its meaning remains elusive.

The linear and rollercoaster cancer journey

It can be argued that the cancer journey is everyone's journey in that its prevention, in terms of genetic makeup and lifestyles, is, or should be, part of the matrix of life. Leydon et al. (2003) argue that the cancer journey has no definitive starting point. However, in reality, the 'presence' of cancer in the psyche begins with the sense that something is wrong, often set against a pre-existing appreciation of personal risk. With this comes immediately the pervasive sense of uncertainty. Delay can occur at this stage if, for that individual, uncertainty may seem better than a certainty they do not want to face. The challenge of this is recognised in the *Cancer Reform Strategy* (DH 2007), which aims, not only to raise public awareness of risk factors and signs and symptoms of early cancer, but also to find effective means of encouraging people to seek help sooner. The journey has fully begun when investigations are carried out towards a diagnosis. The individual is now in the game and it is serious. The game is also new, and support is needed in terms of simple, clear and sensitive communications that meet both informational and emotional needs (McQueen 2009). Fallowfield and Jenkins (Fallowfield et al. 2003; Fallowfield &

Jenkins 2006) are not alone in their exhortations that, despite communication being the heart of nursing and medicine and a core clinical skill, patients, their families and carers still feel let down by less-than-ideal communication at a time when it matters most. The period of waiting for a diagnosis is arguably the hardest time, and often too long, when the person vacillates between hope and fear, bargaining and despair, not daring to accept optimism and fearing pessimism. Drageset and Lindstrom (2003) explored this in women with breast cancer, revealing anxiety that was hard to ameliorate by support mechanisms. Diagnosis can only serve to reinforce the emotions associated with uncertainty and waiting, emotions now replaced by certainty and decisions.

Reactions to a diagnosis are myriad in nature but Greer (1991) identified denial, fighting spirit, stoic acceptance, helplessness/hopelessness and anxiety. Greer argued that the particular responses can, in some cases, influence the course of their disease but in reality one person may move through all such reactions. Hickey (1986) and Hammer et al. (2009), in their respective ways, stress the primacy of 'hope-inspiring nursing' (Hammer et al. 2009: 1) to guard against the sense of hopelessness ever ready to push through and impair healing. Spiegel (2001: 287) looks at hope in relation to having the right attitude to the cancer journey, the "fighting spirit', a kind of realistic optimism . . . determined to make the best of it'. Such an attitude is not to be seen as blind or false hope or an overburdening urge to be positive.

Fallowfield (2008), recognising the above, explores the world of the newly diagnosed patient and their family, the amount of new and possibly alien information to be absorbed, so needed (yet so undesired) and so potent for enabling decisions to be made and for future wellbeing. Nanton et al. (2009) argues that, by skilled and carefully tailored information and communications, not devoid of the gentle use of humour, healthcare professionals could reduce the distress of ongoing uncertainty. Although the emotional labour is recognised (see Chapter 10), if this is done well by both doctor and nurse in their respective roles (Dunniece & Slevin 2000; Quinn 2003), the journey to be faced can at least be cushioned by a trusting relationship with those who may seem at that time to hold their very lives in their hands.

The treatment journey

For a patient who has presented with distressing symptoms or for an emergency cancer treatment (whether surgery, radiotherapy or various forms of chemotherapeutic and other agents), treatment can be seen as a relief despite the diagnosis. However, for many who believed themselves well, or even 'very fit' before diagnosis, treatment makes them ill, often for some time, with spectres of nausea, vomiting, pain and fatigue fixing in the mind (see Chapters 7 and 8). In addition, as some patients find themselves screened for cardiac and renal dysfunction, there comes the realisation that a treatment may damage other organs that indeed, unknown to them or the healthcare professionals, might already be impaired. Even more potent is the reality, for many, of altered appearance, be it through surgical resection, iatrogenically induced loss of hair, weight gain or stress-induced weight loss, all of which can threaten the sense of self (Bredin 2000), and may be considered a form of 'piracy' (Barker 2002).

Decisions have to be made. No longer are such decisions made without close consultation with the patient and the family (DH 2007) but sensitivity on the part of the healthcare professionals is needed to discern just how much involvement is desired. Some family members and carers may find this added responsibility, in the absence of seeing in themselves any real expertise, an extra burden (Fincham et al. 2005). Others, who may have already avidly searched internet sources, value such involvement and appreciate the invaluable partnership when so much that is undesired seems to require acquiescence. Such involvement requires considerable support by the specialist team, particularly the nurse, whose presence is seen as being 24/7, i.e. they are always there (Leyden et al. 2003).

The stress of the cancer diagnosis and treatment journey can manifest itself in both psychological and physiological disturbance, and the coping strategies adopted will be varied (Smith & Fawcett 2006). In terms of giving support, particularly as a nurse, Frank (2002: 45) argues that 'there is no right thing to say to a cancer patient because the cancer patient as a generic entity does not exist. There are only persons who are different to start with, having different experiences according to the contingencies of their diseases'. Some will seek out a new path and, temporarily at least, suspend their 'other' life. Others will look to retain their usual life, minimising any deviation from the norm wherever possible. Kyngas et al. (2000: 11) found this tended to be the case with young people with cancer, where resuming their 'normal life' was seen as 'a source of safety'. Miedema et al. (2007) also found the prevailing aim of young people with cancer was to achieve the 'normalcy' of their pre-cancer lives. This did not mean a denial of the disease; in order for such an aim to be achieved, optimal social, emotional and informational support was needed. For these young people emotional support often comes from the family, as indeed is so often the case whatever the age of the person with cancer.

Families and carers play key roles and they themselves must receive equal support as they travel this cancer journey. These informal carers often feel helpless and uncertain, possibly not knowing what help is available for them (Soothill et al. 2001). Supporting the crucial role of informal carers, family members or not, has to be a key partnership role of the community nurse alongside the specialist team (Wilson et al. 2002; Luker et al. 2003; DH 2007). Koldjeski et al. (2007) demonstrate how family-based oncology nursing can be essential for family wellbeing on the cancer journey. The support and supportive role of families may include children and young people whose needs are often difficult to express, as roles may seem suddenly to change and even to be reversed. Compas et al. (1994) found that the impact of a parent's cancer diagnosis related more to perceived seriousness rather than to the characteristics of the specific cancer, and differed according to the age and gender of both parent and child. Adolescent girls of mothers with cancer were found to experience more significant distress. Thastum explored children's scoping strategies when a parent had cancer and, although finding they 'seemed to manage rather well' (Thastum 2008: 123), it did depend on how well the parent(s) were themselves coping and supported.

Treatments do not always progress smoothly. Side effects can be debilitating (see Chapter 8) and any necessary delay in the next stage of treatment can add yet further stress. The role of the cancer nurse specialist becomes paramount at such times, and the primacy of the therapeutic relationship with the patient and family can positively impact on the maintenance of dignity and wellbeing. Setbacks are hard and treatment decisions may change and, alongside that, the means of coping. Barker (2000: 332) argued that such times can engender a sense of powerlessness, and all in the caring team need to recognise this and provide 'the necessary human, interpersonal and intersubjective conditions for the development of a sense of security that the person not only seeks but needs to continue', even in times of acute uncertainty. He continues that 'maybe one of the virtues of caring is that it focuses the nurse's attention on . . . awareness of the person who is the patient and in so doing fosters an increased awareness of the whole of that experience for the person' (Barker 2000: 332).

Throughout the illness trajectory many decisions will be made as to treatments and their side effects, symptoms and their management where, as Shaha et al. (2008: 61) argue, outcomes are uncertain and 'few guarantees of success are possible'. Uncertainty is multidimensional and as Barker (2000: 332) states, it is part of the human condition. If well supported with information and emotionally, he argues, people have the 'capacity to grow through experience'. The worst of times, with both its certainties and uncertainties, can bring out the best in people.

In the late 1990s the first Cancer Caring Centre was opened in the grounds of Edinburgh's Western General Hospital, the inspiration of Maggie Keswick Jencks, who died of breast cancer in 1995. Her vision was for an environment that would give emotional and psychological support, complementing, but also giving a respite from, the orthodox cancer treatment. It was to be an intimate setting where sufferers could both express, and be helped to manage, their fears and uncertainties, and a place where they and their families could just be themselves: husbands, wives, mothers, with lives to live. Such a setting could also offer means of helping relieve physical and emotional distress through relaxation techniques (Miller 2007). Maggie's Centre, as it became known, offers something that perhaps cannot be offered by the health service, and its success has led to a network of such centres opening across the United Kingdom and even further afield (Miller 2007). The philosophy underpinning such centres can also be seen as facilitating the resilience so needed on the cancer journey by both patient and family. Addressing this notion, Jacelon (1997) identified how some individuals seem to possess resilience to cope with, and 'bounce back' from, life's adversities. Resilience is seen as a 'constellation of traits' (1997: 128), some seemingly inherent in the individual such as a sense of autonomy, enthusiasm or humour; others may be more socially determined and arguably could be learned. Such resilience, if it can be fostered, can counter the sense of fragility and of strained personal resources that can occur on the cancer journey. Nurses and others in the caring team can be key in helping the cancer patient to achieve this or to detect where, on the continuum of response from vulnerability to resilience (Rutter 1985), the cancer patient might be at any one time.

Life after treatment

Following treatment there are new challenges to face as, to some extent, the treatment period, short or extended, provides a 'cocoon' of care that now, if all has progressed optimally, must be left behind. As the time from treatment completion lengthens, the concept of survivorship grows. One of most positive developments in recent years has been that people can and do survive a cancer diagnosis and survivorship is a reality (Doyle 2008). This in itself has necessitated an exploration of what is meant by survivorship (the term first coined in the 1980s), when it begins, and what are the immediate and ongoing needs of those who can describe themselves as cancer survivors. Sontag (2001) was perceptive in her plea not to call those with cancer 'victims'. Mullen (1985) described seasons of survival, beginning at diagnosis, as acute, extended and permanent, but this is a continuous process with needs ebbing and flowing as time passes. More conventionally, survivorship is seen as being disease-free for five years, after which, arguably, the risk of recurrence is less. Survivorship brings with it its own uncertainties and needs that must be specifically understood and provided for (Carter 1989; Vivar & McQueen 2005; Doyle 2008). This is an area for further research, and survivors' needs, although recognised, are not yet fully met (DH 2007).

Doyle (2008: 507) emphasises the need for all nurses to deepen their understanding of cancer survivorship needs and to take a leadership role in 'influencing theory, research and practice' around this 'dynamic concept'. What is recognised is that survivorship has both positive and negative effects. The joy of surviving is tinged with the fear of recurrence, the irreversible and/or ongoing effects of treatments such as body image changes, pain and fatigue (see Chapters 7 and 8). The restoration of 'freedom' may be spoiled by feeling cast adrift from the support of healthcare professionals, who for some may have been like a second family (Rowland 2008). Some will express a sense of growth and new awareness (Barker 2000), but others may remain bitter at having had cancer at all and be unable to move on (Rowland 2008). Yet others sense that, in some ways, though no longer a cancer patient, they do not truly feel a survivor (Doyle 2008). Alongside remain the family and/or the carer who, in many ways, mirror the survivors as they too learn to incorporate this as part of their lives. As normal life resumes, Stott (2008: 61) wonders if the complexity of being a survivor is seen as such, commenting 'Cancer and its effects cast a long shadow' and it must not be assumed that 'patients can just resume their lives as though cancer was just an unfortunate interlude'.

Cancer recurrence

Survivorship can also embrace those who are not disease-free but who, despite treatment, have not seen the cancer eradicated, or for whom it has since recurred, to the same part of the body or spread to other parts of the body as metastases. Reaction to the return of cancer has not been much researched but Griffiths et al. (2008), looking at oral cancer recurrence, identify heightened vulnerability revealed in a mosaic of responses. These were not all negative, and included new-found coping mechanisms and improved relationships. It is undeniable that the return of cancer poses yet further challenges for its clinical and emotional management by the healthcare multidisciplinary team, but with advances in cancer care, many more now live with cancer, rather than see it as immediately mortal. Although the term 'chronic' now has its own critics, cancer can be seen as a chronic illness where, although cure may no longer be possible, quality of life can be maintained for a considerable time in a way that was inconceivable as little as 25 years ago.

Managing metastatic disease is not the same as managing a chronic condition such as diabetes mellitus, and the philosophy of the treatment alters, with the aim of gaining the best control over the cancer whilst not inducing a toxicity that detrimentally affects daily wellbeing. For many, further treatment may require hospital care where the oncology nurse, as a key member of the team, once again guides patients through the decision-making process in relation to the possibilities and realities. Increasingly, however, it is possible for treatments to be based at home (Marsé et al. 2004). Fitch and Maxwell (2008) maintain that nurses are often the most appropriate healthcare providers in supporting patients and their family at home, helping them to understanding their therapy, often able to act as intermediaries in communicating the needs and concerns of patients to their physicians. The patient and family have to acknowledge that some form of treatment will now be a fact of life, for the most part, for the future, however long it may be. Whittemore and Dixon (2008), though not looking specifically at cancer as a chronic illness, explored how people with a chronic illness integrated this reality into their lives. Despite effort and motivation this was found to be hard as they struggled to live life rather than live illness. Such research serves to demonstrate that success in managing formerly life-limiting disorders brings its own challenges for both the participants and all who care for and about them. At this stage of the journey, what might matter most is the ability of healthcare professionals, and particularly the nurse, just to acknowledge a shared humanity and the capacity 'to presence oneself' alongside the patient and family (Benner & Wrubel 1989: 13).

The end of the survival journey

Palliation of symptoms and quality-of-life issues become increasingly the overarching concern for those whose cancer journey moves inexorably towards its end, and where the hope for cure is replaced by a hope for continuance of life. It should be remembered that, for at least 20% of individuals, there is a desired quality of life until the very final days (Lunney & O'Mara 2001). However, for many cancer patients the complexity of physical and emotional symptoms requires specialist clinical, interpersonal, humanitarian and spiritual skills expressed so ideally in the hospice philosophy of care and 'the twin pillars of mind and heart'. Such care is achieved by exquisitely competent symptom manage-ment, combined with 'open, compassionate conversations' (Lunney & O'Mara 2001: 277) with the patient, family and, indeed, close friends. Lunney and O'Mara (2001) suggest that the end-of-life experiences are not entirely new but rather are different expressions of those previously encountered. Hope remains but its complexion has changed. The skill of such care at the end of the journey is explored in several chapters in this text, particularly in Chapters 5, 7, 10 and 12.

The cancer care journey: then and now

So much has changed since Susan Sontag first wrote *Illness as a Metaphor* in the 1970s and openly discussed the association of cancer with death and the sufferers as victims. She believed that when cancer was finally understood, so would the language change and metaphors be rejected (Sontag 1978). Sontag was right in that, as knowledge and scientific understanding has burgeoned and outcomes improved, cancer is more openly discussed and metaphors, if not rejected, have changed, as discussed above, from that of victim to that of survivor on a journey. However, as Mullen (1985) observed, there is no denying that life is forever altered by the experience of cancer and the word still instils fear into most people as the 'diagnosis . . . hits you like a punch in the stomach' (Keswick Jencks 1995: 1). Even at the end of the first decade of the 21st century, cancer is perceived as seriously life-threatening and, in the unexplained symptoms in the 'worried well', it is often what the individual is fearing but avoids voicing (Wick & Zanni 2008). People now expect that the National Health Service will deliver the best and fastest treatment available to save their lives or the lives of those they love, should cancer occur. The current picture in the United Kingdom, however, is not as encouraging as might be believed, comparing poorly in terms of five-year survival with Germany, France and Sweden (Verdecchia et al. 2007). Despite this, the road travelled since the 1970s is worth considering in terms of the cancer experience and the remarkable progress made.

In the 1970s the word cancer was largely taboo; people 'whispered about or alluded to the disease indirectly' (Mayer 2007: 481). In the 1970s, the diagnosis was often missed or made too late, compounded by reluctance of the person to present with the feared symptoms. Diagnostic techniques and treatment were hugely variable between, and even within, different areas of the country. Waiting times for treatment were so long that patients could die before treatment had begun. In terms of treatment, there were few options beyond surgery, usually carried out by generalist surgeons and where, if this did not resolve the problem, life expectancy was limited. Patient and treatment outcomes varied considerably in terms of survival. The concept of specialist services was as yet embryonic. A significant breakthrough for cancer patients' experience occurred with the work of Dr Vicki Clements, based at St Bartholomew's Hospital in London. She herself, diagnosed with ovarian cancer, sought to bring cancer 'out of the closet' and by 1984 had founded the British Association of Cancer United Patients (BACUP) to provide the crucial information, practical support and help that patients and their families so needed. Clements argued that patients deserved honest communications as to their condition and prognosis. Her drive and determination led to what at the time was quite a radical development: that of collaboration between progressive clinicians and patients, with patients recognised, perhaps for the first time, as having their own expertise.

Other major technological advances were occurring in the early 1980s. Computed axial tomography (CAT) was introduced: a scanner allowed a series of cross-sectional scans to be made along a single axis of a body structure or tissue to construct, for the first time, a three-dimensional image. Alongside this, surgical techniques were steadily improving and emerging knowledge of the biological basis of cancer suggested exciting possibilities for the future. Research into the use of radiotherapy and chemotherapeutic agents in the management of cancer was also advancing, although at that time the side effects were significant and hard to alleviate. Nausea and vomiting was an inevitably miserable side effect of most chemotherapeutic agents until the $5HT_3$ receptor antagonist was researched (Marty et al. 1989), developed and introduced in the late 1980s. The drive to improve both cancer prevention and cancer care, in terms of screening equipment and services and specialist centres, gradually gained momentum from both healthcare professionals and the public, and in 1985 led the Minister of Health, Kenneth Clark, to commission an expert working group chaired by Sir Patrick Forrest, to look at breast cancer screening. The Forrest report, published in 1986, recommended breast screening for all women over the age of 50 years (DHSS 1986). The success of this report was reflected in its implementation in full by 1988. Despite these obvious advances, the United Kingdom compared badly with many of its European counterparts in terms of the percentage of gross national product (GNP) spent on health. The computed tomography (CT) scanner was a major and amazing breakthrough, allowing clinicians for the first time to see exactly where a tumour was within the body. It revolutionised detection, diagnosis and subsequent treatment, but this key development was never rolled out by the government, and money for this vital equipment depended on charitable donations and other money-generating appeals.

This could not continue and, by the 1990s, senior clinicians' voices were increasingly heard in the United Kingdom. In 1994 the Chief Medical Officer, Kenneth Calman, chaired the committee that led to the *Calman Hine Report* in 1995 with the recognition, arguably very late, that something must be done for cancer services (DH 1995). This report proved to be the major catalyst for change, leading to the development of cancer specialist centres, where cancer surgery would be performed only by specialists. Resources and priorities were to be so directed that waiting times would be markedly reduced, there would be no socioeconomic disparity and there would be equity of services across the regions (DH 1995). A period of optimism followed as the report impinged on the professional roles and priorities of healthcare professionals and their patients but (although not debated here) the incidence and prevalence of cancer continued to rise and the United Kingdom remained low in the European league tables. In 1999 a group of key cancer experts met with the Prime Minister, Tony Blair, to develop a national cancer plan, and a cancer 'tsar' was created in England to oversee the plan and ensure that resources were in place to improve patient outcomes. In addition to the continuing issues of screening and waiting times, there was to be increased investment into new treatments, the workforce was to be expanded and the infrastructure strengthened (DH 2001). The aim was that by 2010 the picture of cancer survival was to be at least on a par with that of the leading European countries. However, data take time to collect and collate, and the analysis by Verdecchia et al. (2007) still showed a disappointing picture. Mayor (2009) reports that the NHS cancer plan has achieved a tentative increase in survival at one year for many types of cancers but that, until further data are available, such a result should be viewed with a degree of caution.

However, good news is established for breast cancer, where survival rates have been improving for more than 20 years. The estimated relative five-year survival rate for women diagnosed in England and Wales (and other parts of the United Kingdom demonstrate a similar picture) in 2001–3 was 80%, compared with 52% in 1971–5 (Coleman et al. 2004) and the estimated 20-year survival rate has gone from 44% in the early 1990s to 64% for the most recent period (Office of National Statistics 2005).

In 2007 the Cancer Reform Strategy was launched (DH 2007) looking to establish the kind of service seen elsewhere in Europe. It was clearly recognised that many more lives could be saved if the outcomes of the United Kingdom were brought up to the standards of the best countries in Europe and there was little dissent as to what needed to be done. Was this enough to meet the goals? Great credit was given to the involvement of patient groups in this reform strategy, something that would not have been considered or thought possible in the 1970s (DH 2007). Scotland, which continued to have one of Europe's lowest rates for cancer survival, followed a year later with its new cancer plan, entitled *Better Cancer Care*, which aimed to reduce the number of cancer deaths in Scotland (Scottish Government 2008). The common purpose continues to be to improve cancer prevention, detection, treatment options and care and meet head-on the challenges that persist.

Cancer journeys: stories and narratives

Understanding cancer can be seen not as one journey but rather as many different forms of journeys, of suffering, of care and of emotion. There are also the journeys of scientific discovery in the field of cancer, to which this chapter has not done due justice, and journeys of a more sociopolitical nature as to how cancer care has been, and is, seen as a political priority. However, it is the journey of the patient which is the foremost concern of this chapter. Of course, understanding how this journey is experienced depends, to some extent, on understanding the other forms of life journeying. Considerable insight can be gained from the stories that patients, and those who care for them, tell. Many cancer patients feel the need, verbally or in written form, to give a personal narrative of their illness experience. Calman (2000) stated that stories 'help us make sense of the world and able to bear some of the burdens which we face. They give meaning and structure to our daily lives' (Calman 2000: 17). Although the terms are often used interchangeably, 'narrative' looks to go beyond the actual 'story', attempting to capture, investigate and draw out the truth behind the experience for that individual in time, space, personhood and relationships (Clandinin & Connelly 2000).

Repede (2008), telling the story of one woman's journey through metastatic breast cancer, sees such stories as a means of conveying meaning for the reader and healing to the teller. Gaydos (2005) describes the listener or reader as being drawn in and giving their own interpretation, in light of their own unique experiences, which allows the story to become 'a resource and a memory for the listener as well as the narrator' (Gaydos 2005: 256). Gaydos (2005: 257–8) also considers that, as part of the art of nursing, nurses can, through their own skills of 'mutuality', be 'co-creators' of the narratives whereby a shared and more profound meaning of the story is elicited. However, more familiar are the personal accounts read as 'blogs', articles or books. Rachel Clark, in her poignant account of her experience of cancer at the age of 25, speaks directly to healthcare professionals so that they can learn from her words (Clark et al. 2002). In the same vein, Maggie Keswick Jencks gave her inspiring and feisty 'view from the front line' (Keswick Jencks 1995). Lance Armstrong's story is one of the courage and determination of a winning sportsman, with all its metaphors, but it speaks equally for all to hear, of how, for that time in his life, cancer consumed his thoughts before he could once again, with his own altered perspectives on existence, celebrate being alive (Armstrong 2001). Gloria Hunniford, telling the story of her much loved daughter's journey through cancer, writes as a mother walking, not always easily, alongside her daughter, herself also a mother (Hunniford 2005). All such stories speak to everyone but can offer much to healthcare professionals who, despite Gaydos's ideal of being a co-creator of narratives, do not always have the privilege of this opportunity.

The journeys of those who have experienced cancer and who also work as healthcare professionals has a particular poignancy if, as well, their work was in the field of oncology. This was the case for Peter J. Morgan who, about to begin work as an oncologist, was diagnosed with advanced cancer. From that day, continuing his work until his death, he kept a diary, parts of which were made into an educational video (Chabner 1997). His personal narratives and reflections provide a compelling account 'of the survival of the spirit that would not succumb to the "chaos" of cancer' (Chabner 1997: 206) while also relating what in his life was most precious. 'His work as a physician was at the top of his list' (Chabner 1997: 207). Peter J. Morgan epitomises what can be seen as the work and care of a 'wounded healer'.

Wounded healers and the cancer journey

The notion of the wounded healer has its origins in Greek mythology where the centaur, Chiron, was wounded by Herakles's poisoned arrow, a wound that was not to heal and left Chiron in perpetual suffering. Chiron was able to transcend his own suffering and transform it into the capacity, as a wounded healer, to heal others (Conti-O'Hare 2002). The notion of the wounded healer can, to a significant extent, be seen as inherent in all healthcare professionals who, in order to fully 'heal', must have recognised and been immersed in the suffering of others, so much part of the emotional labour of caring. Learning to cope with the inherent stress of others' suffering and transforming it into positivity can then form the basis of a truly healing relationship with the patient (Conti-O'Hare 2002; Dunning 2006). It is not intended to mean that all true 'healers' must themselves have been overtly 'wounded', but many healthcare professionals will attest that only when they had shared similar experiences and become a patient did they fully appreciate, as an insider, the world of the sufferer (Morgan 1984; Dunning 2006). Morgan (1984) argues that as wounded healers, any 'physician or other healthcare worker who . . . had extended hospital care is in a unique position to act as an intermediary between the needs and sensitivities of hospital patients and the rigidities and compulsions of care givers' and 'would have the trust of the patients and the respect of the staff' (Morgan 1984: 1336).

DeMarco et al. (2004) and Picard et al. (2004) explored the world of nurses as cancer survivors and described both the particular vulnerability that insider knowledge gave them and also, despite a sense of role ambiguity, how, as a 'wounded healer' it had deepened the compassion they felt for their own patients on their journey with cancer, acknowledging 'a willingness to accept the vulnerability of both practitioner and patient' (Conti-O'Hara 2002: 33). Mayer (2008) urges nurses as cancer survivors to use their own stories and journeys to enhance the education, interdisciplinary working and research in the field of oncology.

Reflections on the journeys

There cannot really be firm conclusions to a chapter such as this where explorations have no endpoint. The author has looked to illuminate the primacy of the journey as perceived and presented by the traveller. How its stages are perceived, the 'inscape' of the cancer sufferer, before setting out on the road or at journey's close, will depend on many others: journeys by those who care on a personal or professional level, or both; emotional and spiritual journeys; journeys of scientific understanding; journeys of political will. To be human is to journey, and the cancer journey with all its twists and turns, light and shade, is unique to each cancer patient and survivor. For Maggie Keswick Jencks, even in her most difficult times and near the close of her own life, it was that 'above all what matters is not to lose the joy of living' (Keswick Jencks 1995: 13). Surely, for all who participate in and care for those on the journey, we cannot but share the aspirations embedded in this sentiment.

References

Armstrong L (2001) *It's Not About the Bike: My journey back to life*. London: Yellow Jersey Press.

Barker P (2000) Working with the metaphor of life and death. *Journal of Medical Ethics: Medical Humanities* **26**: 97–102.

Barker P (2002) The tidal model: the healing potential within a patient's narrative. *Journal of Psychosocial Nursing and Mental Health Services* **40**(7): 42–50.

Benner P, Wrubel J (1989) *The Primacy of Caring*. Menlo Park, CA: Addison Wesley.

Bredin M (2000) Altered self concept. In: Corner J, Bailey C. *Cancer Nursing Care in Context*. Oxford: Blackwell Science.

Calman KC (2000) *A Study of Story Telling: Humour and Learning in Medicine*. London: The Nuffield Trust/The Stationery Office.

Carter B (1989) Long-term survivors of breast cancer. *Cancer Nursing* **16**(5): 354–61.

Chabner BA (1997) A Personal Journey. Notes from the Edge: the diary of Peter J Morgan. *Oncologist* **2**(4): 206–7.

Clandinin DJ, Connelly FM (2000) *Narrative Inquiry: Experience and Story in Qualitative Research* San Francisco: Jossey Bass.

Clark RN, Jeffries N, Hasler J, Pendleton D (2002) *A Long Walk Home*. Oxford: Radcliffe Publishing.

Coleman MP, Rachet B, Woods LM, et al. (2004) Trends and socioeconomic inequalities in cancer survival in England and Wales up to 2001. *British Journal of Cancer* **90**(7): 1367–73.

Compas BE, Worsham NL, Epping-Jordan JE, et al. (1994) When Mom or Dad has cancer: Markers of psychological distress in cancer patients, spouses and children. *Health Psychology* **13**(6): 507–15.

Conti-O'Hare M (2002) *The Nurse as Wounded Healer: From Trauma to Transcendence*. Boston, MA: Jones & Bartelee.

Crane-Okada R (2007) A compass for the cancer journey: scientific, spiritual, and practical directives. *Oncology Nursing Forum* **34**(5): 945–55.

Davis F (1963) *Passage through Crisis*. Indianapolis: Bobbs-Merril Co.

Department of Health (1995) *A Policy Framework for Commissioning Cancer Services: A report by the Expert Advisory Group on Cancer to the Chief Medical Officers of England and Wales (Calman Hine Report)*. London: DH.

Department of Health (2001) *The NHS Cancer Plan: a plan for investment, a plan for reform*. London: DH (www.dh.gov.uk).

Department of Health (2007) *The Cancer Reform Strategy*. London: DH (www.dh.gov.uk).

Department of Heath and Social Security (1986) *Breast Cancer Screening: Report of the Health Ministers for England, Wales, Scotland and Northern Ireland (The Forrest Report)*. London: HMSO.

DeMarco RF, Picard C, Agretelis J (2004) Nurse experiences of cancer survivors. Part 1: personal. *Oncology Nursing Forum* **31**(3): 523–30.

Doyle N (2008) Cancer survivorship: evolutionary concept analysis. *Journal of Advanced Nursing* **62**(4): 499–509.

Drageset S, Lindstrom TC (2003) The mental health of women with suspected breast cancer: the relationship between social support, anxiety, coping and defence in maintaining mental health. *Journal of Psychiatric and Mental Health Nursing* **10**(4): 401–9.

Dunniece U, Slevin E (2000) Communicating sad, bad and difficult news in medicine. *Lancet* **363** (9405): 312–19.

Dunning T (2006) Caring for the wounded healer – nurturing the self. *Journal of Bodywork and Movement Therapies* **10**(4): 251–60.

Fallowfield LJ (2008) Treatment decision-making in breast cancer: the patient–doctor relationship. *Breast Cancer Research and Treatment* **12**(Suppl 1): 5–13.

Fallowfield LJ, Jenkins V (2006) Current concepts of communication skills training in oncology. *Recent Results in Cancer Research* **168**: 105–12.

Fallowfield LJ, Jenkins V, Farewell V, et al. (2003) Enduring impact of communication skills training: results of a 12-month follow-up. *British Journal of Cancer* **89**(8): 1445–9.

Fincham L, Copp G, Caldwell K, Jones L, Tookman A (2005) Supportive care: experiences of cancer patients. *European Journal of Oncology Nursing* **9**(3): 258–68.

Fitch MI, Maxwell C (2008) Bisphosphonates therapy in metastatic bone disease: the pivotal role of nurses in patient education. *Oncology Nursing Forum* **35**(4): 709–13.

Frank AW (2002) *At the Will of the Body: Reflections on Illness.* Boston, MA: Houghton Mifflin.

Gaydos HL (2005) Understanding personal narratives: an approach to practice. *Journal of Advanced Nursing* **49**(3): 254–9.

Greer S (1991) Psychological response to cancer and survival. *Psychological Medicine* **21**(1): 43–9.

Griffiths MJ, Humphris GM, Skirrow PM, Rogers SN (2008) A qualitative evaluation of patient experiences when diagnosed with oral cancer recurrence. *Cancer Nursing* **31**(4): E11–17.

Hammer K, Mogensen O, Hall EOC (2009) Hope as experienced in women newly diagnosed with gynaecological cancer. *European Journal of Oncology Nursing* **13**(4): 274–9.

Hickey SS (1986) Enabling hope. *Cancer Nursing* **9**(3): 133–7.

Hunniford G (2005) *Next to You.* London: Penguin Books.

Jacelon CS (1997) The trait and process of resilience. *Journal of Advanced Nursing* **25**(1): 123–9.

Keswick Jencks M (1995) *A View from the Front Line.* Edinburgh: Maggie Keswick & Charles Jencks.

Koldjeski D, Kirkpatrick MK, Everett L, Brown S, Swanson M (2007) The ovarian cancer journey of families in the first postdiagnostic year. *Cancer Nursing* **30**(3): 232–42.

Kumar S, Weaver VM (2009) Mechanics, malignancy, and metastasis: the force journey of a tumor cell. *Cancer Metastasis Reviews* **28**: 113–27.

Kyngas H, Mikkonen R, Nousiainen E-M, et al. (2000) Coping with the onset of cancer: coping strategies and resources of young people with cancer. *European Journal of Cancer Care* **10**(1): 6–11.

Lakoff G, Johnson M (1980) *Metaphors We Live By.* Chicago: University of Chicago Press.

Lerner M (1994) *Choices in Health: Integrating the best of conventional and complementary approaches to cancer.* Cambridge, MA: MIT Press.

Leydon GM, Bynae-Sutherland J, Coleman MP (2003) The journey towards cancer diagnosis of people with cancer, their family and carers. *European Journal of Cancer Care* **12**(4): 317–26.

Luker KA, Wilson K, Pateman B, Beaver K (2003) The role of district nursing: perspectives of cancer patients and their carers before and after hospital discharge. *European Journal of Cancer Care* **12**(4): 308–16.

Lunney JR, O'Mara A (2001) The end of the survival journey. *Seminars in Oncology Nursing* **17**(4): 274–8.

Marsé H, Van Cutsom E, Grothey A, Valverde S (2004) Management of adverse events and other practical considerations in patients receiving capecitabine (Xeloda). *European Journal of Oncology Nursing* **8**(Supp1): S16–30.

Marty M, Droz JP, Pouillart P, Paule B, Brion N, Bons J (1989) GR38032F, a 5HT3 receptor antagonist, in the prophylaxis of acute cisplatin-induced nausea and vomiting. *Cancer Chemotherapy and Pharmacology* **23**(6): 389–91.

Mayer DK (2007) Living with Cancer: the journey from victim to survivor. *Clinical Journal of Oncology Nursing* **11**(4): 481–2.

Mayer DK (2008) Wounded healers. *Clinical Journal of Oncology Nursing* **12**(4): 547.

Mayor S (2009) Study shows tentative increase in survival from NHS cancer plan. *BMJ* **333**: b1260.

McQueen A (2009) Waiting for a cancer diagnosis. *Cancer Nursing Practice* **8**(4): 16–23.

Miedema B, Hamilton R, Easley J (2007) From 'invincibility' to 'normalcy': coping strategies of young adults during the cancer journey. *Palliative and Supportive Care* **5**(1): 41–9.

Miller B (2007) Home of inspiration. *Nursing Standard* **22**(8): 22–3.

Morgan PP (1984) 'Wounded healers' can help give hospital patients more humane care. *Canadian Medical Association Journal* **131**(11): 1335–6.

Mullen F (1985) Seasons of survival: reflections of a physician with cancer. *New England Journal of Medicine* **313**(25): 270–3.

Nanton V, Docherty A, Meystre C, Dale J (2009) Finding a pathway: information and uncertainty along the prostate cancer patient journey. *British Journal of Health Psychology* **14**(Pt 3): 437–58.

Office for National Statistics (2005) *Long-term breast cancer survival, England and Wales, up to 2003*. London: ONS (www.statistics.gov.uk).

Picard C, Agretelis J, DeMarco RF (2004) Nurse experiences of cancer survivors. Part II: professional. *Oncology Nursing Forum* **31**(3): 537–42.

Quinn B (2003) Exploring nurses' experiences of supporting a cancer patient in their search for meaning. *European Journal of Oncology Nursing* **7**(3): 164–71.

Reisfield GM, Wilson GR (2004) Use of metaphor in the discourse on cancer. *Journal of Clinical Oncology* **22**(19): 4024–7.

Repede E (2008) All that holds: a story of healing. *Journal of Holistic Nursing* **26**(3): 226–32.

Rowland JH (2008) What are cancer survivors telling us? *Cancer Journal* **14**(6): 361–8.

Rutter M (1985) Resilience in the face of adversity: protective factors resistance to psychiatric disorder. *British Journal of Psychiatry* **147**(6): 598–611.

Scottish Government (2008) *Better Cancer Care, an Action Plan*. Edinburgh: The Scottish Government.

Shaha M, Cox CL, Talman K, Kelly D (2008) Uncertainty in breast, prostate and colorectal cancer: implications for supportive care. *Journal of Nursing Scholarship* **40**(1): 60–7.

Skott C (2002) Expressive metaphors in cancer narratives. *Cancer Nursing* **25**(3): 230–5.

Smith GD, Fawcett TN (2006) Stress. In: Alexander MF, Fawcett JN, Runciman PJ *Nursing Practice: Hospital and Home – The Adult*. Edinburgh: Elsevier.

Sontag S (1978) *Illness as a Metaphor*. New York: Farrer, Straus & Giroux.

Sontag S (2001) *Illness as a Metaphor and AIDS and its Metaphors*. New York: Picador.

Soothill K, Morris SM, Harman JC, Francis B, Thomas C, McIllmurray MB (2001) Informal carers of cancer patients: what are their unmet psychosocial needs? *Health Social Care in the Community* **9**(6): 464–75.

Spiegel D (2001) Mind matters, coping and cancer progression. *Journal of Psychosomatic Research* **50**(5): 287–90.

Stott K (2008) Give me time to heal. *Nursing Standard* **23**(9): 61.

Thastum M (2008) Coping, social relations, and communication: a qualitative exploratory study of children of parents with cancer. *Clinical Child Psychology and Psychiatry* **13**(1): 123–8.

Verdecchia A, Francisci S, Brenner H, et al. (2007) Recent cancer survival in Europe: a 2000–2002 period analysis of EUROCARE-4 data. *Lancet Oncology* **8**(9): 784–96.

Vivar GC, McQueen A (2005) Informational and emotional needs of long-term survivors of breast cancer. *Journal of Advanced Nursing* **51**(5): 520–8.

Whittemore R, Dixon J (2008) Chronic illness: the process of integration. *Journal of Clinical Nursing* **17**(7B): 177–87.

Wick JY, Zanni GR (2008) Hypochondria: the worried well. *Consultant Pharmacist* **23**(3), 192–4, 196–8, 207–8.

Wilson K, Pateman B, Beaver K, Luker KA (2002) Patient and carer needs following a cancer-related hospital admission: the importance of referral to the district nursing service. *Journal of Advanced Nursing* **38**(3): 245–53.

Chapter 2

Integrating cancer genetics into healthcare

Roseanne Cetnarskyj

Cancer genetics is an evolving area of medicine with an impact on patients with common cancers, seen in everyday nursing practice. The identification of genetic variation that affects an individual's risk of developing cancer has driven the development of cancer genetic services. Almost all areas of nursing can involve contact with patients[1] previously diagnosed with a cancer or currently being treated for cancer. Therefore, nurses are ideally placed to identify individuals requiring referral to cancer genetic services, to take a family history and to reassure individuals at low genetic risk.

In the United Kingdom, genetic education is currently not fully integrated into undergraduate programmes for nursing and midwifery students (Kirk and Tonkin 2006). A white paper published by the Department of Health, *Our Inheritance, Our Future: Realising the Potential of Genetics in the NHS*, highlights the need for healthcare professionals to develop genetic knowledge, stating:

> New genetics knowledge and technology has the potential to bring enormous benefits for patients, more personalised prediction of risk, more accurate diagnosis, safer use of medicines and new treatment options.
>
> DH (2003: 22)

Burton (2003) identified the need for all health professionals to have the knowledge and skill to identify individuals at increased risk of any genetic conditions, including cancer, and a recommendation for the creation a NHS genetic education centre to address this educational need was made.

In response to the DH white paper and the Burton report, the National Health Service (NHS) National Genetics Education and Development Centre (NGEDC) was created. The centre's aim is to integrate genetic education for all levels of NHS health professionals, recognising that only limited genetic education was currently provided within United Kingdom undergraduate nursing and midwifery programmes (Kirk & Tonkin 2006). To guide educators, Kirk (2003) published seven competency statements for nurses, from the newly registered nurse to the experienced nurse practitioner.

Using these competencies and findings from other disciplines, the NGEDC developed a United Kingdom workforce document, *Enhancing patient care by integrating genetics in clinical practice* (NGEDC 2007) which includes competencies for all United Kingdom

Perspectives on Cancer Care.   Edited by Josephine (Tonks) N. Fawcett and Anne McQueen
© 2011 Blackwell Publishing Ltd

non-genetics healthcare staff. These competencies are relevant to nurses and are linked to the *NHS Knowledge and Skills Framework* (DH 2004).

The United Kingdom workforce competencies for genetics in clinical practice for non-genetic healthcare staff follow a logical sequence of events in the patient's care pathway, to:

- Identify where genetics is relevant in their area of practice;

- Identify individuals with or at risk of genetic conditions;

- Gather multi-generational family history information;

- Use multi-generational family history information to draw a pedigree;

- Recognise a mode of inheritance in a family;

- Assess genetic risk;

- Refer individuals to specialist sources of assistance in meeting their healthcare needs;

- Order a genetic laboratory test;

- Communicate genetic information to individuals, families and healthcare staff.

NGEDC (2007)

Not all of the competencies are applicable to every healthcare role. This chapter will be structured using the competencies in relation to nursing, and applied to the understanding of cancer genetics.

The relevance of genetics to the nurse's practice

A person's genes have a significant contribution to their health, and increasing knowledge of genetics has an important place in our understanding of diseases, their prevention, diagnosis and treatment. As science and technology advance, our understanding of genetics is further extended and its relevance becomes more pervasive across healthcare. It therefore becomes more and more relevant for nurses in clinical practice to develop the knowledge and skills to be able to provide the necessary practical and supportive care to their patients. It is expected that nurses will be able 'to recognize patterns of disease that may indicate a possible genetic link, educate the family about the implications of a potential genetic susceptibility and refer the family for counselling' (Chapman 2007: 2). Before pursuing, in this chapter, a focus on cancer genetics, a brief section is included on some of the basic concepts relevant to genes and how they operate.

Genes are essentially comprised of deoxyribonucleic acid (DNA) and are carried on the chromosomes in the cell nucleus, each gene at a particular location. As chromosomes are paired (except for the sex chromosomes) there are two copies of each gene. When a gene is 'switched on' it synthesises a protein. This is done via a messenger molecule (messenger ribonucleic acid or mRNA) which travels from the nucleus into ribosomes in the cytoplasm, and here directs specific protein synthesis. This is achieved by a code, determined by the manner in which the chemicals band together. The specific arrangement of the chemicals will influence the particular amino acid formed.

Individuals receive one copy each chromosomes from each of their parents, to give 23 pairs. The first 22 pairs are called autosomes, the 23rd pair are the sex chromosomes. Individuals receive one X chromosome from their mother and either an X or a Y chromosome from their father (XX = female; XY = male).

Genetic disorders can arise when there are abnormalities of the chromosomes, or they may result from a genetic change (mutation)* in a single gene or in several genes. Mutations in genes that can predispose an individual to disease can be inherited at the time of conception, or may occur during an individual's lifetime. Some genetic mutations, of course, do not result in disease. Those that are of significance cause a change in the resulting protein. Inheritance of a disorder depends on how many copies of a gene are necessary to express the disorder. In the case of an autosomal dominant disorder, only one copy is required to manifest the disease; in a recessive disorder two copies of the gene are required – one from the mother and one from the father.

This understanding has been greatly enhanced by the Human Genome Project (HGP), an international project with the primary goal of determining the sequence of chemical base pairs which make up DNA, and identifying and mapping all the 20 000–25 000 human protein coding genes: the human genome.

To understand the implications for the patient with cancer and their family, nurses need to recognise the characteristics of an inherited cancer syndrome.

It is now possible to identify a small number of families that may be at increased risk of developing one of the more common cancers. In the United Kingdom population, certain genetic changes have been identified that will increased a person's risk of breast, ovarian, colorectal or endometrial cancer. A basic understanding of the genetic changes and mode of inheritance will help identify patients requiring referral to a cancer genetic service.

Cancer genetics

The majority of cancers seen are sporadic, and only a small percentage has an inherited component. Inherited cancers are due to a genetic change, a mutation, in specific genes. Although a genetic change is inherited in one copy of the gene, this is not sufficient for development of a cancer. A somatic[2] change in the other copy of the same gene must occur for cancer to develop. The development of a human cancer is a multistep process resulting from a series of genetic changes in a single cell (Fearon & Vogelstein 1990). Inherited genetic changes predominantly occur in tumour suppressor genes, but may also occur in another class of genes, the DNA mismatch repair genes.

Breast and ovarian cancer

There are two tumour suppressor genes in which inherited genetic changes have been identified and predispose an individual to breast or ovarian cancer: *BRCA1* on chromosome 17 (Miki et al. 1994) and *BRCA2* on chromosome 13 (Wooster et al. 1995). Inherited genetic changes within these genes are only responsible for a very small percentage of

---

*Genetic change and mutations are the same.

Table 2.1 Lifetime cancer risk for *BRCA1* and *BRCA2* gene carriers in the UK

Cancer site	BRCA1 risk at age 70	BRCA2 risk at age 70
Breast	87%	84%
Ovarian	44%	27%

Source: Ford *et al.* (1994, 1998).

breast cancer in the United Kingdom population (Peto et al. 1999). It is apparent that *BRCA1* or *BRCA2* genetic changes do not account for all familial breast and ovarian cancers. There are other genes in which a genetic change has a more minor effect, that can interact with environmental factors to cause a cancer to develop.

Individuals with a genetic change in *BRCA1* or *BRCA2* have an increased risk for both breast and ovarian cancer. The lifetime risk of developing cancer to carriers of a genetic change in the *BRCA1* or *BRCA2* gene in the United Kingdom population is shown in Table 2.1.

Male breast cancer is more often reported in families with *BRCA2* genetic changes than in *BRCA1* (Ford et al. 1998). Ovarian cancer related to inherited cancer syndromes is predominantly epithelial. Several mathematical models have been developed to calculate an individual's risk of carrying a *BRCA1* or *BRCA2* genetic change based on specific risk factors (Gail et al. 1989; Claus et al. 1993; Evans et al. 2004), but these are not practical in a non-genetic setting. The cancer genetic service will assess risk using a recommended model, after full investigation of a family history to ascertain risk and eligibility for genetic testing.

Colorectal cancer

There are several genetic changes in genes that can significantly increase the risk of developing colorectal cancer. However, only relatively few families are affected in relation to the general United Kingdom population (Dunlop et al. 2000). The most common conditions associated with such changes are familial adenomatous polyposis (FAP) and attenuated FAP (AFAP), MUTYH-associated polyposis (MAP) and hereditary non-polyposis colorectal cancer (HNPCC) (also known as Lynch syndrome).[3]

FAP results from genetic changes in an autosomal dominant tumour suppressor gene, known as the *APC* gene. Individuals with a genetic change in the *APC* gene have a very high risk of developing colorectal cancer, often in the third decade, of life with approximately 90% before the age of 70 (Vasen et al. 2008). FAP has definitive characteristics on colonoscopy, with more than 100 adenomatous polyps seen in the colon. Cancer is often seen in these families at a young age, but risk can be significantly reduced by effective screening and prophylactic surgery (Bulow et al. 2002). Individuals with FAP also have extracolonic symptoms which further confirm the diagnosis in the absence of a genetic change being identified.

More recently, a milder form of FAP known as attenuated FAP (AFAP) has been identified with genetic changes in a specific region of the *APC* gene. AFAP is characterised by later onset of colorectal cancer and fewer polyps in colon and rectum than FAP (Half et al. 2009).

An autosomal recessive polyposis condition known as MUTYH-associated polyposis (MAP) has been identified (Al-Tassan et al. 2002). On the strength of currently available evidence, it appears that a genetic change in both copies of the *MUTYH* gene is necessary for the risk of developing colorectal cancer to be increased (Sampson et al. 2003). MAP is characterised by the absence of a dominant inheritance pattern, and more than 10 polyps present throughout the colon by age 65 (Neilsen et al. 2009).

Hereditary non-polyposis colorectal cancer (HNPCC) is an autosomal dominant condition due to genetic changes in one of three DNA mismatch repair genes (MMR). The term HNPCC relates to a spectrum of cancers, and individuals with an inherited genetic change in an MMR gene are at risk of developing any of these cancers. HNPCC-related cancer sites include colorectal, endometrium, ovary, stomach, biliary tract, urinary tract and brain. However, the highest risk is for colorectal cancer, which affects 74–82% of males and 30–54% of females with genetic changes in *MLH1* and *MSH2*, by the age of 70. Females also have a 40–60% risk of endometrial cancer (Dunlop et al. 1997; Aarnio et al. 1999).

Tumour material from carriers of a mismatch repair gene genetic change can be identified by immunohistochemistry (IHC) staining for the protein expression of the three major MMR genes and molecular analysis to identify microsatellite instability. Such an examination can be used to direct further genetic testing.

Other cancer syndromes involving the breast and colon

TP53 is a tumour suppressor gene on chromosome 5, encoding a protein, p53, and plays an important role in the regulation of cancer. Germline genetic change in *TP53* leads to Li–Fraumeni syndrome which is associated with a spectrum of cancers, predominantly breast, soft tissue, brain, adrenocortical carcinoma and acute leukaemia, with childhood onset of malignancy commonly affecting at least one family member. A family history should meet stringent guidelines before genetic testing is offered (Chompret et al. 2001).

Juvenile polyposis syndrome (JPS) is the most common hamartomatous polyposis syndrome and is associated with genetic changes in both the *SMAD4* gene, a tumour suppressor gene on chromosome 18, and the *BMPR1A* gene on chromosome 10. The term juvenile relates to the type of polyp and not to the age of onset. JPS is characterised by many hamartomatous polyps in colon and rectum; on colonoscopy examination, individuals may be found to have up to 200 polyps by the age of 20, normally presenting with gastrointestinal bleeding (Desai et al. 1995). Individuals with a genetic change in these genes have a 70% risk of developing colorectal cancer by the age of 60 (Desai et al. 1995).

Peutz–Jeghers syndrome is an autosomal dominant polyposis syndrome with genetic changes in the *STK11* gene on chromosome 19. Genetic changes increase an individual's risk for a number of cancers including breast, lung, oesophageal, colon, pancreas, stomach, small intestine, uterine and ovarian (Giardello et al. 2000). The characteristics of this syndrome are hamartomatous polyposis of the gastrointestinal tract and melanin deposits, most commonly in the perioral region.

Identifying individuals with or at risk of genetic conditions

Only a minority of the United Kingdom population are at a higher risk of developing a cancer at a younger age, because of inherited genetic factors. A broad understanding of cancer genetic syndromes and the indicators of an increased risk shown by the family history can be seen to enhance patient care by nurses. Cancer is a common disease, so chance may account for the apparently high incidence of common cancers such as colorectal or breast cancer in some families. Indicators of a possible genetic predisposition to cancer in patients are:

- Several blood relatives with cancer at the same site;
- A combination of linked cancers, such as breast and ovarian cancer, or colorectal and endometrial cancer, on the same side of the family;
- More than one type of primary cancer in a single patient, or bilateral disease;
- A cancer diagnosed at a younger age than is normal for the population;
- The presence of a rare cancer in several family members;
- Ethnicity, for example, founder[4] genetic changes have been identified in the Ashkenazi Jewish population for breast/ovarian and colorectal cancer.

The nurse should wait until all the facts have been gathered and it is clear that the individual would benefit from referral, before discussing the possibility of referral to a cancer genetic service.

Gathering multi-generational family history information

When referring to cancer genetic services, the required information on the family history should be obtained.

The general public now have an increased awareness regarding a family history of cancer and it is anticipated that, in the future, taking a three-generation family history may become a routine part of the nurse's role.

Therefore, having the ability to ask the appropriate questions relating to a cancer family history, the ability to construct a family tree and knowledge of local cancer genetic services will prove to be valued skills for the nurse. Including a family tree with the referral will enable the genetic counsellor to begin their consultation from a sound knowledge base.

Confirmation of cancer

However, there is substantial evidence that family history information initially given by patients may not be accurate, and the further removed from the person providing the information, the less accurate the information is likely to be (Douglas et al. 1999; Ivanovich et al. 2002; Mitchell et al. 2004; Murff et al. 2004). Because of this, when a significant family history is suspected by the genetic counsellor, it is important that tumour site, tumour type and age at diagnosis for each cancer in a family tree is properly confirmed before making a final assessment of risk, offering clinical surveillance or genetic testing. It is very important that cancers reported are confirmed, to ensure appropriate surveillance.

Cancers can be confirmed via pathology reports, if the individual concerned is still living. The genetic counsellor will request a signed consent from the affected person (usually via the patient seen in the clinic) to access this information. An individual with cancer who would benefit from a more comprehensive risk assessment by the cancer genetic service should be asked for consent to include pathology reports with the referral.

The genetic service will confirm any relevant cancers via other sources such as hospital records, GP notes, death certificates and entries in the Cancer Registry and in Registers of Births, Deaths and Marriages. There are twelve cancer registry centres in the United Kingdom which provide an information service to the cancer genetic services (UKACR 2009).

Any information relating to a relative's cancer diagnosis is useful to the consultation in genetics. Asking patients to bring any relevant information concerning cancers in their family may speed up the risk assessment process. Providing privacy for the session gathering information on family history is very important, as it is not unusual for a patient to become very emotional due to the sensitivity of the information being discussed. They may also become anxious as they realise that they or their close family members may be at an increased risk of developing cancer (Schneider 2002).

Using family history information to draw a pedigree

Discussing the family history information is the first step in the process of constructing a family tree. After asking a patient about family history, it is important that the record of information is in a readable format. To enable family trees to be understood by health professionals, Bennett et al. (1995) published a set of recommended family history (pedigree)[5] symbols which are now used universally. It is standard in genetic practice to construct a three-generation family tree and, ideally, nurses will develop their skills to provide this information.

Construction of a family tree

Construction of a family tree is essential to identify any potential inheritance patterns. Family history enquiry should include the health of the patient's brothers, sisters, children,

---

Box 2.1   First- and second-degree relatives

1st-degree relatives are:	2nd-degree relatives are:
Mother	Grandparents
Father	Aunts and uncles
Brothers and sisters	Half-brothers and -sisters
Children	Grandchildren
	Nieces and nephews

parents, aunts, uncles and grandparents. Ideally a record should be obtained of all first- and second-degree relatives (see Box 2.1). Information on more distant relatives such as cousins is also important, if they are known to have had cancer.

For each person included in a family tree, it is important to record the following information:

- Full name (including maiden names and previous married or known names);
- Date of birth (if available); if not available, record current age;
- Date of death (if applicable);
- Type of cancer diagnosed (recorded for each cancer diagnosed in an individual);
- Age at diagnosis (recorded for each cancer diagnosed in an individual).

A key is generated for the known cancers in the family, and dating and signing the family tree is good practice. Symbols and relationship lines used in the construction of the family tree are shown in Figure 2.1.

Constructing a family tree is like any other nursing skill. It requires knowledge and practice to become competent. Several resources are suggested at end of this chapter to allow nurses to deepen and develop their knowledge and skills. Examples of a three-generation family tree are seen in Figures 2.2 and 2.3.

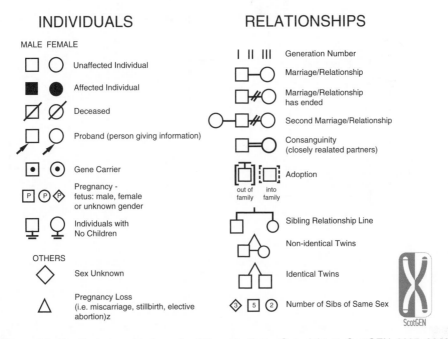

Figure 2.1 Family tree symbols and relationship lines. Copyright © ScotGEN 2007–2010, reproduced with permission.

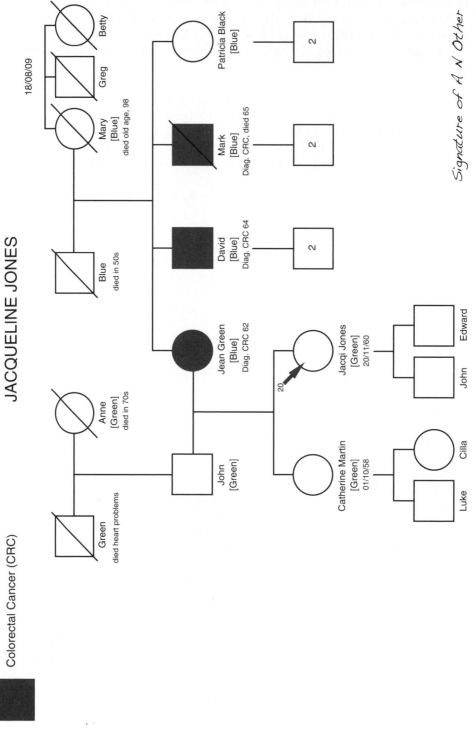

Figure 2.2 Example of a recessive family tree.

Methods of collecting family history

As cancer genetic services have evolved, so the methods of collecting a family history may vary between centres. Different methods of obtaining a family history are detailed below:

- A face-to-face appointment in a clinic.
- A form used to collect family history information: a family data collection form. This form is sent to the patient for completion. When returned, a family tree can be constructed on the basis of the information supplied, and the patient may be sent an appointment, or a letter of explanation if they are not eligible for an appointment.
- A telephone call to the patient to obtain the family history information.

Each method has advantages and disadvantages, and to date there is little published research on the quality of data obtained using each method. Cancer genetic services often utilise a combination of these methods, though nurses are more likely to have the opportunity to collect the family history information in a face-to-face interview. Genetic departments will normally use a pre-printed family history form to draw the family tree.

Most genetic healthcare professionals still draw family history freehand. There are also computer programs available to construct family trees but, currently, these tend to be used after a consultation, for families where more work is being undertaken.

Recognising a mode of inheritance in a family

A basic understanding of autosomal dominant and autosomal recessive inheritance is required in order to understand the meaning of the information recorded in the family tree.

Autosomal dominant inheritance

The autosomes are the 22 pairs of chromosomes found in each somatic cell. The pair of sex chromosomes are not autosomes. Autosomal relates to a gene located on one of the autosomes. Dominant means that a genetic change in a single copy of the particular gene will be sufficient to cause the condition. An example would be a *BRCA1* or *BRCA2* genetic change. An individual with an autosomal dominant genetic change will have a high risk of developing the condition. Their children will have a 50% risk of inheriting the same genetic change. An example of a dominant family history is shown in Plate 1.

Two factors that affect dominant inheritance are incomplete *penetrance* and variable *expressivity*.

The penetrance of a disorder relates to the number of people that have the genetic change for that particular disorder and then go on to develop the condition. Penetrance can vary from nearly 100%, as in individuals with an *APC* genetic change causing familial adenomatous polyposis, to around 40% for ovarian cancer in women with a *BRCA1* genetic change. Penetrance will differ with each dominant disorder.

Expressivity relates to how the condition manifests in an individual. Some cancer syndromes, such as FAP, present with a variety of symptoms; individuals with an *APC* genetic change may have the spectrum of symptoms. In addition to their proliferation of colorectal polyps or cancer, they may also have desmoid cysts, pigmented lesions of the retina, jaw cysts, sebaceous cysts or benign tumours of the bone (osteomas). It is not unusual for individuals with the *APC* gene, within the same family, to have a different spectrum of symptoms. There can be great variability in the severity of a condition between individuals within the same family.

When an autosomal dominant condition is suspected, several family members in more than one generation will normally be seen to be affected. Unfortunately, this pattern for a dominant family history is not always obvious, due to incomplete penetrance and variable expressivity. This is a reason for referring an individual to cancer genetic services or seeking advice from them. When several family members have cancer but are not first-degree relatives to each other, it can be the result of incomplete penetrance. Genetic counsellors will offer guidance to nurses encountering difficult family histories.

Autosomal recessive inheritance

Recessive inheritance relates to inheriting a genetic change on both copies of an autosomal gene. A person requires two copies of a recessive genetic change to develop a particular condition. In other words, a genetic change is inherited from each parent. If only one copy is inherited it would not normally affect health. In a recessive condition, there would normally be several affected members in one generation. An example of a recessive family history can be seen in Figure 2.2.

Understanding these two modes of inheritance will enable a judgement to be made on the likely chance that the patient's cancer or their family history of cancer is the result of an inherited genetic change. Knowledge of modes of inheritance allows the identification of other individuals within a family tree who may also be at increased genetic risk.

Assessing genetic risk

We know that environmental factors contribute to the risk of developing cancer. These environmental risk factors are better understood in some cancers than in others. The environmental risk factors can interact with an underlying genetic susceptibility; for example, individuals who smoke and have genetic change in the *TP53* gene have a threefold higher risk of developing lung cancer compared to those who do not smoke (Le Calvez et al. 2005).

Non-genetic healthcare staff would not be expected to make an accurate assessment of genetic risk. Their role should be to have an understanding of basic family history assessment and the local evidence-based guidelines.

It is acknowledged that many referrals to cancer genetic services are not necessary, and such referrals can cause additional anxiety to patients, as well as increasing the waiting time (Lucassen et al. 2001; Wonderling et al. 2001; McDonald et al. 2008). If non-genetic healthcare staff were confident in their knowledge and could apply the guidelines to a family history to help them make an assessment of risk, it is expected that the number of unnecessary referrals to the cancer genetic services would decrease. In many cases a nurse with the correct knowledge and skill could reassure the patient that a referral was not required, and relieve some of their anxiety.

Guidelines for health professionals

Assessing risk from family history information can be complex and there are now published guidelines to assist health professionals with the risk assessment in cancer families (SIGN 2003; NICE 2006; Scottish Executive 2009). It is likely that these will continue to be refined in the coming years and it is important that nurses have access to current local guidelines.

It is not possible to provide an exhaustive list of current guidelines. By way of illustration, in Scotland the four cancer genetic services use one set of guidelines for individuals with a breast, ovarian or colorectal cancer family history. Individuals with other cancer family histories are seen on request, and their risk is assessed using guidance from current literature. The Scottish guidelines provide guidance to non-genetic health professionals on the family histories that warrant referral to cancer genetic services. They are also used by health professionals specifically trained in cancer genetics, to guide them as to which patients should be offered entry into a clinical surveillance programme and/or which families can be offered genetic testing due to their significantly increased family history risk.

The breast cancer family guidelines are available via the Scottish Government Health Directorates on the website (Scottish Executive 2009). Many women with a family history of ovarian cancer also meet the criteria for breast screening; therefore, these guidelines should also be considered for women with a family history of ovarian cancer.

Table 2.2 provides an example of the criteria for referral to the cancer genetic service in Scotland, for an individual with family history of breast cancer.

The Scottish guideline used for individuals with a family history of colorectal cancer is the no. 67 SIGN guideline (SIGN 2003). This guideline provides information for either a suspected FAP or an HNPCC family history. All Scottish guidelines for individuals with a family history of cancer are available via the Scottish Genetics Education Network website (scotgen.org.uk) and should be checked regularly for updates.

In England and Wales, most cancer genetic services will use the NICE CG 41 guideline (NICE 2006) for risk assessment of breast cancer families. The British Society of Gastroenterology and Association of Coloproctology for Great Britain and Northern Ireland (BSGAC) guidelines (Cairns et al. 2009) for families with colorectal cancer will be used in some United Kingdom cancer genetic services. Most United Kingdom genetic centres support the use of the modified Amsterdam criteria (Vasen et al. 1999) as surveillance and testing criteria for high-risk families (see Box 2.2).

The evidence for surveillance is less strong for families not meeting these criteria. It is now common practice for cancer genetic services to offer microsatellite instability (MSI) and immunohistochemistry (IHC) screening on tumour material from an affected family

Table 2.2　Moderate, high risk and very high breast cancer guidelines in Scotland

Moderate risk	High risk	Very high risk
One 1st-degree relative with breast cancer (BRCA) under age 40	Four or more relatives affected with either breast cancer at age 60 or ovarian cancer at any age, in three generations	Female carriers of a mutation in *BRCA1*, *BRCA2* or *TP53*
One 1st-degree relative with male breast cancer	One individual that has both breast and ovarian cancer	50% risk of having a mutation in *BRCA1*, *BRCA2* or *TP53*
Two 1st-degree or one 1st- and one 2nd-degree relative with BRCA under age 60, or ovarian cancer at any age, on the same side of the family	Families where there is the 20% likelihood of a *BRCA1*, *BRCA2* or *TP53* mutation	
Three 1st- or 2nd-degree relatives with BRCA or ovarian cancer on the same side of the family where one is 1st-degree to the proband or the proband's father		

Source: Scottish Executive (2009).

Box 2.2　Modified amsterdam criteria

All criteria must be met

At least three relatives with an HNPCC-associated cancer (colorectal, endometrial, small bowel, ureter or renal pelvis).
One person should be a first-degree relative of the other two.
At least two successive generations affected.
At least one person should be diagnosed with their cancer before the age of 50.
Familial adenomatous polyposis (FAP) should be excluded in the cases with colorectal cancer.
Tumours should be verified by pathological examination.

Source: Vasen et al. (1999)

member, as a method of more accurate risk assessment for surveillance and testing. However, guidelines on family history criteria for these families are not universally agreed in the United Kingdom due to the current lack of research evidence. This supports the need for healthcare professionals to confirm local guidelines as a means of assisting referral decision making.

Referring individuals to specialist sources

To refer and provide a patient with accurate information about cancer genetic services requires a full understanding of the aims of the service. Regional cancer genetic services aim to:

- Identify, in their own population, those individuals who are at a moderate or significant increased risk of developing cancer,
  - through education of appropriate health professionals and development of clear guidelines for referral.
- Reduce the mortality rate from common cancers such as breast, ovarian and colorectal cancer,
  - through accurate risk assessment and appropriate screening or offer of prophylactic surgery for those at the relevant increased risk for their cancer type;
  - by offering genetic testing within a family (where available) and delivering the results promptly.
- Discharge those not at increased risk compared to the general population risk from current screening programmes,
  - through identification of individuals currently in a surveillance programme due to inaccurate risk assessment, non-adherence to published guidelines or as a result of current guidelines being changed and updated;
  - by dissemination of current guidelines to all health professionals that are involved in provision of surveillance programmes.
- Reduce the number of low-risk referrals to the genetic service,
  - through education of health professionals to enhance their family history skills, and by promoting the use of current guidelines and the development of knowledge on risk assessment.

Regional cancer genetic services offer local and outreach clinics throughout the United Kingdom. Information on United Kingdom genetics services is available via the Genetic Interest Group website (http://www.geneticalliance.org.uk/). These services are mainly under the auspices of the National Health Service. However, some areas in England and Wales offer private genetic services.

The use of cancer genetic services has dramatically increased in recent years due to the identification of genetic changes in cancer-predisposing genes and the improvement in technology. Therefore, cancer genetic services have evolved and developed to meet the demand from the general public, due to increased awareness, often from personal stories in the media.

Patients should be shown the local guidelines when discussing their eligibility for referral. There are also resources available on cancer websites to which patients can be directed, where information can help them understand why referral to cancer genetic services is not required (see Box 2.3).

Consent for referral

Any referral to the cancer genetic service must always be with the consent of the patient, and they must be allowed to make an informed choice about referral. They may have a

---

Box 2.3   Additional resources for healthcare professionals and patients

Detailed fact sheets on autosomal dominant and recessive inheritance: www.genetics.com.au

Fact sheets to aid understanding or to aid explanation on dominant and recessive inheritance to a patient: www.scotgen.org.uk

An excellent animation on 'pathways to cancer': www.insidecancer.org

Publications with detailed information and resources on a variety of aspect relating to family history and construction of family tree: www.geneticseducation.nhs.uk

Learning material to enhance the knowledge and skill for constructing a family tree: www.scotgen.org.uk

Information relating to the role of UK cancer registries, the services offered and the consent require before information will be released: www.isdscotland.org and the United Kingdom Association of Cancer Registries (UKACR) at http://82.110.76.19/

Referral and surveillance guidelines for Scotland, England and Wales: www.sign.ac.uk/, www.sehd.scot.nhs.uk/mels/HDL2007_08.pdf, www.scotgen.org.uk, www.nice.org.ukand local genetic departments

A talking glossary of terms that will be useful when identifying unfamiliar terminology: www.genome.gov/glossary

Actual case patients discussing their own experience: www.geneticseducation.nhs.uk/tellingstories/genetic_results.asp?condition=18

Information on ethical issues in genetics can be found at: http://www.hgc.gov.uk/Client/Content.asp?ContentId=793

Patients can find more information on genetic testing and insurance at: http://www.abi.org.uk/Information/Consumers/Health_and_Protection/499.pdf

Information on cancer genetics and written for the general public is available at: http://www.macmillan.org.uk/Cancerinformation/Causesriskfactors/Genetics/Cancergenetics/Cancergenetics.aspx

http://breakthrough.org.uk/breast_cancer/family_history/

http://www.cancerhelp.org.uk/about-cancer/cancer-questions/genetics-and-cancer-risk

http://www.beatingbowelcancer.org/Content/269/Family-history

Access to an online learning module on cancer genetics: http://learning.bmj.com/learning/search-result.html?moduleId=10010136

Association of British Insurers: http://www.abi.org.uk/Information/Consumers/Health_and_Protection/499.pdf

---

high-risk family history but choose not to seek further information from cancer genetic services (O'Neil et al. 2006). If appropriately detailed information has been provided to make this choice, their choice is always respected, but they might be advised to find information on their local cancer genetic service and be encouraged to discuss things further with their own GP should they subsequently change their mind.

On occasions the problem may arise where a family member has been referred to cancer genetic services in their own area but, due to different guidelines used for the risk assessment, the patient is not eligible for referral in their own area. The reality that practice may vary across the country must be honestly and openly explained. The patient should be clear that they are being referred for risk assessment in the first instance and that at this stage genetic testing is not, as yet, being offered. The genetic healthcare professionals will discuss the availability of either surveillance screening and/or genetic testing.

Surveillance screening

Surveillance screening is offered to an individual when the family history risk is assessed as indicating a moderate, high or significantly increased risk that a genetic change is contributing to the cancers in the family. The frequency and screening modality will depend on:

- the level of risk assessment;
- whether a genetic change has been identified in the family;
- the site of cancers in the family;
- the age of onset of cancer in the family;
- the age of the person eligible for screening;
- the availability of screening modality in the local area.

The surveillance screening modalities that may be offered to an individual with an increased cancer risk are:

- Females within breast/ovarian cancer families are offered annual mammography (unless under age of 40, when it is every two years) and an annual clinical breast examination. This is reassessed at the age of 50.
- Families with FAP confirmed or suspected will be offered a combination of flexible sigmoidoscopy and colonoscopy.
- Families with confirmed HNPCC or increased colorectal cancer risk will be offered colonoscopy.

Currently no effective screening is available for ovarian or endometrial cancer, and such individuals need to discuss the options with gynaecologist. Prophylactic surgery is currently the most effective method of reducing ovarian cancer (Rebbeck et al. 2009). Equally the risk of endometrial cancer is thought to be reduced by prophylactic surgery, but the evidence is limited.

As indicated, the patient being referred to a cancer genetic service should be aware that the initial appointment will be to undertake a risk assessment on the family history. At this appointment the genetic healthcare professional will discuss the availability of either surveillance screening and/or genetic testing based on the information that is confirmed in the family history and further discussion with the patient.

Genetic laboratory testing

An inherited predisposition to cancer can be confirmed in some families if a genetic change within a gene which predisposes to cancer is detected in an *affected* family member. Such testing is generally activated by staff in the cancer genetics centre. When a genetic change that increases the risk of developing cancer is identified in a research setting, it can take several years for these research findings to be translated into an NHS genetic test. Public expectation of genetic testing may at times be unrealistic. Currently, genetic testing has little to offer except in rare families who have a family tree which suggests a 'cancer syndrome'.

Genetic testing

Some individuals can be tested for genetic changes in *BRCA1* and *BRCA2* genes, *APC* and *MHL1*, *MSH2* and *MSH6*. The first stage of genetic testing in families is to find a genetic change in a family member with the cancer, known as 'mutation analysis'; it can take a significant time to identify a genetic change. Even though the family history meets high-risk criteria and thereby the individual may be eligible for genetic testing, with the exception of *APC* genetic changes the chance of identifying a genetic change in these families is not high. The availability of genetic testing in a family depends on several factors:

- The family history meets the laboratoriy' criteria for testing;
- There is a living family member with cancer;
- A family member with cancer is willing to undergo genetic counselling to ensure informed consent and provide a blood sample for testing.

If a genetic change in a gene which may predispose to cancer is identified in a family member, genetic testing can be offered to relevant unaffected family members. This is known as 'direct gene testing', the result of which will predict if a person has inherited the known genetic change in the family. It does not mean that they will definitely develop cancer. These individuals undergo a series of genetic counselling appointments before informed consent for testing is taken. This is to that ensure individuals have had optimal time to ask questions, explore relevant issues and process information. Knowing they have a genetic change does help some individuals make important health and lifestyle decisions such as considering prophylactic surgery, having children sooner than planned and perhaps reflecting on career decisions (Schwartz et al. 2009).

It is important to be aware, when discussing genetic testing, that identical twins share the same DNA, so if one twin is identified to have a genetic change this will also give a genetic test result to the other twin. However, twin studies have shown that, even though they have the same genetic change, identical twins are unlikely to develop a cancer at the same site or at the same time (Lichtenstein et al. 2001). This reflects the role of environmental factors in the development of cancer in the individual.

Although the NHS can control access to genetic testing and provide genetic counselling services to support those having genetic testing, individuals can potentially access genetic testing via the Internet. Genetic testing is offered on the Internet with little or no support services, and quality control of the laboratories that undertake the testing may well be inadequate (Human Genetic Commission 2007).

Communicating with individuals, families and healthcare staff

Communication of genetic information can be difficult. Discussing diseases of family members can be distressing for patients; they can become quite emotional and may find it awkward discussing trends through their family line. It is important that the nurse is sensitive to the patient's feelings, that language is tailored to enable the unique patient to understand the information given, and time allowed to address questions and correct any misunderstandings. The nurse can also inform patients of the useful and clearly written resources they can access. These are accessible through most large cancer charity websites. Nurses may equally find it useful to access this material to develop their awareness of information available to the general public. Guidance is given in Box 2.3.

Ethical issues

Ethical issues in genetic medicine are among the most complex encountered in healthcare practice. This is mainly due to the dynamics involving perhaps many family members rather than a single individual (Morrison 2005). In order to address some of these ethical issues, genetic departments provide full information, offer counselling and have rigorous consenting procedures in place, usually ensured over more than one appointment.

Genetic testing and insurance

Patients may ask whether referral to a genetic department will affect their insurance prospects. Any current insurance policy is not affected, as long as, if asked, any cancers in the family at the time of taking the policy out have been declared.

For any new policy for life insurance or critical illness cover, patients must inform the insurance company of the cancers in the family. However, since October 2000, there has been a moratorium on the accessing of applicants' genetic test results by insurance companies that are members of the Association of British Insurers (ABI).

A person that has taken a genetic test does not need to declare this to an insurance company and the insurance company cannot ask them to take a genetic test. At the time of writing, they can apply for up to £500 000 of life insurance cover, £300 000 of critical illness insurance and income protection cover up to £30 000 annually without informing the insurance company about a genetic test for a known genetic change that would increase their risk of cancer (ABI 2008).

Rare cancer syndromes

There are many rare cancer syndromes that are seen within a cancer genetic service. Non-genetic nurses are less likely to see these cancers unless working in a specialist area, where they will probably be aware of the conditions relevant to their practice. The local genetic department will be willing to discuss any queries nurses may have regarding a patient's family history. Some rare syndromes do have a known genetic change identified, and testing is available.

Conclusion

This chapter has sought to provide an overview of the currently available information in cancer genetics relevant to non-genetic nurses. This is a new area of knowledge for many nurses caring for people with cancer. In order to gain further understanding of cancer genetics, the reader is referred to case studies 2.1 and 2.2, which illustrate the nurse's role in supporting patients. In addition the reader is encouraged to explore the material in Box 2.3.

Case study 2.1   Mrs L

Mrs L is a 40-year-old woman who has just been given a diagnosis of breast cancer following a mammogram and biopsy. Mrs L is naturally upset; she then informs you that she is the fourth person in her family to develop breast cancer. Her mother and maternal aunt both developed breast cancer at ages 50 and 52, respectively. Mrs L's older sister was diagnosed with breast cancer last year, at age 46. She asks you if there could be something causing this in her family.

The nurse's response and support

As a nurse you will need to explain to Mrs L that in a small number of families there can be a genetic change in a gene that can increase the risk of breast cancer in the family.

Take as much family history information as is possible and construct a family tree. If Mrs L does not feel able to do this at this appointment, arrange to see her when she feels better able to give her family history, or you can give her a family history data collection form to take away and return to you.

Check the local cancer referral guidelines and your local policy for referral. If Mrs L is eligible for referral, ask her if this is what she would prefer. With this level of family history, Mrs L would be eligible for referral at United Kingdom centres.

Mrs L will benefit from seeing the guidelines for her referral to the genetics department. Offer further information but allow her time to understand the situation and to ask whatever questions she might find helpful.

You can show Mrs L the guidelines, to let her see that she can be referred to the genetic department. It is likely that Mrs L will ask questions about what will happen at the genetic appointment.

Remembering that Mrs L will also need to have several appointments to discuss her options, which would very likely to include surgery and chemotherapy, she may be reluctant to be referred to the genetic department. There are occasions when the genetic counselling appointment may inform decision making for surgery; for example, prophylactic surgery of the unaffected breast, due to the increased risk of developing cancer.

You can explain that her family history will be discussed, confirmed and a risk assessment made at the genetics department. Take time to do this, as it may be hard at first for Mrs L to absorb this information. She will then have the opportunity to discuss her risk assessment in relation to her current diagnosis of breast cancer, and also begin to discuss and understand the risks for other family members.

If Mrs L chooses not to be referred at this time, reassure her that she can discuss this again at any time with her consultant, a nurse on the ward or her GP, to request a referral to the genetics department.

You could also inform Mrs L of the cancer charity websites where she would be able to access information to help her with her decision making.

Case study 2.2

Mr J

Mr J is a 59-year-old man who is in the ward following surgery for colorectal cancer. He tells you that he is a little worried about his children's risk of developing colorectal cancer as his wife's mother has colorectal cancer too.

The nurse's response and support

As a nurse you can explain to Mr J that in a small number of families there can be a genetic cause of colorectal cancer.

More information can be obtained from Mr J on his family history, and his wife's family history can also be explored. This gives more information and reveals that Mr J is the only person in his family to have had colorectal cancer. His father had lung cancer at age 65 and was a heavy smoker. Mr J's mother-in-law developed colorectal cancer at age 81; and he was not aware of any other cancers on his wife's maternal family history.

You could offer support by directing Mr J to any of the cancer charity websites, where he would be able to access information to reassure him that his children are not at an increased risk with the family history disclosed to you. He can also use this resource to help him discuss further family history information with his wife.

Notes

Acknowledgement: The author would very much like to thank Professor Mary Porteous for being a critical reader for her chapter.

1. In this chapter the term 'patient' has been used to represent a person that is seen or cared for by a nurse.
2. A somatic cell is any cell of the body except sperm and egg cells.
3. HNPCC and Lynch syndrome are used interchangeably in the literature.

4. Founder genetic changes or mutations have been identified in several populations.
5. In this chapter the term 'family tree' is used. However, in some literature the term 'pedigree' is found. Both family tree and pedigree are used interchangeably.

References

Aarnio M, Sankila R, Pukkala E, et al. (1999) Cancer risk in mutation carriers of DNA-mismatch-repair genes. *International Journal of Cancer* **81**(2): 214–18.

Al-Tassan N, Maynard J, Fleming N, Hodges AK, Sampson JR, Cheadle JP (2002) Inherited variants of MYH associated with somatic G:C → T:A mutations in colorectal cancer. *Nature Genetics* **30**(2): 227–32.

Association of British Insurers (2008) Genetic tests and insurance: what you need to know. http://www.abi.org.uk/Information/Consumers/Health_and_Protection/499.pdf.

Bennett RL, Steinhaus KA, Uhrich SB, et al. (1995) Recommendations for standardized human pedigree nomenclature. Pedigree Standardization Task Force of the National Society of Genetic Counselors. *American Journal of Human Genetics* **56**(3): 745–52.

British Society of Gastroenterology (2009).

Bulow C, Vasen H, Jarvinen H, et al. (2002) Ileorectal anastomosis is appropriate for a subset of patients with familial adenomatous polyposis. *Gastroenterology* **119**: 1454–60.

Burton H (2003) *Addressing genetics, delivering health: A strategy for advancing the dissemination and application of genetics knowledge throughout our health professions*. Cambridge: Public Health Genetics Unit.

Cairns S, Scholefield J, Steele M, et al. (2010) United Kingdom guidelines for colorectal cancer screening and surveillance in high risk groups (update from 2002). *Gut* **59**(5): 666–89.

Chapman DD (2007) Cancer genetics. *Seminars in Oncology Nursing* **23**(1), 2–9.

Chompret A, Abel A, Stoppa-Lyonnet D, et al. (2001) Sensitivity and predictive value of criteria for p53 germline mutation screening. *Journal of Medical Genetics* **38**(1): 43–7.

Claus EB, Risch N, Thompson WD (1993) The calculation of breast cancer risk for women with a first degree family history of ovarian cancer. *Breast Cancer Research and Treatment* **28**(2): 115–20.

Department of Health (2003) Our Inheritance, *Our Future: Realising the Potential of Genetics in the NHS*. London: TSO Publishing.

Department of Health (2004) *NHS Knowledge and Skills Framework*. London: TSO Publishing.

Desai DC, Neale KF, Talbot IC, Hodgson SV, Phillips RKS (1995) Juvenile polyposis. *British Journal of Surgery* **82**(1): 14–17.

Douglas FS, O'Dair LC, Robinson M, Evans DG, Lynch SA (1999) The accuracy of diagnoses as reported in families with cancer: a retrospective study. *Journal of Medical Genetics* **36**(4): 309–12.

Dunlop MG, Farrington SM, Carothers A, et al. (1997) Cancer risk associated with germline DNA mismatch repair gene mutations. *Human Molecular Genetics* **6**(1): 105–10.

Dunlop MG, Farrington SM, Nicholl I, et al. (2000) Population carrier frequency of hMSH2 and hMLH1 mutations. *British Journal of Cancer* **83**(12): 1643–5.

Evans DGR, Eccles DM, Rahman N, et al. (2004). A new scoring system for the chances of identifying a BRCA1/2 mutation outperforms existing models including BRCAPRO. *Journal of Medical Genetics* **41**(6): 474–80.

Fearon ER, Vogelstein B (1990) A genetic model for colorectal tumorigenesis. *Cell* **61**(5): 759–67.

Ford D, Easton D, Bishop D, Narod S, Goldgar D, and the Breast Cancer Linkage Consortium (1994) Risks of cancer in BRCA1-mutation carriers. *Lancet* **343**(8899): 692–5.

Ford D, Easton DF, Stratton M, et al. and the Breast Cancer Linkage Consortium (1998) Genetic heterogeneity and penetrance analysis of the *BRCA1* and *BRCA2* genes in breast cancer families. The Breast Cancer Linkage Consortium, *American Journal of Human Genetics* **62**(3): 676–89.

Gail MH, Brinton LA, Byar DP, et al. (1989) Projecting individualized probabilities of developing breast cancer for white females who are being examined annually. *Journal of the National Cancer Institute* **81**(24): 1879–86.

Giardello FM, Brensinger JD, Tersmette AC, et al. (2000) Very high risk of cancer in familial Peutz–Jeghers syndrome. *Gastroenterology* **119**(6): 1447–53.

Half E, Bercovich D, Rozen P (2009) Familial adenomatous polyposis. *Orphanet Journal of Rare Diseases* **12**(4), 22.

Human Genetic Commission (2007) *More Genes Direct.* http://www.hgc.gov.uk/Client/document. asp?DocId=139&CAtegoryId=10.

Ivanovich J, Babb S, Goodfellow P, et al. (2002) Evaluation of the family history collection process and the accuracy of cancer reporting among a series of women with endometrial cancer. *Clinical Cancer Research* **8**(6): 1849–56.

Kirk M (2003) *Fit for Practice in a Genetic Era: A competence-based education framework for nurses, midwives and health visitors.* Wales: Public Policy Unit.

Kirk M, Tonkin E (2006) *Survey of practice and needs of UK educators in delivering a genetic competence framework.* Birmingham: NHS National Education and Development Centre.

Le Calvez F, Mukeria A, Hunt JD, et al. (2005) *TP53* and *KRAS* mutation load and types in lung cancers in relation to tobacco smoke: distinct patterns in never, former, and current smokers. *Cancer Research* **65**(12): 5076–83.

Lichtenstein P, Holm NV, Verkasalo PK, et al. (2000) Environmental and heritable factors in the causation of cancer – analyses of cohorts of twins from Sweden, Denmark, and Finland. *New England Journal of Medicine* **343**(2): 78–85.

Lucassen A, Watson E, Harcourt J, Rose P, O'Grady J (2001) Guidelines for referral to a regional genetics service: GPs respond by referring more appropriate cases. *Family Practice* **18**(2): 135–40.

McDonald K, Iredale R, Higgs G (2008) Primary care referrals to a British regional cancer genetics service. *Journal of Clinical Nursing* **17**(22): 3074–6.

Miki Y, Swensen J, Shattuck-Eidens D, et al. (1994) A strong candidate for the breast and ovarian cancer susceptibility gene BRCA1. *Science* **266**(5182): 66–71.

Mitchell RJ, Brewster D, Campbell H, et al. (2004) Accuracy of reporting of family history of colorectal cancer. *Gut* **53**(2): 291–5.

Morrison JP (2005) The ethical and insurance issues of cancer genetics. In: Lalloo F, Kerr B, Friedman J, Evans G (eds) *Risk Assessment and Management in Cancer Genetics.* Oxford: Oxford University Press.

Murff HJ, Spigel DR, Syngal S (2004) Does this patient have a family history of cancer? An evidence-based analysis of the accuracy of family cancer history. *Journal of the American Medical Association* **292**(12): 1480–9.

National Health Service National Genetics Education and Development Centre (2007) *Enhancing patient care by integrating genetics in clinical practice.* Birmingham: NHS National Education and Development Centre.

National Institute for Health and Clinical Excellence (2006) *Familial Breast Cancer: The Classification and Care of Women at Risk of Familial Breast Cancer in Primary, Secondary and Tertiary Care.* London: NICE.

Nielsen M, Joerink-van de Beld MC, Jones N, et al. (2009) Analysis of MUTYH genotypes and colorectal phenotypes in patients with MUTYH-associated polyposis. *Gastroenterology* **136**(2): 471–6.

O'Neill SM, Peters JA, Vogel VG, Feingold E, Rubinstein WS (2006) Referral to cancer genetic counseling: Are there stages of readiness? *American Journal of Medical Genetics Part C Seminars in Medical Genetics* **142C**(4): 221–31.

Peto J, Collins N, Barfoot R., et al. (1999) Prevalence of BRCA1 and BRCA2 gene mutations in patients with early-onset breast cancer. *Journal of the National Cancer Institute* **91**(11): 943–9.

Rebbeck TR, Kauff ND, Domcheck SM (2009) Metaanalysis of risk reduction estimates associated with risk-reducing salpingo-oophorectomy in BRCA1 or BRCA2 mutation carriers. *Journal of the National Cancer Institute* **101**(2): 80–7.

Sampson JR, Dolwani S, Jones S, et al. (2003) Autosomal recessive colorectal adenomatous polyposis due to inherited mutations of MYH. *Lancet* **362**(9377): 39–41.

Schneider K (2002) *Counselling about Cancer*, 2nd edn. New York: John Wiley & Sons.

Schwartz MD, Valdimarsdottir HB, DeMarco TA, et al. (2009) Randomized trial of a decision aid for BRCA1/BRCA2 mutation carriers: impact on measures of decision making and satisfaction. *Health Psychology* **28**(1): 11–19.

Scottish Executive (2009) *Cancer Genetic Services in Scotland: Management of women with a family history of breast cancer.* http://www.sehd.scot.nhs.uk/mels/CEL2009_06.pdf.

Scottish Intercollegiate Guideline Network (2003) *Management of Colorectal Cancer.* Edinburgh: SIGN Publication.

United Kingdom Association of Cancer Registries (UKACR) UK cancer registries (online) at http://82.110.76.19/.

Vasen HF, Watson P, Mecklin JP, Lynch HT (1999) New clinical criteria for hereditary nonpolyposis colorectal cancer (HNPCC, Lynch syndrome) proposed by the International Collaborative group on HNPCC. *Gastroenterology* **116**(6): 1453–6.

Vasen HF, Möslein G, Alonso A, et al. (2008) Guidelines for the clinical management of familial adenomatous polyposis (FAP). *Gut* **57**(5): 704–13.

Wonderling D, Hopwood P, Cull A, et al. (2001) A descriptive study of UK cancer genetics services: an emerging clinical response to the new genetics. *British Journal of Cancer* **85**(2): 166–70.

Wooster R, Bignell G, Lancaster J, et al. (1995) Identification of the breast cancer susceptibility gene BRCA2. *Nature* **378**(6559): 789–92.

Further reading

Benjamin C, Gamet K (2005) Recognising the limitation of your genetics expertise. *Nursing Standard* **20**(6): 49–54.

Bennett RL (1999) *The Practical Guide to the Genetic Family History.* New York: John Wiley & Sons.

Bexfield A, Nigam Y (2008) Genes and chromosomes. Part 2: Cell division and genetic diversity. *Nursing Times* **104**(24): 24–5.

Bexfield A, Nigam Y (2008) Genes and chromosomes. Part 3: Genes, proteins and mutations *Nursing Times* **104**(25): 26–7.

Bradley A (2005) Utility and limitations of genetic testing and information. *Nursing Standard* **20**(5): 52–5.

Gaff C (2005) Identifying clients who might benefit from genetic services and information. *Nursing Standard* **20**(1): 49–53.

Haydon J (2005) Genetics: uphold the right of all clients to informed decision-making and voluntary action. *Nursing Standard* **20**(3): 48–51.

Kirk M (2005) Introduction to the genetics series. *Nursing Standard* **20**(1): 48.

Kirk M (2005) The role of genetic factors in maintaining health. *Nursing Standard* **20**(4): 50–4.

Lalloo F, Kerr B, Friedman J, Evans G (eds) (2005) *Risk assessment and management in cancer genetics*. Oxford: Oxford University Press.

Middleton A, Ahmed M, Levene S (2005) Tailoring genetic information and services to clients' culture, knowledge and language level. *Nursing Standard* **20**(2): 52–6.

Morrison PJ, Hodgson SV, Haites NE (eds) (2002) *Familial Breast and Ovarian Cancer*. Cambridge: Cambridge University Press.

Nigam Y, Bexfield A (2008) Genes and chromosomes. Part 1: An introduction. *Nursing Times* **104** (23): 22–3.

Skirton H, Barnes C (2005) Obtaining and communicating information about genetics. *Nursing Standard* **20**(7): 50–3.

Chapter 3

'Being with woman': the care of the childbearing woman with cancer

Rosemary Mander

Through the medium of this chapter, I intend to open up a topic which rarely sees the light of day. Cancer in the childbearing woman for whom the midwife provides care tends to be disregarded by the midwifery literature, even though its occurrence (at least regular, if not frequent) is widely recognised. The reason for this disregard is uncertain, but I would suggest that it may constitute a serious omission.

This disregard is significant for two interrelated reasons. First, due to a number of demographic and other factors, an increasing number of women are choosing to delay their childbearing until their more mature years. Hence, it is likely that the health problems of maturity, such as cancer, will feature more commonly in childbearing and in midwifery practice than was previously the case (Leslie 2005).

The second reason for the significance of the midwife's disregard of cancer in childbearing probably follows on from the first. As Leslie et al. observe: 'Most reproductive-aged women who have cancer are . . . able to conceive at any time' (2005: 627). The woman of childbearing age with cancer is unlikely to be deterred from her childbearing plans by the onset of the malignant condition. In fact, the reverse may be the case, when the woman finds that her cancer persuades her that her plans for a family are rendered more urgent. While the cancer diagnosis may not diminish the woman's 'maternal instinct', what is the midwife's view? The reasons for midwives giving so little attention to life-threatening conditions, such as cancer, may relate to the, generally correct, traditional assumption that childbearing happens to young women who are well. This assumption has been dubbed 'the healthy pregnant woman effect' (Ronsmans et al. 2004: 277).

It is possible, though, that there may be something more underpinning this omission. In preparing for a study of the midwife's experience of providing care for the woman who dies, I found that some midwives hold superstitious beliefs that are profoundly disconcerting. These are more fundamental than believing that 'bad things come in threes' or that red-haired women are prone to poor outcomes. The midwives with whom I explored my plans were all too clear in their views: I would be 'tempting fate' by going forward with this study. The perception that 'saying it will make it so' came through, loud and clear. I consider that a similar concern may prevent midwives from addressing the issues raised

Perspectives on Cancer Care. Edited by Josephine (Tonks) N. Fawcett and Anne McQueen
© 2011 Blackwell Publishing Ltd

by cancer in childbearing. While I probably should not generalise on the basis of my personal experience, such 'superstitious thinking' features prominently among those occupational groups whose work is intimately involved with birth and death (Pilette 1983).

For the purposes of this chapter, I am focusing on the woman who is already pregnant, rather than the woman with cancer contemplating childbearing; this means that I will not be addressing the subject of fertility preservation (King et al. 2008). In this chapter, I aim to begin with a picture of the significance of cancer in childbearing, including the numerical significance and the interaction between the pregnancy and the cancer. This is followed by consideration of the conflicts of interest or paradoxes which face both the childbearing woman with cancer and the midwife and others who provide care for her and her family. Such conflicts of interest clearly carry serious implications for decisions about the timing or implementation of treatment, and issues relating to the mother's survival. I then move on to explore the implications for staff of providing such care. This will lead into a comparison of the role of the midwife with the palliative care team, in situations where end-of-life care is required and the woman's quality of life is of paramount importance. This discussion leads us to recognise that the underlying ethos of midwifery resonates with that of palliative care; both feature a focus on the woman/patient and the reality of her situation. In this way they both address her specific needs, without undue medical intervention to work against the reality of the situation the woman faces. I will conclude with a more reflective contemplation of the midwife's role in providing care for the childbearing woman with cancer, particularly for the woman whose cancer has been such that she is nearing the end of her life.

Significance of cancer in childbearing

Having argued already the personal and professional significance of cancer, it may be helpful to put cancer in pregnancy into context by considering its frequency. We are often reminded that cancer is the major non-traumatic cause of death in women of childbearing age (Rayburn 2005). The North American literature suggests that cancer complicates approximately one in 1000 pregnancies (Leslie 2005). Drawing on a United Kingdom perspective, Lewis et al. (2007) translate this into one case per 6000 live births. These authors warn, though, that this figure may be misleadingly lowered by the difficulty in diagnosing certain forms of cancer during pregnancy. It is necessary to bear in mind that cancer does not discriminate: all types of cancers can present during pregnancy.

The work of Lewis et al. (2007) focuses on the Confidential Enquiries into maternal deaths in the United Kingdom. This, in itself, clearly demonstrates the crucially important significance of cancer in childbearing. Although this observation may serve as a serious reflection of why cancer in childbearing matters, the dire consequences of these women's conditions may be compounded by the complex social and personal situations in which they find themselves. This may serve to emphasise the complexity of the lives of childbearing women, to the extent that the diagnosis of cancer may be perceived as little more than yet another tribulation. For example, the situation for one young foreign woman was that she was seeking asylum, having been raped and impregnated by enemy soldiers in a conflict zone (Lewis et al. 2007); hence, she was profoundly stigmatised in her home country. Because of her perception of dishonour, she did not seek healthcare when she came to the United Kingdom, resulting in neither her pregnancy nor her cancer being recognised until she went into labour.

Throughout this chapter, I tend to focus on the possibility of a poor outcome for the childbearing woman. Although not invariably applicable (Stensheim et al. 2009), this approach is appropriate in view of the difficulty of diagnosing many cancers during pregnancy due to physiological changes (Shepherd 1990). This difficulty, which may be exacerbated by the focus on the pregnancy, means that the diagnosis is likely to be made at a later stage in the development of the cancer than would happen outwith pregnancy. My attention to poorer outcomes is also an accurate reflection of the rather limited literature on cancer in childbearing.

Interaction of the cancer with the pregnancy and childbirth

For most women with cancer, the pathology of their condition and its prognosis will not be directly affected by a pregnancy (Stensheim et al. 2009). There are some malignancies, though, which will be affected by the pregnancy. These conditions include the cancers which are hormone-dependent, such as those affecting the breast or reproductive organs. Similarly, cancers involving the blood, brain or skin are also likely to have their growth accelerated by the pregnancy. There is one cancer which is directly caused by pregnancy; this is choriocarcinoma, which develops from trophoblastic cells of the placenta (Lewis et al. 2007).

While the direct effects of the pregnancy on the cancer may be limited, the literature indicates that there may be serious consequences due to indirect effects (Mander & Haraldsdottir 2002). These effects are likely to be due to delay in the diagnosis of the woman's condition. This delay may, in turn, be attributable to the pregnancy masking certain symptoms, or other more obvious symptoms being misattributed to the pregnancy itself. Alternatively, invasive diagnostic tests may need to be postponed because of the presence of the pregnancy.

In terms of the effects of the cancer on the pregnancy, cancers of the pelvis and reproductive tract have the capacity to affect, that is obstruct, the progress of physiological labour. The fetus is surprisingly well protected from any adverse effects which may result from any malignant tumour. This is due to the placental barrier effectively minimising the risk of metastases crossing over to affect the fetus (Hacker & Jochimsen 1986). If, however, the tumour has reached an advanced stage, because of the woman's generally poor health, there is an increased risk of intrauterine growth retardation; this carries with it the likelihood of low birth weight, neonatal problems and even fetal or neonatal death (Zemlickis et al. 1996).

Cancer, childbearing and conflicts of interest

The treatment and care of the woman with cancer is rife with conflicts. Some of these paradoxes may affect practitioners, such as the possibility of termination of pregnancy.

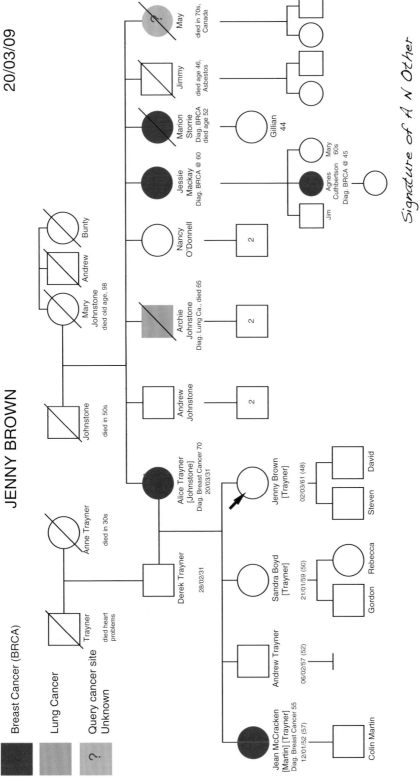

Plate 1 An example of an autosomal dominant family tree.

The Pathobiology of Mcuositis – 5 Phases

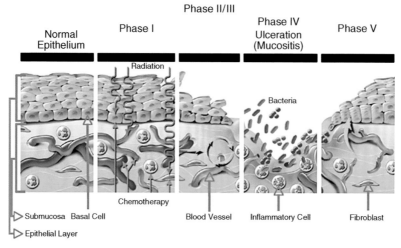

Plate 2 Pathobiology. Copyright © Stephen T. Sonis, reproduced with permission.

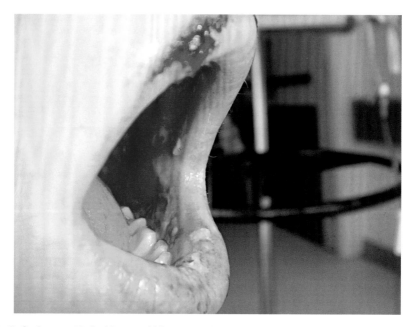

Plate 3 Oral mucositis in 13-year-old boy post-chemotherapy.

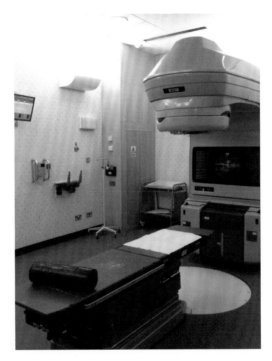

Plate 4 External beam radiotherapy.

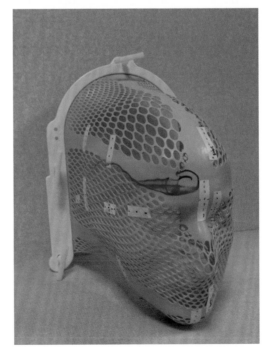

Plate 5 A thermoplastic shell.

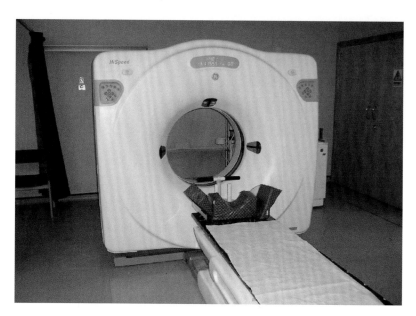

Plate 6 A computed tomography simulator.

Most of the bio/medico/ethical issues, however, relate to the comparative welfare of the mother and the fetus (Oduncu et al. 2003). The ultimate paradox, which faces the mother, is the absolute opposites of a life-threatening condition (malignant disease) coexisting with a life-giving process (pregnancy).

Interventions

The basis of these conflicts of interest tends to be related to the interventions which would benefit the mother. Whereas these interventions are able to reduce the severity of the woman's condition and possibly prolong her life, anti-cancer agents carry the risk of 'more severe fetal effects' (Leslie et al. 2005: 627), by which is meant teratogenesis, in the first trimester of pregnancy. The effects on the fetus are less at a later stage of pregnancy. These conflicts of interest do not cease with the birth. In their analysis of the effects of chemotherapeutic agents in pregnancy, Leslie et al. go on to consider their effects during lactation. These researchers demonstrate caution by acknowledging the lack of empirical data on the effects of chemotherapeutic agents during breast-feeding; however, they remind the reader that approximately 5% of any drug is excreted via the breast milk. Despite the lack of evidence, it is possible that this excretion may render this breast-fed baby vulnerable to increased risks of neutropenia, bone marrow suppression and restricted growth (Leslie et al. 2005).

As well as the nature of the interventions carrying the potential for fetal and/or neonatal damage, it is essential for consideration to be given to the timing of any therapeutic interventions. As well as the teratogenetic and other risks to be considered in early pregnancy, in later pregnancy the administration of pharmacological or other agents needs to be related to the planned timing of the birth of the baby.

The timing of the birth

The actual timing of the birth of the baby will be determined by the mother's condition, the need for therapy being balanced against the need for the baby to be born at as mature a gestational age as possible. The rationale would be to minimise the almost inevitable complications accompanying the birth of a preterm, low birth-weight baby. Thus, the costs and benefits of delaying treatment for the mother on one hand must be weighed against the multiplicity of risks of low birth weight due to prematurity (Farine & Kelly 1996). As Leslie et al. (2005) discuss, the birth of the baby may be brought forward to as early as 34 weeks' gestation, to allow the mother then to be treated with chemotherapeutic drugs. These researchers consider that, at this gestation, the neonatal/infant outcomes approximate to those of a term infant, as long as steroid therapy has been administered to the woman prior to the birth, to enhance fetal/neonatal lung maturation. If the decision is made that an early delivery by caesarean is necessary, any required chemotherapy would be delayed until full postoperative healing had occurred.

Decision making: mother and baby

In the light of this considerable potential for conflict of interest, the process of decision making assumes even more importance than is usually the case. This decision making may prove problematic when care providers may have ceased to be aware of the assumptions which are inherent among their professional colleagues. This problem emerged in the practice of Iseminger and Lewis (1998), who found that the professionals had seriously underestimated the capacity of the woman and her family to dispute the unrecognised and unacknowledged assumptions made by care providers. In a case study, these authors describe as a 'no brainer' (1998: 279) the assumption by oncology staff that a woman diagnosed with breast cancer when 15 weeks pregnant would opt for termination. This particular couple's belief system, however, meant that they could neither comprehend nor agree to this course of action.

The decision about whether, when and how aggressively to treat the childbearing woman's malignant condition should ideally be made jointly between the woman, her family and her care providers. If there is to be any possibility of achieving this ideal arrangement, honesty about the diagnosis and prognosis is paramount. At the same time, though, sensitivity to the current needs of all involved is essential. The possibility may also need to be taken into account that the woman's condition may in itself affect her ability to participate in such decisions. This may require frequent assessment which is both ongoing and individual (Iseminger & Lewis 1998).

The fundamental basis of client or patient decision making rests on the provision of reliable evidence-based information. Such information facilitates consideration of the advantages and shortcomings of the various routes available, in the light of the woman and her family's personal value systems. These considerations 'drive the medical management' (Koren et al. 1996a: ix). Koren and colleagues, while recognising the crucial input of the woman and her family, warn that such involvement may be little more than pious rhetoric. Thus, the idealised form of patient/client involvement mentioned above appears likely to be unrealistic, not only because of its rhetorical nature, but also because of the impracticability of organising well-designed trials to provide answers to the really challenging therapeutic questions (Oduncu et al. 2003). Thus, the conclusion must be drawn that evidence in this context is deficient to the point of being 'sparse or missing' (Koren et al. 1996a: ix).

Decision making clearly assumes even greater significance in rapidly changing situations, such as the diagnosis of, for example, breast cancer in the middle trimester of pregnancy. The woman and those caring for her would be required to contemplate delaying treatment, with serious consequences for the woman, or facilitating the birth of a severely preterm infant, with all of its associated threats to neonatal survival (Farine & Kelly 1996).

Implications for the midwife and other staff

For maternity staff who find themselves providing care for the childbearing woman with cancer, many would say that a huge change in mindset is needed. This change may be said to verge on a major reorientation from their usual approach to care. Whereas many staff are said to choose to practise in maternity because it is a relatively 'happy' environment, providing care for a woman with cancer demands that such practitioners redirect their way of thinking. Thus, staff are required to turn away from the usual focus of maternity, which has a tendency to be perceived as reflecting a healthy, cheerful and optimistic outlook.

Their focus has to be changed to embrace care of the pregnant woman with cancer; this may include her end-of-life care and the implications for the partner and family of life without the baby's mother. As this chapter unfolds, I hope that the argument I put forward will show how, and to what extent, the midwife is required to make such significant adjustments in her attitude to care.

Ethical issues

The midwife and her colleagues caring for the childbearing woman with cancer are likely to be faced with an excess of ethical dilemmas. This difficult situation, though, is further compounded by the fact that the dilemmas are not for the staff to address, contend with or try to resolve. These dilemmas are, primarily, for the woman to struggle with, it is hoped, with the support of those who are near to her. The staff may find that they are in the unenviable position of, effectively, 'sitting on the sidelines' while the woman and her family are agonising over crucial value-laden personal decisions. These decisions may have been facilitated by the staff having 'prepared the ground' by giving the woman and her family all the relevant information which is available. The fundamentally important concept of autonomy, though, means that the woman, having been given the information, must then be allowed the freedom to choose between the alternative therapeutic courses of action (Oduncu et al. 2003).

Maternal autonomy

The crucial ethical principle of maternal autonomy is enshrined in the legal system of the United Kingdom. In this country this principle is closely linked with the premise that the fetus is not recognised as an individual and thus has none of the rights of a human being until it becomes independent from the mother at birth (Beauchamp & Childress 2001).

Personhood

Personhood, as a term, may be used in certain other countries where fetal rights may be ascribed at an earlier, or later, stage of gestation (Iseminger & Lewis 1998). The literature on this confusing situation is astutely summarised by Oduncu et al. (2003: 135): '[there are] at least as many different concepts of "person" as there are authors'. More disconcertingly, though, in some situations differing interpretations of 'personhood' have been shown to jeopardise the autonomy of the childbearing woman (Cahill 1999; Blackwell et al. 2000).

Beneficence

As well as the concept of maternal autonomy, the ethical principle of beneficence (including, necessarily, non-maleficence) to the fetus features prominently in this scenario. While some may assume that these two ethical principles are in conflict, I see no reason why such an assumption should be made. This assumption manifests itself in the work of Oduncu et al. (2003: 137), who write 'the *physician* has to consider the well-being of the fetus' (emphasis added).

This quotation might seem to imply that the woman only considers her own health, rather than considering the wellbeing of her unborn baby. Although the work of Iseminger and Lewis (1998) carries overtones of a very different ethos, one of their case reports shows that such an assumption is certainly not safe. The possibility that the woman may decide to sacrifice her own life in the interests of her baby's survival must be recognised. I venture to suggest that the ethical conflict which Oduncu et al. (2003) advance, with maternal autonomy counter to fetal beneficence, is more apparent than real.

Decisions

As briefly mentioned above, there are many conflicts which affect decision making. These conflicts may cause difficulties for the midwife within her role as a practitioner. As Blackwell et al. (2000) indicate, the pivotal role of the practitioner is to support the woman in making her unenviable decisions. This support is likely to involve encouraging a profound level of self-exploration on the part of the childbearing woman. She may need to take a long hard look at her support systems, and at her beliefs and values. A person such as a practitioner, who is not a part of those systems, beliefs or values, would be best positioned to facilitate such a long hard look. There exists the possibility that the woman's decisions may conflict with the practitioner's own personal value system; this might demand of the practitioner herself some difficult soul searching. If the woman is taking what may be regarded by some as an inappropriate decision, though, she is likely to need more support from the practitioner rather than less.

Provision of care

The care provided for the childbearing woman with cancer will require the skills of specialists; these may include the palliative care nurse, the oncologist, the pharmacist, the dietitian, the perinatologist, the faith leader, perhaps the surgeon and the radiologist, as well as the midwife and the obstetrician. The extent to which the members of this multidisciplinary team are able to cooperate will determine the quality of care offered to this woman and her baby. In view of the relative infrequency of cancer manifesting itself during pregnancy, Blackwell et al. (2000) are right to identify that the team members may know little about each other on either a professional or, even less, a personal basis. Thus, a steep learning curve may face many of the team members. Blackwell and colleagues argue that the different team members may be required to educate each other about their own specific areas of expertise and perspective. Thus, it is possible that some unanticipated benefits may accrue from this woman's experience.

Organisational issues

Bearing in mind the heterogeneity of the multidisciplinary team providing care for the childbearing woman with cancer, it is inevitable that organisational matters will feature. The 'glitches' that happen all too frequently in the provision of daycare, such as appointments being allowed to run late, documents being mislaid or investigation results not being available, may become serious obstacles to timely decision making in this woman's case. Because of the paucity of literature on this topic (Koren et al. 1996b), a major resource on the quality of this woman's care is found in the United Kingdom Confidential Enquiries into maternal deaths (Lewis 2007). This authoritative report, which investigates all maternal deaths in the United Kingdom, found that for many such women with cancer, care is of a high quality. The assessors for the Confidential Enquiries, however, found it necessary to draw attention to the fact that some issues raised in previous reports had not been addressed by service providers. Examples of the issues which had been disregarded included the investigation of seriously abnormal symptoms, such as severe pain of a continuing nature. This appears to have been mistaken for the intermittent pain which is characteristic of certain 'minor disorders' of pregnancy (see Chapter 7).

This, perhaps unlikely, source provides an example of the high standard of care which is possible. The report for 2003–5 includes a case study (Lewis et al. 2007) which began with the rapid diagnosis of the pregnant woman's cancer. This was followed up with seamlessly organised care involving the named midwife, the obstetrician, the oncologist and the palliative care nurse in a 'one stop shop' arrangement. By attending the birth and making the postnatal visits, the midwife ensured 'continuity of carer' (McCourt et al. 1998: 1) throughout the woman's childbearing experience. The midwife maintained personal contact with the woman and her family for the rest of the woman's life and, together with the obstetrician and the palliative care nurse, attended the woman's funeral. One of the assessors, whose role it is to judge whether any avoidable factors had contributed to the death, and who for obvious reasons are not known for their tender-heartedness, was moved to observe 'the midwifery commitment made me cry' (Lewis et al. 2007).

Risk status

In more specific terms, the midwifery care of the childbearing woman with cancer will feature many interventions often regarded as specific to the 'high-risk' pregnancy. Probably because there is a risk of intrauterine growth retardation, Blackwell et al. (2000) concentrate on the monitoring of fetal growth and wellbeing. They suggest that 'testing', which presumably includes assessment of the biophysical profile, should begin as early as 26 weeks, that is, very shortly after the fetus is legally considered viable. Writing from a North American perspective, these nurses recommend weekly 'testing'. As possible side effects of any cancer therapy, Blackwell and colleagues point out the risk of bone marrow depression causing the woman to develop a range of blood cell disorders. The anaemia encountered by many childbearing women is a particular problem for the woman with cancer. Thus, these conditions render the childbearing woman more likely to develop infections and bleeding disorders.

The childbirth education which is routinely offered to all childbearing women would need to be particularly tailored to meet the needs and to address the particular risks to which this woman is vulnerable. Maintaining her nutritional status and the avoidance of infections will feature more prominently in this woman's childbirth education (Blackwell et al. 2000). It should go without saying that the participation of this woman's 'significant other' is even more important in this situation than is usually the case. The childbirth education of the woman with cancer would be provided on a one-to-one basis, possibly by the midwife or the small team of midwives providing all of the woman's midwifery care.

The place of care

Where the woman's care will happen will vary according to her condition. The multi-disciplinary nature of her care, though, is probably a reason for her antenatal care being provided at, or at least by, a tertiary centre offering perinatal and neonatal services. While the woman is mobile and sufficiently well to attend, there is a strong argument for her care being provided on an outpatient or daycare basis. This may involve attendance at a dedicated daycare unit. Alternatively, monitoring at home may be possible, either by midwifery staff visiting her or else by the use of 'telemedicine' technology (Twaddle & Young 1999). Heaman (1998) reviewed the evidence on hospitalisation of the woman with a high-risk pregnancy, and concluded that admission is not invariably in the woman's or the baby's best interests. Hospitalisation is likely to engender in the woman 'feelings of helplessness and loss of control' (Heaman 1998: 627). This researcher also identified an issue which is particularly important for the woman with cancer; that is, the adverse effects of antenatal hospitalisation on interpersonal relationships within the family. In view of the potential for this woman's life to be foreshortened, the maintenance of these relationships is crucial, not least for the wellbeing of the baby.

Support for the childbearing woman with cancer and her family

Although the support provided for the childbearing woman with cancer and her family carries many implications for the midwife, I consider that it is sufficiently important to deserve attention in its own right. The evidence base relating to social support in high-risk childbearing is not strong. This is partly because, as Hodnett (1993) pointed out, the outcomes which are measured tend to be those which are most easily measurable, such as birth weight. The other aspects of support, which may be relatively intangible (such as satisfaction or self-confidence), have received less research attention. It may be that these less tangible outcomes are more likely to matter to the woman and her family.

As well as support from the 'formal' carers, which is the main focus here, a number of web-based sources of support are available to people with cancer. These include more generic websites, as well as those specific to the childbearing woman, such as Support for Cancer in Pregnancy (http://www.sfcip.org/julie-exp.htm). The support provided by sources such as this may be helpful to those who access it. It may be necessary to mention, though, the lack of research evidence endorsing such interventions to help people who are distressed (Mander 2006).

While, as mentioned already, the literature relating to the woman with cancer is limited, some of the material on the experience of the woman with a high-risk pregnancy may be relevant. In her North American study, Vercler (2006) was able to identify the 'significant role' which healthcare providers played in helping women who were experiencing the stress-related emotions associated with high-risk childbearing. The first and most important finding of this research was the need for staff to make time for communicating with, and particularly listening to, the woman. Unlike the work of Blackwell et al. (2000), Vercler's research emphasised the need to consider the woman as an individual in her own right, with all her unique concerns and needs, rather than just as a 'vessel' for a baby. It is to be hoped that such a plea for the individualisation of care may not be necessary in the present context, but the literature does have a tendency to focus on the baby, the conflicts and the treatments, with little regard for how the woman does or does not fit in to this scenario. Unsurprisingly, in view of her study's focus on 'family-centered care', Vercler points up the crucial involvement of the family in the care of the woman with a high-risk pregnancy. For all too obvious reasons, the family's involvement in the care of the woman with cancer becomes particularly significant. Thus, the midwife is likely to find herself providing support, not only for the woman and her baby, but also for all those who will, eventually, be taking responsibility for caring for and raising the 'baby'.

A slightly earlier North American study, which is also likely to be relevant to the support of the childbearing woman with cancer, involved a group of women who were doubly disadvantaged (Coffman & Ray 2002). These researchers used a grounded theory approach to explore the support needs of African American women experiencing a high-risk pregnancy. The findings of this study resonate particularly powerfully with the midwifery model of care (Wagner 2005). The model or theory, which arose out of Coffman and Ray's work (2002: 536), is known as the theory of 'mutual intentionality'. As well as comprising 'caring', 'knowing' and 'believing in', this theory includes 'being there', 'sharing information' and 'doing for the other'. Terms such as these are familiar to midwives and nurses as they echo the fundamental precepts of all that midwifery and nursing practice strives to achieve. There exists a particularly close alignment with the idealised form of midwifery practice which has been summarised in the 'partnership model' (Guilliland & Pairman 1995; Fleming 2000).

The fundamentally important role of the midwife is encapsulated in her name. The word 'midwife' is derived from the Old English term meaning 'with woman'. Understanding this basic meaning is becoming increasingly important as the midwife may have other calls on her attention, such as the management of technological devices. Similarly, there may be other occupational groups who have agendas which differ from the welfare of the childbearing woman (Mander 1993; 1994); in such circumstances the midwife becomes the woman's advocate. As Leap (2000: 3) has explained, this 'with woman' relationship benefits the woman in ways which extend far beyond the woman's birth experience. The midwife should be able to engage with the woman at such a profound level that mutual respect and trust is engendered. On the basis of this mutuality, learning about their strengths and any weaknesses ensues. The midwife is able to facilitate the woman's learning, not only about childbearing, but also about any longer-term aspects of her life. This long-term learning serves to empower the woman to cope more effectively with the challenges which are likely to face her. For the vast majority of women, childbirth and motherhood constitute the major challenges. Leap spells out the nature of these challenges as being not only physical, but also 'intellectual, social and spiritual' (2000: 4). The support provided by the midwife being 'with woman' in this way will be of particular benefit to the childbearing woman with cancer. As mentioned by Leap, and as manifested in the case study mentioned above, continuity of carer facilitates the development of the relationship which she advocates. The extent to which such a relationship is facilitated by health systems such as the UK National Health Service may be debatable; the case study to which I have referred establishes, however, that it may be achievable.

The midwife's role in caring for the childbearing woman with cancer

In the previous section, the appropriateness of the traditional midwifery role in the context of end-of-life care has been proposed. In order to further advance this line of reasoning, I would like to consider whether there is any comparability, or even similarity, between the midwife and her role in caring for this woman and that of a more conventional cancer carer. The care provider with whom I would like to draw comparisons is the palliative care nurse. The role of the nurse in palliative care is addressed in depth in Chapter 12, so my focus is purely for purposes of comparison (Mander & Haraldsdottir 2002).

The first aspect of comparability relates to a point which I have mentioned already, which is the role of the midwife as being 'with woman' (Leap 2000). One of the essential 'capacities' of the palliative care nurse is 'being with' (Rushton 2005: 316). Along the same lines, Benner (1984) coined the term 'presence', to indicate the profound level of engagement of the nurse with the other (see Chapters 1 and 10). Used as an active verb, 'presencing' involves psychic effort to still the mind, focus it totally on the here and now and accept the status quo, as well as physical actions. The physical activities serve to enhance the psychic endeavours through touching and other interpersonal contact.

Whereas Benner (1984) sought to distinguish the 'being with' aspect of 'presence' from the 'doing for', Rushton argues that there is some common ground between these concepts and they are not mutually exclusive. These observations contrast with the work of Haraldsdottir (2007), which was undertaken in a United Kingdom hospice setting. This phenomenological study suggested that many palliative care practitioners considered themselves to achieve both 'being with' and 'doing for', concurrently.

On the basis of this brief consideration of the input of the palliative care nurse, I contend that, at least in this respect, the midwifery role bears comparison. Midwives' 'with woman' concept and practice equates to a large extent with the 'being with' sought after in palliative care. This similarity is found in the oft-used phrase coined by midwife, Hazel Smith: 'the less we do, the more we give' (Leap 2000: 2).

This telling aphorism summarises a fundamental principle of midwifery practice. Where midwives practise in a culture of intervention and medicalisation, the opportunity or the ability to do 'less', though, is a rare achievement. This need to 'do' things has been seriously criticised as the 'doing for' or 'doing to' mentality which, effectively, reduces the childbearing woman to a passive role in her own birthing experience. The concept of being 'with woman' is assuming greater significance as midwives are managing to regain control over 'normality' in childbearing (Downe 2008).

The other aspect of potential similarity between palliative care nurses and midwives which may affect their care of the childbearing woman with cancer is found in the care provider's ability to cope with uncertainty. In the case of the palliative care nurse, the uncertainty is likely to relate to the person's prognosis. This means not knowing when death may occur. Such uncertainty may make it difficult for the affected person as well as those close to them to prepare themselves for what may be a longer or shorter illness trajectory. Rushton writes about such uncertainty in positive terms, recommending that it should be 'honoured rather than extinguished' (2005: 321). Such a recommendation may not be easily accepted by personnel who are accustomed to interventions to limit unpleasant phenomena, such as pain and anxiety. Rushton suggests that an openness among staff may assist those who are less comfortable with uncertainty, to be able to at least tolerate the 'not knowing' (2005: 321). For the midwife, the uncertainties which are now starting to attract research attention are particularly found in relation to the woman's labour (M. Page 2009, personal communication). The progress and course of labour, which determine its duration and outcome, are widely regarded as unpredictable. This unpredictability has led to the notorious medical maxim that 'labour is only normal in retrospect' (Percival 1970: 1222).

For some who are involved in labour, its inherent uncertainty may be perceived negatively. This perception often manifests itself in the form of risk (Mead & Kornbrot 2004). Almost inevitably, such risk carries the imperative to reduce it. It was this way of thinking which led to the current overwhelming vogue for interventive practice in the form of 'active management of labour' (O'Driscoll and Meagher 1986; O'Driscoll & Meagher 1986). In their authoritative research, Mead and Kornbrot suggest that the extent of either uncertainty acceptance or aversion in a particular clinical setting may be a function of the culture of the people who practise there.

On the basis of this discussion, it is argued that there are powerful similarities between the different practitioners' ability to 'be with' the childbearing woman with cancer and their ability to tolerate the uncertainty which is inherent in the condition. In this way, it may be that midwives and palliative care nurses may possess more skills in common than is at first apparent. Such similarities may be of particular value in the care of women who develop cancer during childbearing, in the future. For this reason, the change in mindset required of midwives, mentioned earlier, may not be as great as some believe.

Thus, it can be seen that the philosophy of the midwife is to embrace the uncertainty which physiological childbearing brings with it. The midwife's focus is on support of the childbearing woman. An important example of this philosophy is the need for the midwife and the woman to function as a team in order to 'work with' the woman's labour. This strategy may be contrasted with the usual, more medicalised approach to managing labour (Leap & Anderson 2004). This philosophy of childbirth resonates powerfully with that of palliative care practitioners where the aim is the holistic care of the individual whereby, in the context of the reality of terminal illness, the patient's quality of living is maintained while a peaceful and meaningful death is facilitated (Cain 2001). Thus, the midwife, both in general and in the particular context of cancer, and the palliative care practitioner can be seen to share a common aim, that of working with the reality of the situation in which the woman finds herself, rather than in opposition to that reality in an attempt to correct or remedy it.

Conclusion

Although the literature on the midwifery care of the woman with cancer is particularly deficient, the comparison I have drawn between the care provided in childbearing and in palliative care is not entirely novel. In his contemplation of the service provided by the family physician during pregnancy, Clark (2008) likens his work to that of the palliative care consultant. These similarities include the essential importance of open and honest communication and the need for a continuing trusting relationship. Both forms of care are, arguably, under threat from intrusive technology, the benefits of which have been inadequately established. Clark argues that offering pregnancy care is a good preparation for providing palliative care.

Despite mention of the Confidential Enquiries (Lewis 2007), maternal death has not featured prominently in this chapter. Obviously, this prospect must be a consideration in those caring for the childbearing woman with cancer. In my research on the midwife's experience of caring for the woman who dies, deaths from cancer were not a major component (Mander 2001). The findings of this study, however, may be relevant in terms of the midwives' powerful need for support at the time of a maternal death, be it from those who have attended the woman who died and shared the experience of the loss, or from others who have had to face a similar experience. The support needs of the midwife caring for a woman with cancer need greater attention to facilitate 'space' for contemplation, reflection and insights into their experiences of providing what may be, effectively, palliative care. Rushton (2005: 316) referred to this as 'human homework', allowing the midwife time to contemplate the very personal and potentially painful issues which caring for the childbearing woman cancer will raise. The provision of such 'space' will also ensure that the care which the midwife provides is as compassionate and competent as this woman deserves and needs.

Acknowledgements

I would like to thank Pam Smith and Joan Hemphill for their contributions.

References

Beauchamp TL, Childress JF (2001) *Principles of Biomedical Ethics*, 5th edn. Oxford: Oxford University Press.

Benner P (1984) *From Novice to Expert: Excellence and Power in Clinical Nursing Practice*. Menlo Park, CA: Addison-Wesley.

Blackwell DA, Elam S, Blackwell JT (2000) Cancer and pregnancy: a health care dilemma. *Journal of Obstetric Gynecologic and Neonatal Nursing* 29(4): 405–11.

Cahill H (1999) An Orwellian scenario: court ordered caesarean section and women's autonomy. *Nursing Ethics* 6: 6494–505.

Cain JM (2001) End of life care: history and the role of the obstetrician and gynaecologist. *Best Practice and Research in Clinical Obstetrics and Gynaecology* 15(2): 195–201.

Clark D (2008) Pregnancy care: an apprenticeship for palliative care? *Journal of the American Board of Family Medicine* 21(1): 63–4.

Coffman S, Ray MA (2002) African American women describe support processes during high-risk pregnancy and postpartum. *Journal of Obstetric, Gynecologic, and Neonatal Nursing* 31(5): 536–44.

Downe S (2008) *Normal Childbirth: Evidence and Debate*, 2nd edn. Edinburgh: Churchill Livingstone.

Farine D, Kelly EN (1996) *The pregnant patient with malignant disease: maternal-fetal conflict*. In: Koren G, Lishner M, Farine D (eds) *Cancer in Pregnancy: Maternal and Fetal Risks*. Cambridge: Cambridge University Press, pp. 15–26.

Fleming V (2000) *The midwifery partnership in New Zealand: past history or a new way forward?* In: Kirkham M (ed.) *The Midwife–Mother Relationship.* London: Macmillan, pp. 193–206.

Guilliland K, Pairman S (1995) *The Midwifery Partnership: A model for practice.* Wellington, New Zealand: Department of Nursing and Midwifery, Victoria University of Wellington.

Hacker NF, Jochimsen PR (1986) *Common malignancies among women: sites and treatment.* In: Andersen BL (ed.) *Women with Cancer: Psychological Perspectives.* New York: Springer-Verlag.

Haraldsdottir E (2007) The Constraints of the Ordinary: 'Being with' patients in a hospice in Scotland. PhD thesis, University of Edinburgh, Edinburgh.

Heaman M (1998) Psychosocial impact of high-risk pregnancy: hospital and home. *Clinical Obstetrics and Gynecology* **41**(3): 626–39.

Hodnett E (1993) Social support during high-risk pregnancy: does it help? *Birth* **20**(4): 218–19.

Iseminger KA, Lewis MA (1998) Ethical challenges in treating mother and fetus when cancer complicates pregnancy. *Obstetrics and Gynecology Clinics of North America* **25**(2): 273–85.

King L, Quinn GP, Vadaparampil ST, et al. (2008) Oncology social workers' perceptions of barriers to discussing fertility preservation with cancer patients. *Social Work Health Care* **47**(4): 479–501.

Koren G, Lishner M, Farine D (eds) (1996a) *Cancer in Pregnancy: Maternal and Fetal Risks.* Cambridge: Cambridge University Press.

Koren G, Lishner M, Zemlickis D (1996b) Cancer in pregnancy: identification of unanswered questions on maternal and fetal risks. In: Koren G, Lishner M, Farine D (eds) *Cancer in Pregnancy: Maternal and Fetal Risks.* Cambridge: Cambridge University Press, pp. 1–15.

Leap N (2000) The less we do, the more we give. In: Kirkham M (ed.) *The Midwife–Mother Relationship.* London: Macmillan, pp. 1–17.

Leap N, Anderson T (2004) The role of pain in normal birth and the empowerment of women. In: Downe S (ed.) *Normal Childbirth: Evidence and Debate.* Edinburgh: Churchill Livingstone, pp. 25–40.

Leslie KK (2005) Cancer complicating pregnancy. *Obstetrics and Gynecology Clinics of North America* **32**(4): xv–vi.

Leslie KK, Koil C, Rayburn WF (2005) Chemotherapeutic drugs in pregnancy: cancer complicating pregnancy. *Obstetrics and Gynecology Clinics of North America* **32**(4): 627–40.

Lewis G (ed.) (2007) *The Confidential Enquiry into Maternal and Child Health (CEMACH) Saving Mothers' Lives: Reviewing maternal deaths to make motherhood safer – 2003–2005. The Seventh Report of the Confidential Enquiries into Maternal Deaths in the United Kingdom.* London: CEMACH.

Lewis G, Drife J, de Swiet M (2007) *Cancer and other tumours.* In: Lewis G (ed.) *The Confidential Enquiry into Maternal and Child Health (CEMACH) Saving Mothers' Lives: Reviewing maternal deaths to make motherhood safer – 2003–2005. The Seventh Report of the Confidential Enquiries into Maternal Deaths in the United Kingdom.* London: CEMACH, pp. 212–21.

Mander R (1993) Epidural analgesia 1: recent history. *British Journal of Midwifery* **1**(6): 259–64.

Mander R (1994) Epidural analgesia: 2. research basis. *British Journal of Midwifery* **2**(1): 12–16.

Mander R (2001) The midwife's ultimate paradox: a UK-based study of the death of a mother. *Midwifery* **17**(4): 248–59.

Mander R (2006) *Loss and Bereavement in Childbearing,* 2nd edn. London: Routledge.

Mander R, Haraldsdottir E (2002) Care for the dying mother-to-be. *European Journal of Palliative Care* **9**(6): 240–2.

McCourt C, Page L, Hewison J, Vail A (1998) Evaluation of one-to-one midwifery: women's responses to care. *Birth* **25**(2): 73–80.

Mead MMP, Kornbrot D (2004) The influence of maternity units' intrapartum intervention rates and midwives' risk: perception for women suitable for midwifery-led care. *Midwifery* **20**(1): 61–71.

O'Driscoll K, Meagher D (1986) *Active Management of Labour,* 2nd edn. London: Baillière Tindall.

Oduncu FS, Kimmig R, Hepp H, Emmerich B (2003) Cancer in pregnancy: maternal-fetal conflict. *Journal of Cancer Research and Clinical Oncology* **129**(3): 133–46.

Percival RC (1970) Management of normal labour. *Practitioner* March: 1221–4.

Pilette WL (1983) Magical thinking by inpatient staff members. *Psychiatric Quarterly* **55**(4): 272–4.

Rayburn WF (2005) Cancer complicating pregnancy. *Obstetrics and Gynecology Clinics of North America* **32**(4): xiii–xiv.

Ronsmans C, Lewis G, Hurt L, Physick N, Macfarlane A, Abrahams C (2004) Mortality in pregnant and non-pregnant women in England and Wales 1997–2002: Are pregnant women healthier? In: Lewis G (ed.) *Why Mothers Die 2000–02. The Sixth Report of the Confidential Enquiries into Maternal Deaths in the United Kingdom.* London: RCOG Press, pp. 272–8.

Rushton CH (2005) A framework for integrated pediatric palliative care: being with dying. *Journal of Pediatric Nursing* **20**(5): 311–25.

Shepherd J (1990) *Cancer complications in pregnancy.* In: Shepherd J, Monaghan J (eds) *Clinical Gynaecological Oncology.* Oxford: Blackwell Scientific Publications.

Stensheim H, Møller B, van Dijk T, Fossa SD (2009) Cause-specific survival for women diagnosed with cancer during pregnancy or lactation: a registry-based cohort study. *Journal of Clinical Oncology* **27**(1): 45–51.

Twaddle S, Young D (1999) The economics of maternity care. In: Marsh G, Renfrew M (eds) *Community-based Maternity Care.* Oxford: University Press Oxford, pp. 119–36.

Vercler L (2006) Family-Centered Care and High-Risk Pregnancy. http://www.pressganey.com/galleries/default-file/patient_4.pdf (accessed 29.01.09).

Wagner M (2005) Midwifery and international maternity care. *Midwifery Today* **75**(12). http://www.midwiferytoday.com/articles/maternitycare.asp (accessed 29.06.09).

Zemlickis D, Lishner M, Koren G (1996) Review of fetal effects of cancer chemotherapeutic agents. In: Koren G, Lishner M, Farine D (eds) *Cancer in Pregnancy: Maternal and Fetal Risks.* Cambridge: Cambridge University Press, pp. 168–80.

Chapter 4

Mucositis and the development of a new instrument for the measurement of oral mucositis in children

Deborah Tomlinson and Lillian Sung

Mucositis is the injury that occurs to the mucosal barrier of the gastrointestinal tract, particularly to oral and oropharyngeal mucosa, as a result of radiation therapy or chemotherapy. Mucositis describes a clinical condition that is characterized by oral erythema, ulceration and pain (Scully et al. 2003). Oral mucositis-related symptoms are common, distressing consequences of such cancer therapies (Sonis 2004a). At least 40% and up to 70% of patients treated with standard chemotherapy protocols can develop mucositis (Scully et al. 2003). From the patient's perspective, mucositis is important because it is painful, affects quality of life, may prevent eating and drinking, and can result in hospitalisation for hydration or pain control (Meurman et al. 1997; Scully et al. 2003; Sonis 2007). From the health authority perspective, increased costs are associated with duration of any hospitalisation and treatment of infection which may occur in the presence of mucositis (Sonis 2004b). Mucositis is one of the most frequent and treatment-limiting toxicities associated with cancer therapy protocols (Treister & Sonis 2007). Despite this there are currently no standard effective treatments (Scully et al. 2003).

In addition, the incidence of this disabling, almost invariable side effect of cancer therapy is considered to be under-reported (Sonis 2007). Reasons for this may include the variability of the severity of mucositis, and failed consensus on the assessment of oral mucositis. Fortunately, however, research activity in oral mucositis is growing as the recognition of its importance increases (Scully et al. 2003).

Mucositis is a particularly important consequence of chemotherapy in children and, in fact, the risk of mucositis may even be higher in children than in adults. This may be related to a higher proliferative index of basal epithelial cells in children, the high incidence of haematological malignancies, and the tendency to use more intensive therapies (Parulekar et al. 1998).

Effective oral assessment is fundamental when an attempt is being made to compare management strategies for oral mucositis (Brown & Wingard 2004). In order to conduct clinical trials of mucositis prevention and treatment, reliable, valid, sensitive and easy-to-use instruments are required (Eilers & Epstein 2004).

Perspectives on Cancer Care.   Edited by Josephine (Tonks) N. Fawcett and Anne McQueen
© 2011 Blackwell Publishing Ltd

Although researchers have developed many oral mucositis assessment scales for use in adults, there remains a paucity of validated instruments for assessing mucositis in children (Tomlinson et al. 2007). As a result, oral mucositis research in children receiving cytotoxic therapy has been impeded by the lack of an acceptable, appropriate assessment scale. To this end, a group of experts has been working on producing an oral mucositis assessment scale appropriate for use in children, and this is the principal perspective of this chapter. The reader should not look to this chapter for details of direct nursing care but rather be enabled, by understanding the pathophysiological reality of oral mucositis and the research process involved in the development of a mucositis evaluation scale, to discern the implications for improving nursing care of this distressing experience for the child, the child's family and all involved in the child's care.

Pathophysiology of oral mucositis

The development of mucositis is the result of a complex series of events that mainly occurs in the submucosa, with epithelium being the target tissue (Sonis 2004b). The sequence of events occurs in five stages: initiation, primary damage response, signal amplification, ulceration and healing (Plate 2).

Initiation

Cytotoxic therapy causes damage throughout the cell, affecting both DNA and non-DNA structures. Initial direct damage can lead to immediate cell death in basal epithelial and submucosal cells. However, this direct injury accounts only for a small number of injured cells and does not account for the magnitude of clinical symptoms associated with mucositis (Sonis 2007; Treister & Sonis 2007). Importantly, chemotherapeutic agents and radiation trigger the production of reactive oxygen species (ROS). The ROS are initiators of a series of events that includes damage to connective tissue, DNA and cell membranes, stimulation of macrophages, and a series of critical biological mechanisms, molecules and pathways, including p53, nuclear factor kappa-B (NF-κB) and the ceramide pathway (Scully et al. 2003; Sonis 2007; Treister & Sonis 2007). These pathways assist in control of cell proliferation, differentiation and cell survival, programmed cell death and apoptosis. At this stage the mucosa has a normal appearance despite the underlying biological havoc.

Primary damage response

The activation of signalling pathways by radiation, chemotherapy, ROS, damaged cells and their damaged DNA begins the processes that result in mucosal injury. Activated transcription factors that impact the viability of the basal epithelia include NF-κB, which is considered one of the most significant transcription factors in the development of mucositis (Sonis 2007). NF-κB regulates the expression of approximately 200 genes, many of which have important roles in the development of mucositis; NF-κB is a regulator of proinflammatory cytokines such as tumour necrosis factor (TNF), interleukin

(IL)-6 and IL-1β. These proteins are thought to produce early damage that ultimately results in apoptosis of epithelial basal cells (Treister & Sonis 2007). NF-κB also impacts the *BCL2* genes and a mechanism is provided that can directly promote apoptosis (Sonis 2007).

Signal amplification

In this phase, many of the molecules produced during the primary response phase provide positive feedback to destructive pathways. For example, the proinflammatory cytokines such as TNF-α cause the activation of several mechanisms that may lead to over-expression of protein-regulating genes, apoptosis and destruction of the epithelial basement membrane. Positive feedback loops magnify the initial injury and also prolong the damage by continuing to provide signals for several days after the patient has received cancer therapy (Sonis 2007).

Ulceration

The culmination of the previous stages is the development of ulcers that penetrate through the epithelium into the submucosa (Plate 3). This is the most significant phase for the patient, due to the clinical symptoms of pain and loss of function (Sonis 2004a). Ulceration is often characterised by depth and joining, with a pseudomembrane covering the lesion. The pseudomembrane often contains a multitude of oral bacteria that may potentially invade the blood vessels of the submucosa, causing bacteraemia. Neutropenic and myeloablated patients have significant risk of developing sepsis (Sonis 2007; Treister & Sonis 2007).

Healing

Mucositis lesions normally heal spontaneously within two to three weeks of completion of cytotoxic therapy, in the absence of infection. This final stage in the development of mucositis is the least understood. However, signalling from submucosal mesenchyme to the epithelium controls the migration, differentiation and proliferation of new tissue (Treister & Sonis 2007). Interestingly, the reconstituted submucosa is not identical to its state before mucosal injury (Sonis 2007).

Advanced understanding of the biological complexity of mucositis following cytotoxic therapy can begin to provide information that may assist in the development of pharmacological agents for its prevention and treatment. Therefore an accurate measurement of oral mucositis will be required to reflect and record the potential efficacy of treatments.

Measuring oral mucositis in adults

Oral mucositis assessment tools

A variety of mucositis scoring systems have been developed for a range of uses, from measurement of mucosal damage for routine mouth care to sophisticated clinical research studies. Scoring systems can aid in the evaluation of interventions that may be considered

Table 4.1 World Health Organization (WHO) scoring criteria for oral mucositis

Grade	0	1	2	3	4
Description	Normal	Soreness with or without erythema	Ulceration and erythema; patient can swallow a solid diet	Ulceration and erythema; patient cannot swallow a solid diet	Ulceration and pseudomembrane formation of such severity that alimentation is not possible

in the treatment or prevention of oral mucositis. However, no scale is universally acceptable (Sonis 2004a). The reasons for this are explained below.

Oral assessment following cancer therapy has been considered for three decades (Beck 1979; Eilers et al. 1988). Oral assessment tools were often implemented to assess the impact of emerging oral care protocols, often without reliability and validity data (Eilers et al. 1988). However, several instruments have been developed that have been useful, in varying degrees, in mucositis research within the population of adults with cancer (Donnelly et al. 1992; Cox et al. 1995; Dibble et al. 1996; Dodd et al. 1996; Tardieu et al. 1996; Riesenbeck & Dorr 1998; Andersson et al. 1999). Generally, there have been three types of scales: simple instruments, objective instruments and combined instruments.

Simple instruments

These are single scales that typically range from 0 (no symptoms) to 4 or 5 (worst symptoms possible) and include the World Health Organization (WHO) Grading System (Table 4.1) and the National Cancer Institute (NCI) common Toxicity Criteria (CTC) (Table 4.2) based upon the ability to eat and drink, combined with objective signs of mucositis (WHO 1979; NCI 2003). These two scales are considered most clinically relevant on the basis that a global score is readily available (Sonis et al. 2004). The scoring of mucositis is sometimes

Table 4.2 National Cancer Institute Common Toxicity Criteria (NCI-CTC) version 3 scoring criteria for oral mucositis

Mucositis functional/symptomatic score					
Grade	0	1	2	3	4
Description	No mucositis	Able to eat solids	Requires liquid diet	Alimentation not possible	Symptoms associated with life threatening consequences
Mucositis/stomatitis clinical score					
Description	No mucositis	Erythema of the mucositis	Patchy ulceration or pseudome-mbranes	Confluent ulcerations or pseudome-mbranes	Tissue necrosis

included as part of toxicity criteria instruments that have been developed by various oncology groups, for example the Radiation Therapy Oncology Group (RTOG) (Cox et al. 1995).

Objective scales

These are instruments based upon what an examiner can observe. They were developed originally for research purposes when it was recognised that the WHO and other functional scales, that reflect limitations in activities such as eating and drinking, may under-report mucositis if effective analgesia is provided (Sonis et al. 1999). The Oral Mucositis Rating Scale (OMRS) was developed as a comprehensive measurement of a broad range of oral mucosa changes associated with cancer therapy (Schubert et al. 1992), and consisted of 91 items that focused on 13 areas of the mouth. The scale was evaluated in 188 adult bone marrow transplant patients (Schubert et al. 1992), and the information gained was used to develop an Oral Mucositis Index (OMI) with 34 items (Schubert et al. 1992). With reliability and construct validity demonstrated, an abbreviated, 20-item version was then developed (McGuire et al. 2002).

The Oral Mucositis Assessment Scale (OMAS) was designed by a panel of experts and provided an objective, simple and reproducible tool that could be applied specifically to multicentre clinical trials (Sonis et al. 1999). The OMAS measured the degree of ulceration or pseudomembrane formation and mucosal erythema in nine sites of the mouth. Following testing with 188 patients receiving chemotherapy and 56 receiving radiotherapy, the OMAS was reported to be reliable, valid and easy to use; however, for those patients with severe mucositis, undergoing repeated examinations was difficult (Sonis et al. 1999).

Combined scales

These are scales in which objective and subjective experiences and functional dimensions are assessed in one instrument; their development and evaluation has been led primarily by the nursing discipline, with its focus on oral care.

The Oral Assessment Guide (OAG) (Eilers et al. 1988) was developed primarily as a clinical tool but was then found valuable as a research instrument. The OAG consists of eight categories with three descriptors for each category. The original study consisted of 20 adult patients undergoing bone marrow transplant. Content validity of the descriptors was supported, by review of nursing and dental literature and by obtaining written evaluative validation of the eight categories by four experts (Eilers et al. 1988). Registered nurses and an investigator established inter-rater reliability of the instrument.

A patient-reported 10-item (6 questions) oral mucositis daily questionnaire (OMDQ) was developed and used in adult bone marrow transplant patients as a result of focus groups and one-to-one interviews with adult cancer patients (Stiff et al. 2006). To assess the reliability and validity of the OMDQ, 212 patients were included in a phase III study to determine the efficacy of palifermin (a recombinant keratinocyte growth factor used to reduce the duration and severity of mucositis) compared to placebo in reducing bone marrow transplant-related oral mucositis. Test-retest reliability was acceptable. Validity was demonstrated as the questions in the OMDQ that related to mouth and throat soreness correlated with the WHO, RTOG and Western Consortium for Cancer Nursing Research (WCCNR) scales (Stiff et al. 2006).

Utilisation of oral mucositis assessment tools

The tools discussed above have been used in a number of studies, with variable outcomes.

Puyal-Casado et al. (2003) designed a protocol for the evaluation and treatment of oral mucositis that used the WHO grading system to determine treatment, but unfortunately no data were provided on the effectiveness of the protocol itself. Dodd et al. (1996) compared various methods of determining oral mucositis, in 127 adult patients, including the Chemotherapy Knowledge Questionnaire, Behaviour Checklist, self-care behaviour (SCB) logs, the OAG, interviews and medical record review; however, the results, disappointingly, demonstrated a wide range in mucositis prevalence (30% to 69%) within the same sample (Dodd et al. 1996). A larger study, of 199 patients, also used the OAG as part of the design to assess the occurrence of oral mucositis in patients receiving chemotherapy, and concluded that the OAG was more useful as a general oral assessment tool, as only one item was concerned with the mucosa (Dodd et al. 2000). The OMAS scoring system was used to evaluate oral mucositis in 92 haematopoietic stem-cell transplantation patients (Sonis et al. 2001), and was found to be a significant predictor of outcomes in blood and bone marrow transplant patients. Sixty adult patients admitted to bone marrow transplantation units were examined for oral ulcerative lesions and graded on a scale (0–4) that accounted for size and number of lesions (Woo et al. 1993). No other aspect of mucositis was reported.

Etiz and colleagues (2002) evaluated the validity and reproducibility of five different mucositis scoring systems to evaluate 43 patients with head and neck malignancies who had received radiation therapy (Etiz et al. 2002). The five systems were the WHO, RTOG, Hickey, Van der Schueren and Makkonen, all using similar descriptive terminology, but varying in their grading. Forty-three patients were included in the study. The authors point out that the terminology used to describe the mucositis was limiting, preventing inter-changeability, e.g. slight erythema versus pronounced erythema, spotted mucositis versus 'confluent' mucositis versus ulcer. Despite this, the study results implied that all the scoring systems were valid (Etiz et al. 2002).

The above may seem over-complex and complicated to those unfamiliar with oral assessment, but it serves to confirm that there is no ideal, universally acceptable scale for use in the adult population.

Measuring oral mucositis in children

A number of studies have provided some better understanding of oral mucositis in children (Williams & Martin 1992; Kennedy & Diamond 1997; Levy-Polack et al. 1998; Nelson et al. 2001; Costa et al. 2003; Chen et al. 2004; Cheng et al. 2004; Aquino et al. 2005; Pereira Pinto et al. 2006; El-Housseiny et al. 2007). Before looking closely at these studies, it is useful to reflect on the distress mucositis can cause, particularly to the child, who cannot so readily rationalise or intellectualise the experience. Box 4.1 highlights the lived experience of mucositis for the child and for the family.

Box 4.1   The lived experience of oral mucositis for children and their parents

Children's Experience

Pain – described as the worst symptom of oral mucositis:

- I couldn't talk, eat or swallow anything. Even swallowing saliva gave me great pain.
- I wanted to talk but I couldn't.
- When I chewed it was like I had bitten my own tongue.
- Seriousness on a scale of 1 to 10 – I'd say 11.

Negative emotional outcomes:

- It was hard and I felt unhappy.
- I didn't want to be unable to speak, so I lost my temper and hit my mother.

The dilemma of eating:

- I couldn't eat and I was hungry.
- I didn't want to eat, but I still had to eat because I felt hungry.

Challenges in oral care:

- Yes, my Dad often forced me to do it. Mum also forced me to do it.
- When the pain was really bad, I cried while rinsing my mouth.

Parents' Experience

Pain:

- Sometimes the pain was so intense it made my daughter tremble. When she trembled she tugged me.
- My son even gave up on video games. He wasn't in the mood for them and he was just lying there.
- There're pros and cons of using morphine. It relieved the pain, but it made my son kind of confused and clumsy. I was worried whether he might fall out of the bed.

Negative emotional outcomes:

- I didn't like to see her crying. When she cried I felt heartbroken.
- I was worried and sad, so I wasn't able to eat either.

The dilemma of eating:

- I was worried she might be starving.
- You wouldn't be happy seeing her losing so much weight.

Challenges in oral care:

- Sometimes my son doesn't cooperate with mouth rinsing. That's the main problem.

Source: Cheng (2009)

Various studies have investigated oral mucositis in children. However, few of these studies are comparable due to the variety of assessment scales used (Tomlinson et al. 2008a). There has been little focus on work conducted to assess the measurement properties of oral mucositis scales in children (Tomlinson et al. 2007). Kennedy and Diamond reported on a basic tool, which graded mucositis on a scale of 0 to 4, as an example of how to assess and subsequently manage chemotherapy-induced mucositis in children (Kennedy & Diamond 1997). However, reliability or validity considerations with use of the scale were not reported and there was no discussion of this scale being implemented.

Implementation of a calendar to record oral mucositis in 16 children and 8 adults used a Modified Eastern Co-operative Oncology Group grading system (Anderson et al. 1998). The severity of painful mucositis was related to dietary intake ability, e.g. score 2 corresponded to painful mucositis with soft foods only but, again, the scale was not examined for reliability or validity. Aquino et al. (2005) studied the effectiveness of oral glutamine on mucositis in children undergoing bone marrow transplantation. This study used a modified Walsh scale (Walsh 1990) to grade the oral mucositis in a total of 120 patients (Aquino et al. 2005). The modified scale removed the scoring of 'voice' and 'swallow' from the original scale, and added further descriptors to some categories. However, the properties of the modified Walsh scale were not examined.

Two instruments that have recently received limited paediatric evaluation, in terms of psychometric properties, are the OMAS and the OAG. The OMAS was demonstrated to display construct validity in children at least 6 years of age (Sung et al. 2006). The OMAS was measured in 16 children during 45 cycles of chemotherapy, for a total of 156 assessments.

The OAG was implemented in one study in order to develop an oral care algorithm for children receiving cytotoxic therapy (Nelson et al. 2001). Nurses, in this study, reported confusion with the numerical scoring regarding the teeth category, where babies without teeth scored 0 or 'not applicable'. As a result the overall score was inaccurate (Nelson et al. 2001). In addition, the pain status was an important consideration that was lacking from the assessment. Changes were made to the OAG to score no teeth as 1 (normal for that particular child), the gag reflex test was omitted, signs and symptoms of teething were included, as was space to document pain assessment. Finally the instrument was reworded to make it more understandable to scorers. Useful lessons had been learnt.

Chen and colleagues used an adapted OAG to assess 30 children with leukaemia and lymphoma undergoing chemotherapy who experienced oral complications (Chen et al. 2004). The opinions of five experts demonstrated content validity of the OAG in this study. Another study also investigated the validity of a modified OAG for children and, by using a judgement quantification process that included the opinions of 19 experts, content validity was established for the items of the OAG instrument (Gibson et al. 2006). Chen et al. used the OAG assessment in nine paediatric patients, carried out by a dentist and registered nurse, to establish inter-rater reliability (Chen et al. 2004). The limitations of the OMAS and the OAG for use with children are discussed in the next section.

There is little in the literature on the unique challenges of measuring mucositis in young children. Most studies have excluded very young children (Tomlinson et al. 2007). Practical aspects must be addressed such as feasible lighting sources, ensuring optimal visualisation of the smaller oral cavity, and approaching children unable to report subjective and functional domains reliably, who may be (understandably) uncooperative.

Development of children's international mucositis evaluation scale

Following previous experience of the study of oral mucositis assessment in children, our opinion was that an ideal mucositis assessment instrument had not been developed for this population (Sung et al. 2007a; 2007b; Tomlinson et al. 2008b).

The development of instruments (Siminoff et al. 2006; 2008; Hodgkinson et al. 2007; Kushner et al. 2008; Schmidt et al. 2008) generally includes:

1. Item generation;
2. Refinement of wording of items to develop the instrument;
3. Testing of the psychometric properties of the instrument.

The development of any measurement instrument for use in the paediatric setting is often only briefly reported to include the generation of items. However, a series of steps are often followed (Smith et al. 2005; Butt et al. 2009). Sources for item generation can include previously published reliable and valid instruments, research studies, the use of focus groups of healthcare experts, and focus groups or semi-structured questionnaires involving parents of children within the considered population (Lin et al. 2007; Butt et al. 2009). Reports of refinement vary from asking opinion of the understandability of the instrument to assessing reliability and validity (Heyland & Tranmer 2001; Smith et al. 2005).

To develop a scale that was appropriate and easy to use in the paediatric population, a sequential process was followed that led to the development of the Children's International Mucositis Evaluation Scale (ChIMES). The series of steps which were implemented is illustrated in Figure 4.1.

Step 1: Literature review

Almost no standardisation in the measurement of oral mucositis is available, even within the adult literature. Many studies that developed or evaluated oral mucositis scales included small sample sizes of 20 or fewer adult patients (Beck 1979; Eilers et al. 1988; Spijkervet et al. 1989; Dibble et al. 1996; Tardieu et al. 1996; McGuire et al. 1998).

As previously discussed, the only two mucositis assessment instruments evaluated with children, in terms of psychometric properties, are the OMAS and OAG instruments. While these two instruments were found to be valid in the paediatric population, both have limitations. For example, while the OMAS appears to have excellent measurement properties in cooperative patients, it is unlikely that very young children will be able to cooperate with the examination, as it requires careful observation of nine different oral sites. The main criticism of the OAG is that, while it may be a very good measure for assessing oral hygiene, many of the items are not specific for mucositis. For example, attributes not correlated with mucositis include deeper or raspy voice, lips that are dry or cracked, or a coated or cracked tongue, which increase the score of the OAG. Also, the OAG score increases in the presence of teeth debris, which is neither sensitive nor specific for oral mucositis. Finally, there is an item for decreased saliva production, scored from 1 to 3. In children, severe mucositis typically is not associated with decreased saliva

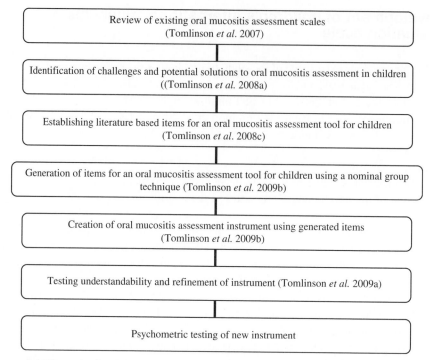

Figure 4.1 Steps in the development of the Child International Mucositis Evaluation Scake (Tomlinson et al. 2009b).

production and, in fact, most of these children drool as they are unable swallow their saliva (Tomlinson et al. 2007).

A limitation of all scoring systems in which an overall numeric evaluation of mucositis is obtained is that a given score can be obtained in a number of ways. The score may stay the same for a single patient but some aspects of the mucositis may have varied considerably over the course of evaluation. Some of the scoring systems, particularly those with many items, are lengthy and time-consuming (Tomlinson et al. 2007). The difficulty and the time factor may increase when assessing children whose cooperation may be challenging to obtain. In the study by Chen et al. (2004), the age range of children included was 2 to 17 years. However, there was no discussion as to the ease or appropriateness of using the OAG in this age group. Additionally, if repetitive examinations are necessary, this may be problematic and result in poor recruitment to a study. A measurement tool must be tolerable for patients, not cause increased pain or fatigue (Eilers & Epstein 2004; Jaroneski 2006).

Reviewing the literature on the use and limitations of various scales assists understanding of the need for the continuing development of different scales, but fails to identify systematically the challenges to the assessment of mucositis in children. In an attempt to describe these challenges and potential solutions, we convened a focus group of experts with knowledge of mucositis assessment, paediatric cancer and paediatric mucositis to discuss issues relevant to mucositis assessment in children undergoing cancer chemotherapy (Tomlinson et al. 2008a).

Step 2: Using focus group methodology

The focus group consisted of nine healthcare professionals with expertise in mucositis assessment, oral assessment in children and paediatric cancer. Participants were invited, based on their previous work in research and clinical practice in this field. A tenth participant who was a clinical epidemiologist, who did not have content expertise in paediatric cancer or mucositis, moderated the discussions. The moderator had previous experience using focus group techniques. Among the nine content experts, there was representation from medicine (n = 2), nursing (n = 5) and dentistry (n = 2). Participants were from Canada (n = 6), the United States (n = 2) and the United Kingdom (n = 1) (Tomlinson et al. 2008a). The focus group convened at the Hospital for Sick Children, Toronto, Canada.

We considered that valuable data regarding opinions and experiences could be obtained quickly and inexpensively from a focus group (Parahoo 2006). Focus groups have high validity; participant comprehension of concepts can be easily accomplished, and the results are credible to readers (Marshall & Rossman 2006). Focus group interviews typically include opinions and experiences of 5 to 15 people simultaneously (Polit & Tatano Beck 2005). Standard and well-described procedures for managing a focus group were followed (Morgan & Krueger 1998); the process followed a series of methodologically developed semi-structured questions that highlighted the challenges and possible solutions to mucositis assessment in children aged 2 to 18 years. Flexibility in phrasing was acceptable, and the moderator was able to probe for clarification when necessary (Parahoo 1997).

Four main areas of concerns had been identified from the literature (Tomlinson et al. 2008a):

1. The challenges in oral assessment in children, related to age and cooperation;
2. The need for proxy responses, while recognising the challenges of reporting pain and function attributed to oral mucositis;
3. The need for an instrument that is simple, quick to complete, and easy to use in almost all children;
4. Educational considerations.

The challenges in oral assessment in children

Most of the discussion focused on the fact that children present challenges for oral assessment because of their physical size, their potential inability to cooperate with oral examination, and their actual and potential inability to communicate symptoms, dependent on age. The focus group participants agreed that devices such as tongue depressors were undesirable for use in children and suggested that, when needed, a toothbrush may be suitable as an instrument to facilitate oral examination.

The need for proxy responses

While there have been several studies on the results of parent proxy-reports and self-reports from children, the emphasis is often on quality of life (QOL) (Jokovic et al. 2004; Yeh et al. 2005; Felder-Puig et al. 2006; Davis et al. 2007; Varni et al. 2007a; 2007b). Often there is some discordance with the results between the parent proxy and child self-report groups in these QOL studies. The difference in reports is often in terms of rating and in terms of the reason for the given answers. However, it was found that both children and parents interpreted the meaning of items in a QOL scale similarly (Davis et al. 2007). There have been few studies that have reported on child and parent perceptions of oral health-related QOL (Locker et al. 2002; Jokovic et al. 2003a; 2003b; 2004). There is also paucity in the literature regarding child and parent-proxy reports for oral assessment scales (Tomlinson et al. 2008a). Several scales, for example, the OMAS (Sonis et al. 2001), WHO and RTOG (Etiz et al. 2002), all include an objective component which requires accurate visual examination of the oral cavity, identified above as problematic. Other assessment scales, such as OAG (Eilers et al. 1988), a combined scale, and the OMI (Schubert et al. 1992; McGuire et al. 2002), an objective symptom scale, were used in a study by McGuire and colleagues (1998). The assessment of pain due to oral mucositis was debated regarding the appropriateness of such an assessement tool for oral mucositis. Some studies suggest that, because pain is one of the most distressing symptoms experienced by such patients, the inclusion of a pain scale is essential in any assessment tool (Jaroneski 2006). Others argue that, because pain can be affected by the use of analgesics, the assessment may not be a true reflection of the actual severity. The opinion of the focus group was that pain assessment should be recorded concurrently with administered pain medications and the reasons for which the pain medications were administered (Tomlinson et al. 2008a).

The need for an instrument that is simple, quick to complete, and easy to use

A one-page assessment tool was considered to be ideal. The assessment would include objective findings, but the emphasis would not be heavily weighted on the physical examination, thereby enhancing consistency in the assessment of variably cooperative children. A short assessment form would also reduce assessment time for proxy respondents and help ensure more accurate real-time reports of oral assessment (Tomlinson et al. 2008a).

Educational considerations

Issues concerning education include promoting awareness of the importance of regular oral assessments, demonstrating the utility of the scale in clinical research, and training staff on the practice of oral assessment and use of the assessment scale. Nurses are known to place high priority on oral care for patients with cancer (Miller & Kearney 2001; Southern 2007). Much of the adult literature regarding oral assessment concludes that nurses require an extensive knowledge of oral mucositis, its assessment and its management (Miller & Kearney 2001; Brown & Wingard 2004; Daniel et al. 2004; Eilers & Epstein 2004; Jaroneski 2006; Southern 2007). However, there is little suggestion about how this knowledge should be attained or how training should be conducted. Daniel et al. commented on the need for academic institutions that train oncology professionals to include oral care issues in their curricula (Daniel et al. 2004). In 2004, the Multinational Association for Supportive Care in Cancer/International Society of Oral Oncology (MASCC/ISOO) disseminated mucositis management guidelines for those caring for adults (Rubenstein et al. 2004). A survey conducted in 2005 concluded that there was little awareness of these guidelines among cancer healthcare professionals (McGuire et al. 2006). In 2006, the UKCCSG-PONF (United Kingdom Childhood Cancer Study Group and Paediatric Oncology Nurses Forum) produced evidence-based guidelines on mouth care for children with cancer (UKCCSG-PONF 2006) that, in light of findings by Glenny et al. (2004) of a significant variation in preventive oral care therapies, focused on preventive strategies.

Step 3: Establishing literature-based items for an assessment tool for children

In order to determine whether existing scales can be satisfactorily modified for use in children, or whether a new scale needed to be developed in this population, identification of items that should be included in a paediatric mucositis scale was an early step in the process (Tomlinson et al. 2008c). The first and main objective was to describe literature-based items that should be considered for a paediatric mucositis scale. The second objective was to describe other issues that should be considered when assessing mucositis in children.

To achieve the first objective, in relation to a paediatric scale, the items were divided into objective items, subjective items and functional items (Tomlinson et al. 2008c) (see Table 4.3).

None of the scales available in the literature were developed specifically for use in children. Various studies showed little consistency in the scales or items used in the assessment of oral mucositis in children, with exception of those studies by Cheng and colleagues (Cheng et al. 2001;2002; 2004; Cheng & Chang 2003).

Table 4.3 Items used in the assessment of oral mucositis

Objective	Subjective	Functional
Erythema/redness of the mucosa	Pain/soreness	Difficulty eating or drinking
Ulcers/pseudomembranes	Mouth dryness	Difficulty swallowing
Plaques/white patches	Taste changes	Respiration affected
Necrosis		Problems with talking/changes in voice
Haemorrhage		Difficulty sleeping
Lesions (undefined)		Unable to wear dentures
Oedema		
Altered papilli on tongue		
Plaque or debris on teeth/denture bearing line		
Atrophy of mucosa		
Amount and viscosity of saliva		
Dryness/changes to lips		
Dry mouth		
Changes in voice quality		

Source: Tomlinson et al. (2008c)

Objective items

Objective elements are commonly included on scales; a wide variety of specific signs have been measured. Several instruments have either included or focused specifically on visible mouth lesions. For example, the OMAS scoring system examines ulcers on a scale from 0 to 3, and erythema on a scale from 0 to 2, within the oral cavity. The WHO scale combines objective and functional symptoms; the objective elements include erythema and ulcers, and functional symptoms (e.g. the inability to eat or drink), similarly graded.

The OAG (Eilers et al. 1988) assesses objective, subjective and functional symptoms and the OMI (Schubert et al. 1992; McGuire et al. 2002) is solely an objective symptom scale. The OAG contained multiple objective elements which included oedema, papillary loss and teeth debris. The OMI included objective elements such as erythema, oedema and ulceration. It has always to be recognised that even careful examination and recording of multiple sites in the oral cavity can be problematic in light of the burden on patients who may also be experiencing other side effects of chemotherapy (McGuire et al. 1998).

Another important issue to consider for objective oral assessment is that assessments may be performed by several observers and, as was noted previously, interpretation of oral lesions may vary. Adequate training of assessors is required to ensure inter-rater reliability (Stokman et al. 2005). This also highlights the value of using a simple, straightforward tool that leaves little room for interpreter variability. However, this still cannot control for the problem of optimal visualisation of the oral cavity in order to make such an assessment.

Subjective items

In our review, we found that all the scales that include subjective items also include objective items, with the exception of OMDQ (Stiff et al. 2006); as discussed, despite controversy around its inclusion in the instruments used, the common symptom identified is pain. Few studies have considered the difficulties in monitoring pain in young children with mucositis (Etiz et al. 2002). Since pain is best described by the individual experiencing it (McGuire et al. 1998, Etiz et al. 2002), the best assessor should be the child. However, this may just not be possible in young children. Tomlinson et al. (2008a) argue that, where possible, despite this, pain should be evaluated, either within a specific mucositis instrument or as a separate evaluation; and to resolve the influence of analgesic use on pain scores, the use of analgesics should be recorded concurrent with a pain assessment, to provide a more global view of the patient's experiences (Tomlinson et al. 2008a).

Other subjective symptoms assessed have been changes in taste and mouth dryness. For example, Levy-Polack et al. (1998) evaluated mouth dryness from both the subjective perspective of the patient or caregiver, and an objective perspective of clinical examination, but did not discuss the effectiveness of either method of evaluation or its usefulness.

Functional items

Functional items, reflecting limitations in activities related to oral mucositis that have been included in many previous scales, are the ability to eat and drink, swallow, speak and sleep.

However, the assessment of the ability to eat and drink may be problematic, particularly in children. Young children refuse to eat and drink for many reasons including anorexia, nausea and childhood distress. It may be impossible to determine whether these functional limitations are related to mucositis rather than to other causes (Tomlinson et al. 2008a). Once again, the administration and effectiveness of analgesics may affect scoring of functional scales.

This literature review facilitated the first steps in generating items for a scale. Additional items were obtained by a focus group approach, discussed below.

Step 4: Generating items for an oral mucositis assessment scale for children

The nominal group technique (NGT) is a structured process developed in the 1960s when Andre Delbecq and Andrew Van de Ven noted that the analysis from decision-making groups in areas of industry, aerospace and environmental studies could be applied to healthcare (Van de Ven & Delbecq 1972). The main aim of the NGT is to ensure that all participants receive equal opportunity to express their opinions (Hall 1983). A short-coming of non-structured focus groups is for discussions to become dominated by the opinions of the most confident personalities in the group. The NGT aims to limit this potential by ensuring equal opportunities for each participant to express their opinion (Carney et al. 1996). Participants were those experts who had participated in the previously discussed focus group. Therefore, moderation of the NGT was not research-er-led, which avoided domination of the leader's opinions rather than those of the participants.

The nominal group process consisted of a series of steps shown in Box 4.2.

The NGT question addressed to the group was: 'For the purpose of clinical trials, in the evaluation of oral mucositis in children, what items do you think should be included in an

---

Box 4.2   Steps involved in the nominal group process

1. Introduce the nominal group process (NGT) to the group, including the purpose and description of the process.
2. Opening statement consisting of the NGT question that is developed in advance of the meeting.
3. Individual, silent generation of ideas in writing.
4. A round-robin recording of ideas on a flip chart.
5. Discussion of these ideas for clarification.
6. Preliminary vote (rank order) on the importance of items generated.
7. Discussion of the preliminary vote.
8. Final vote to establish importance of each item.
9. Conclusion.

Source: Tomlinson et al. (2009b)

Table 4.4 Items generated by nominal group technique that are important in a paediatric oral mucositis assessment tool

Suggested item (n = 30)	Number of votes
Presence of ulcers	11
Pain assessment	11
Effect on eating	9
Drooling/pooling of saliva	7
Amount of pain medication received	7
Effect on drinking	3
Rationale for not eating	0
Capacity to open mouth (how much)	0
Size and number of ulcers	0
Saliva production	0
Redness	0
Distinct versus coalesced	0
Throat pain/pain when swallowing	0
Parent's perception of pain	0
What does mouth feel like? (verbal child)	0
Voice changes	0
Infant scale for non-verbal – sucking	0
Swelling	0
Won't open mouth versus too sore to open	0
Presence of thrush	0
Weight loss	0
Plaque accumulation on teeth	0
Bleeding	0
Hydration/total parenteral nutrition	0
Oral microbiological cultures	0
Reasons for nutritional supplementation	0
Parent's evaluation of oral health	0
Assessor's global score	0
Effect on sleep	0
Lip description	0

Source: Tomlinson et al. (2009c)

assessment tool?' The list of generated items and the final assigned votes are shown in Table 4.4.

Step 5: Creation of oral mucositis assessment instrument

The generated items identified in Table 4.4 can be grouped into three main areas:

1. Pain: pain assessment, amount of pain medication received;
2. Function: effect on eating, drooling/pooling of saliva, effect on drinking;
3. Appearance: presence of ulcers.

Following further discussion by the expert group, a draft of a newly developed Children's International Mucositis Evaluation Scale (ChIMES) was created.

Consideration had been given to the appropriateness of a single assessment scale for children of any age. It was considered that a single version of a self-report instrument should be tested in this initial phase (Tomlinson et al. 2009b) and, as discussion had included doubts concerning the ability of younger children to answer this type of questionnaire, a parent 'proxy' version was created.

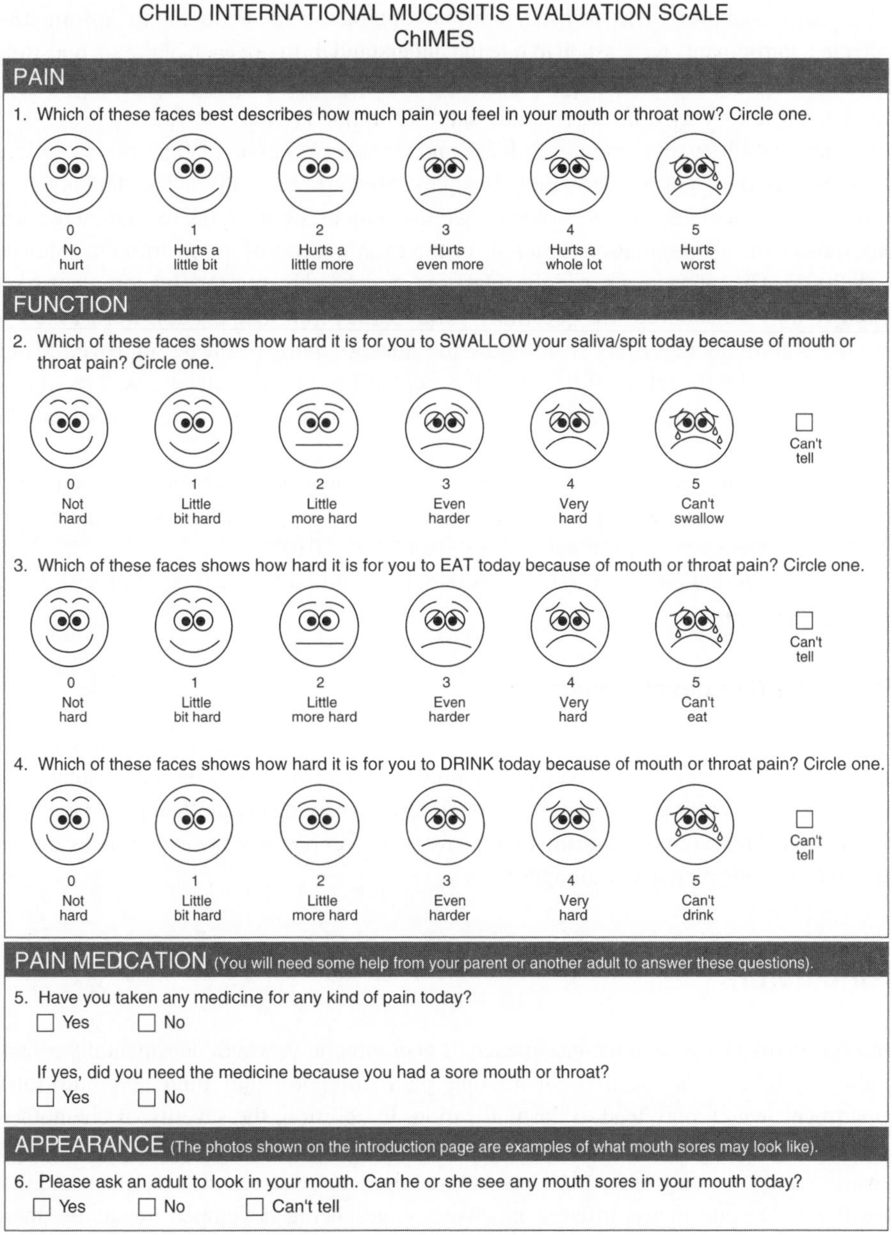

CHILD INTERNATIONAL MUCOSITIS EVALUATION SCALE
ChIMES

PAIN

1. Which of these faces best describes how much pain you feel in your mouth or throat now? Circle one.

0	1	2	3	4	5
No hurt	Hurts a little bit	Hurts a little more	Hurts even more	Hurts a whole lot	Hurts worst

FUNCTION

2. Which of these faces shows how hard it is for you to SWALLOW your saliva/spit today because of mouth or throat pain? Circle one.

0	1	2	3	4	5	☐ Can't tell
Not hard	Little bit hard	Little more hard	Even harder	Very hard	Can't swallow	

3. Which of these faces shows how hard it is for you to EAT today because of mouth or throat pain? Circle one.

0	1	2	3	4	5	☐ Can't tell
Not hard	Little bit hard	Little more hard	Even harder	Very hard	Can't eat	

4. Which of these faces shows how hard it is for you to DRINK today because of mouth or throat pain? Circle one.

0	1	2	3	4	5	☐ Can't tell
Not hard	Little bit hard	Little more hard	Even harder	Very hard	Can't drink	

PAIN MEDICATION (You will need some help from your parent or another adult to answer these questions).

5. Have you taken any medicine for any kind of pain today?
☐ Yes   ☐ No

If yes, did you need the medicine because you had a sore mouth or throat?
☐ Yes   ☐ No

APPEARANCE (The photos shown on the introduction page are examples of what mouth sores may look like).

6. Please ask an adult to look in your mouth. Can he or she see any mouth sores in your mouth today?
☐ Yes   ☐ No   ☐ Can't tell

Figure 4.2 Final version, Child International Mucositis Evaluation Scale.

Step 6: Understandability, content validity and acceptability

To ensure that the ChIMES is understandable, it was considered that information should be obtained from both the parents and children wherever possible (Sweeting & West 1998; Varni et al. 1998; 2007b; Eiser & Morse 2001; Schilling et al. 2007). To this end, parents, children and teenagers in a paediatric oncology setting were asked for their views on ChIMES and their recommendations (Tomlinson et al. 2009a).

Purposive sampling was utilised, consent obtained and demographic information collected. Participants were asked to rate the understandability of each of the six questions included in the instrument, on a five-point ordinal scale that ranged from 0 'very easy to understand' to 5 'very difficult to understand' (Tomlinson et al. 2009a).

Content validity using parents, children and teenagers as content experts was derived from the experience of Stewart and colleagues (Stewart et al. 2005). The data obtained from children and teenagers ensures that instrument items reflected language and experiences of this population targeted for the eventual use of the instrument (Stewart et al. 2005). The interviewer read the questions, recorded responses and comments, and asked if they considered the question 'good', 'okay' or 'bad'. They were asked to provide comments regarding if and how the questionnaire could be improved (Tomlinson et al. 2009a). Rating of the overall acceptability of the scale also was rated on a five-point ordinal scale ranging from 1 'very difficult to complete' to 5 'very easy to complete'.

Generally, results were positive, but several comments made led to the development of further drafts and their testing, until the final instrument appeared to contain the correct content that was easy to understand (Tomlinson et al. 2010).

A final version of ChIMES was developed for both child self-report (see Figure 4.2) and parent proxy-report.

Step 7: Further development

The only way to ensure the usefulness of any new instrument is by its evaluation in practice. The next step in the development process of ChIMES is its current evaluation in an international multicentre large cohort of children receiving chemotherapy. At the heart of any clinical research is the desire to improve wherever possible the experiences and the outcomes for our patients of all ages.

Conclusion

Oral mucositis is a common consequence of chemotherapy, which detrimentally affects quality of life. It can lead to distressing pain, infection and fluid and nutritional impairment, which may lead to hospitalization. In addition, the severity of chemotherapy-induced oral mucositis may limit delivery of anti-cancer therapy. Reliable, valid, sensitive and easy-to-use instruments are required to assess and treat the condition effectively. Despite many different mucositis scales being developed for adults, there has previously been limited evaluation of instruments that were appropriate for children.

It is hoped that this chapter has been able to demonstrate the process of developing a simple, feasible and reliable instrument to measure oral mucositis in children. With increased clinical research investigating interventions to reduce and prevent oral mucositis, such an instrument will be critical to effective conduct of this research in children.

References

Anderson PM, Schroeder G, Skubitz KM (1998) Oral glutamine reduces the duration and severity of stomatitis after cytotoxic cancer chemotherapy. *Cancer* **83**(7): 1433–9.

Andersson P, Persson L, Hallberg IR, Renvert S (1999) Testing an oral assessment guide during chemotherapy treatment in a Swedish care setting: a pilot study. *Journal of Clinical Nursing* **8**(2): 150–8.

Aquino VM, Harvey AR, Garvin JH, et al. (2005) A double-blind randomized placebo-controlled study of oral glutamine in the prevention of mucositis in children undergoing hematopoietic stem cell transplantation: a Pediatric Blood and Marrow Transplant Consortium Study. *Bone Marrow Transplantation* **36**(7): 611–16.

Beck S (1979) Impact of a systematic oral care protocol on stomatitis after chemotherapy. *Cancer Nursing* **2**(3): 185–99.

Brown CG, Wingard J (2004) Clinical consequences of oral mucositis. *Seminars in Oncology Nursing* **20**(1), 16–21.

Butt ML, Pinelli J, Boyle MH, et al. (2009) Development and evaluation of an instrument to measure parental satisfaction with quality of care in neonatal follow-up. *Journal of Developmental and Behavioral Pediatrics* **30**(1): 57–65.

Carney O, McIntosh J, Worth A (1996) The use of the Nominal Group Technique in research with community nurses. *Journal of Advanced Nursing* **23**(5): 1024–9.

Chen CF, Wang RH, Cheng SN, Chang YC (2004) Assessment of chemotherapy-induced oral complications in children with cancer. *Journal of Pediatric Oncology Nursing* **21**(1), 33–9.

Cheng KK (2009) Oral mucositis: a phenomenological study of pediatric patients' and their parents' perspectives and experiences. *Supportive Care in Cancer* **17**(7): 829–37.

Cheng KK, Chang AM (2003) Palliation of oral mucositis symptoms in pediatric patients treated with cancer chemotherapy. *Cancer Nursing* **26**(6): 476–84.

Cheng KK, Molassiotis A, Chang AM, Wai WC, Cheung SS (2001) Evaluation of an oral care protocol intervention in the prevention of chemotherapy-induced oral mucositis in paediatric cancer patients. *European Journal of Cancer* **37**(16): 2056–63.

Cheng KK, Molassiotis A, Chang AM (2002) An oral care protocol intervention to prevent chemotherapy-induced oral mucositis in paediatric cancer patients: a pilot study. *European Journal of Oncology Nursing* **6**(2): 66–73.

Cheng KK, Chang AM, Yuen MP (2004) Prevention of oral mucositis in paediatric patients treated with chemotherapy; a randomised crossover trial comparing two protocols of oral care. *European Journal of Cancer* **40**(8): 1208–16.

Costa EM, Fernandes MZ, Quinder LB, de Souza LB, Pinto LP (2003) Evaluation of an oral preventive protocol in children with acute lymphoblastic leukemia. *Pesquisa Odontologica Brasileira* **17**(2): 147–50.

Cox JD, Stetz J, Pajak TF (1995) Toxicity criteria of the Radiation Therapy Oncology Group (RTOG) and the European Organization for Research and Treatment of Cancer (EORTC). *International Journal of Radiation Oncology, Biology, Physics* **31**(5): 1341–6.

Daniel BT, Damato KL, Johnson J (2004) Educational issues in oral care. *Seminars in Oncology Nursing* **20**(1): 48–52.

Davis E, Nicolas C, Waters E, et al. (2007) Parent-proxy and child self-reported health-related quality of life: using qualitative methods to explain the discordance. *Quality of Life Research* **16**(5): 863–71.

Dibble SL, Shiba G, MacPhail L, Dodd MJ (1996) MacDibbs Mouth Assessment: a new tool to evaluate mucositis in the radiation therapy patient. *Cancer Practice* **4**(3): 135–40.

Dodd MJ, Facione NC, Dibble SL, MacPhail L (1996) Comparison of methods to determine the prevalence and nature of oral mucositis. *Cancer Practice* **4**(6): 312–18.

Dodd MJ, Miaskowski C, Dibble SL, Paul SM, MacPhail L, Greenspan D, Shiba G (2000) Factors influencing oral mucositis in patients receiving chemotherapy. *Cancer Practice* **8**(6): 291–7.

Donnelly JP, Muus P, Schattenberg A, De Witte T, Horrevorts A, De Pauw BE (1992) A scheme for daily monitoring of oral mucositis in allogeneic BMT recipients. *Bone Marrow Transplantation* **9**(6): 409–13.

Eilers J, Epstein JB (2004) Assessment and measurement of oral mucositis. *Seminars in Oncology Nursing* **20**(1): 22–9.

Eilers J, Berger AM, Petersen MC (1988) Development, testing, and application of the oral assessment guide. *Oncology Nursing Forum* **15**(3): 325–30.

Eiser C, Morse R (2001) Can parents rate their child's health-related quality of life? Results of a systematic review. *Quality of Life Research* **10**(4): 347–57.

El-Housseiny AA, Saleh SM, El-Masry AA, Allam AA (2007) The effectiveness of vitamin 'E' in the treatment of oral mucositis in children receiving chemotherapy. *Journal of Clinical Pediatric Dentistry* **31**(3): 167–70.

Etiz D, Orhan B, Demirustu C, Ozdamar K, Cakmak A (2002) Comparison of radiation-induced oral mucositis scoring systems. *Tumori* **88**(5): 379–84.

Felder-Puig R, di Gallo A, Waldenmair M, et al. (2006) Health-related quality of life of pediatric patients receiving allogeneic stem cell or bone marrow transplantation: results of a longitudinal, multi-center study. *Bone Marrow Transplantation* **38**(2): 119–26.

Gibson F, Cargill J, Allison J, et al. (2006) Establishing content validity of the oral assessment guide in children and young people. *European Journal of Cancer* **42**(12): 1817–25.

Glenny AM, Gibson F, Auld E, et al. (2004) A survey of current practice with regard to oral care for children being treated for cancer. *European Journal of Cancer* **40**(8): 1217–24.

Hall RS (1983) The Nominal Group Technique for planning and problem solving. *Journal of Biocommunication* **10**(2): 24–7.

Heyland DK, Tranmer JE (2001) Measuring family satisfaction with care in the intensive care unit: the development of a questionnaire and preliminary results. *Journal of Critical Care* **16**(4): 142–9.

Hodgkinson K, Butow P, Hunt GE, et al. (2007) The development and evaluation of a measure to assess cancer survivors' unmet supportive care needs: the CaSUN (Cancer Survivors' Unmet Needs measure). *Psycho-Oncology* **16**(9): 796–804.

Jaroneski LA (2006) The importance of assessment rating scales for chemotherapy-induced oral mucositis. *Oncology Nursing Forum* **33**(6): 1085–90; quiz 1091–3.

Jokovic A, Locker D, Stephens M, Guyatt G (2003a) Agreement between mothers and children aged 11–14 years in rating child oral health-related quality of life. *Community Dentistry and Oral Epidemiology* **31**(5): 335–43.

Jokovic A, Locker D, Stephens M, Kenny D, Tompson B, Guyatt G (2003b) Measuring parental perceptions of child oral health-related quality of life. *Journal of Public Health Dentistry* **63**(2): 67–72.

Jokovic A, Locker D, Guyatt G (2004) How well do parents know their children? Implications for proxy reporting of child health-related quality of life. *Quality of Life Research* **13**(7): 1297–307.

Kennedy L, Diamond J (1997) Assessment and management of chemotherapy-induced mucositis in children. *Journal of Pediatric Oncology Nursing* **14**(3): 164–74; quiz 175–7.

Kushner JA, Lawrence HP, Shoval I, et al. (2008) Development and validation of a Patient-Reported Oral Mucositis Symptom (PROMS) scale. *Journal/Canadian Dental Association. Journal de l Association Dentaire Canadienne* **74**(1): 59.

Levy-Polack MP, Sebelli P, Polack NL (1998) Incidence of oral complications and application of a preventive protocol in children with acute leukemia. *Special Care in Dentistry* **18**(5): 189–93.

Lin FR, Ceh K, Bervinchak D, Riley A, Miech R, Niparko JK (2007) Development of a communicative performance scale for pediatric cochlear implantation. *Ear and Hearing* **28** (5): 703–12.

Locker D, Jokovic A, Stephens M, Kenny D, Tompson B, Guyatt G (2002) Family impact of child oral and oro-facial conditions. *Community Dentistry and Oral Epidemiology* **30**(6): 438–48.

Marshall C, Rossman GB (2006) Designing Qualitative Research. Thousand Oaks, CA: Sage Publications.

McGuire DB, Yeager KA, Dudley WN, et al. (1998) Acute oral pain and mucositis in bone marrow transplant and leukemia patients: data from a pilot study. *Cancer Nursing* **21**(6): 385–93.

McGuire DB, Peterson DE, Muller S, Owen DC, Slemmons MF, Schubert MM (2002) The 20 item oral mucositis index: reliability and validity in bone marrow and stem cell transplant patients. *Cancer Investigation* **20**(7–8): 893–903.

McGuire DB, Johnson J, Migliorati C (2006) Promulgation of guidelines for mucositis management: educating health care professionals and patients. *Supportive Care in Cancer* **14**(6): 548–57.

Meurman JH, Pyrhonen S, Teerenhovi L, Lindqvist C (1997) Oral sources of septicaemia in patients with malignancies. *Oral Oncology* **33**(6): 389–97.

Miller M, Kearney N (2001) Oral care for patients with cancer: a review of the literature. *Cancer Nursing* **24**(4): 241–54.

Morgan DL, Krueger RA (1998) *The Focus Group Kit.* Thousand Oaks, CA: Sage Publications.

National Cancer Institute (2003) *Common Toxicity Criteria V3.0.* Bethesda, MD: National Cancer Institute.

Nelson W, Gibson F, Hayden S, Morgan N (2001) Using action research in paediatric oncology to develop an oral care algorithm. *European Journal of Oncology Nursing* **5**(3): 180–9.

Parahoo K (2006) *Nursing Research: Principles, Process and Issues.* London: Macmillan.

Parulekar W, Mackenzie R, Bjarnason G, Jordan RC (1998) Scoring oral mucositis. *Oral Oncology* **34**(1): 63–71.

Pereira Pinto L, de Souza LB, Gordon-Nunez MA, et al. (2006) Prevention of oral lesions in children with acute lymphoblastic leukemia. *International Journal of Pediatric Otorhinolaryngology* **70** (11):1847–51.

Polit DF, Tatano Beck C (2005) *Essentials of Nursing Research: Methods, Appraisal and Utilization.* Philadelphia: Lippincott, Williams & Wilkins.

Puyal-Casado M, Jiménez-Martinez C, Chimenos-Küstner E, López-López J, Juliá A (2003) A protocol for the evaluation and treatment of oral mucositis in patients with hematological malignancies. *Medicina Oral,* **8**(1), 10–8.

Riesenbeck D, Dorr W (1998) Documentation of radiation-induced oral mucositis. Scoring systems. *Strahlentherapie und Onkologie* **174** (Suppl 3): 44–6.

Rubenstein EB, Peterson DE, Schubert M, et al. (2004) Clinical practice guidelines for the prevention and treatment of cancer therapy-induced oral and gastrointestinal mucositis. *Cancer* **100** (9 Suppl): 2026–46.

Schilling LS, Dixon JK, Knafl KA, Grey M, Ives B, Lynn MR (2007) Determining content validity of a self-report instrument for adolescents using a heterogeneous expert panel. *Nursing Research* **56** (5): 361–6.

Schmidt S, Thyen U, Chaplin J, Mueller-Godeffroy E, Bullinger M (2008) Healthcare needs and healthcare satisfaction from the perspective of parents of children with chronic conditions: the DISABKIDS approach towards instrument development. *Child: Care, Health and Development* **34**(3): 355–66.

Schubert MM, Williams BE, Lloid ME, Donaldson G, Chapko MK (1992) Clinical assessment scale for the rating of oral mucosal changes associated with bone marrow transplantation: Development of an oral mucositis index. *Cancer* **69**(10): 2469–77.

Scully C, Epstein J, Sonis S (2003) Oral mucositis: a challenging complication of radiotherapy, chemotherapy, and radiochemotherapy: part 1, pathogenesis and prophylaxis of mucositis. *Head and Neck* **25**(12): 1057–70.

Siminoff LA, Rose JH, Zhang A, Zyzanski SJ (2006) Measuring discord in treatment decision-making; progress toward development of a cancer communication and decision-making assessment tool. *Psycho-Oncology* **15**(6): 528–40.

Siminoff LA, Zyzanski SJ, Rose JH, Zhang AY (2008) The Cancer Communication Assessment Tool for Patients and Families (CCAT-PF): a new measure. *Psycho-Oncology* **17**(12): 1216–24.

Smith SR, Highstein GR, Jaffe DM, Fisher EB, Strunk RC (2005) Refinement of an instrument to evaluate parental attitudes about follow-up care after an acute emergency department visit for asthma. *Journal of Asthma* **42**(7): 587–92.

Sonis ST (2004a) A biological approach to mucositis. *Journal of Supportive Oncology* **2**(1): 21–32; discussion 35–6.

Sonis ST (2004b) The pathobiology of mucositis. *Nature Reviews Cancer* **4**(4): 277–84.

Sonis ST (2007) Pathobiology of oral mucositis: novel insights and opportunities. *Journal of Supportive Oncology* **5** (9 Suppl 4): 3–11.

Sonis ST, Eilers JP, Epstein JB, et al. (1999) Validation of a new scoring system for the assessment of clinical trial research of oral mucositis induced by radiation or chemotherapy. Mucositis Study Group. *Cancer* **85**(10): 2103–13.

Sonis ST, Oster G, Fuchs H, et al. (2001) Oral mucositis and the clinical and economic outcomes of hematopoietic stem-cell transplantation. *Journal of Clinical Oncology* **19**(8): 2201–5.

Sonis ST, Elting LS, Keefe D, et al. (2004) Perspectives on cancer therapy-induced mucosal injury: pathogenesis, measurement, epidemiology, and consequences for patients. *Cancer* **100** (9 Suppl): 1995–2025.

Southern H (2007) Oral care in cancer nursing: nurses' knowledge and education. *Journal of Advanced Nursing* **57**(6): 631–8.

Spijkervet FK, van Saene HK, Panders AK, Vermey A, Mehta DM (1989) Scoring irradiation mucositis in head and neck cancer patients. *Journal of Oral Pathology and Medicine* **18**(3): 167–71.

Stewart JL, Lynn MR, Mishel MH (2005) Evaluating content validity for children's self-report instruments using children as content experts. *Nursing Research* **54**(6): 414–18.

Stiff PJ, Erder H, Bensinger WI, et al. (2006) Reliability and validity of a patient self-administered daily questionnaire to assess impact of oral mucositis (OM) on pain and daily functioning in patients undergoing autologous hematopoietic stem cell transplantation (HSCT). *Bone Marrow Transplantation* **37**(4): 393–401.

Stokman MA, Sonis ST, Dijkstra PU, Burgerhof JG, Spijkervet FK (2005) Assessment of oral mucositis in clinical trials: impact of training on evaluators in a multi-centre trial. *European Journal of Cancer* **41**(12): 1735–8.

Sung L, Tomlinson GA, Greenberg ML, et al. (2006) Validation of the oral mucositis assessment scale in pediatric cancer. *Pediatric Blood & Cancer* **49**(2): 149–53.

Sung L, Tomlinson GA, Greenberg ML, et al. (2007a) Serial controlled N-of-1 trials of topical vitamin E as prophylaxis for chemotherapy-induced oral mucositis in paediatric patients. *European Journal of Cancer* **43**(8): 1269–75.

Sung L, Tomlinson GA, Greenberg ML, et al. (2007b) Validation of the oral mucositis assessment scale in pediatric cancer. *Pediatric Blood & Cancer* **49**(2): 149–53.

Sweeting H, West P (1998) Health at age 11: reports from schoolchildren and their parents. *Archives of Disease in Childhood* **78**(5): 427–34.

Tardieu C, Cowen D, Thirion X, Franquin JC (1996) Quantitative scale of oral mucositis associated with autologous bone marrow transplantation. *European Journal of Cancer Part B Oral Oncology* **32B**(6): 381–7.

Tomlinson D, Judd P, Hendershot E, Maloney AM, Sung L (2007) Measurement of oral mucositis in children: a review of the literature. *Supportive Care in Cancer* **15**(11): 1251–8.

Tomlinson D, Gibson F, Treister N, et al. (2008a) Challenges of mucositis assessment in children: Expert opinion. *European Journal of Oncology Nursing* **12**(5): 469–75.

Tomlinson D, Isitt JJ, Barron RL, et al. (2008b) Determining the understandability and acceptability of an oral mucositis daily questionnaire. *Journal of Pediatric Oncology Nursing* **25**(2): 107–11.

Tomlinson D, Judd P, Hendershot E, Maloney AM, Sung L (2008c) Establishing literature-based items for an oral mucositis assessment tool in children. *Journal of Pediatric Oncology Nursing* **25** (3):139–47.

Tomlinson D, Gibson F, Treister N, et al. (2009a) Understandability, content validity and overall acceptability of the Children's International Mucositis Evaluation Scale (ChIMES): Child and parent reporting. *Journal of Pediatric Hematology/Oncology* **31** (6): 416–23.

Tomlinson D, Gibson F, Treister N, et al. (2009b) Designing an oral mucositis assessment instrument for use in children: generating items using a nominal group technique. *Supportive Care in Cancer* **17**(5): 555–62.

Tomlinson D, Gibson F, Treister N, et al. (2010) Refinement of the Children's International Mucositis Evaluation Scale (ChIMES): Child and parent perspectives on understandability, content validity and acceptability. *European Journal of Oncology Nursing* **14**(1): 29–41.

Treister N, Sonis S (2007) Mucositis: biology and management. *Current Opinion in Otolaryngology & Head and Neck Surgery* **15**(2): 123–9.

UK Childhood Cancer Study Group-Paediatric Oncology Nurses Forum (2006) Mouth Care for Children and Young People with Cancer: *Evidence-based Guidelines*. Vol. 2008.

Van de Ven A, Delbecq A (1972) The nominal group as a research instrument for exploratory health studies. *American Journal of Public Health* **62**(3): 337–42.

Varni JW, Katz ER, Seid M, Quiggins DJ, Friedman-Bender A, Castro CM (1998) The Pediatric Cancer Quality of Life Inventory (PCQL). I. Instrument development, descriptive statistics, and cross-informant variance. *Journal of Behavioral Medicine* **21**(2): 179–204.

Varni JW, Limbers CA, Burwinkle TM (2007a) How young can children reliably and validly self-report their health-related quality of life?: an analysis of 8,591 children across age subgroups with the PedsQL 4. 0 Generic Core Scales. *Health and Quality of Life Outcomes* **5**: 1.

Varni JW, Limbers CA, Burwinkle TM (2007b) Parent proxy-report of their children's health-related quality of life: an analysis of 13,878 parents' reliability and validity across age subgroups using the PedsQL 4. 0 Generic Core Scales. *Health and Quality of Life Outcomes* **5**: 2.

Walsh LJ, Hill G, Seymour G, Roberts A (1990) A scoring system for the quantitative evaluation of oral mucositis during bone marrow transplantation. *Special Care Dentistry* **10**(6): 190–5.

Williams MC, Martin MV (1992) A longitudinal study of the effects on the oral mucosa of treatment for acute childhood leukaemia. *International Journal of Paediatric Dentistry* **2**(2): 73–9.

Woo SB, Sonis ST, Monopoli MM, Sonis AL (1993) A longitudinal study of oral ulcerative mucositis in bone marrow transplant recipients. *Cancer* **72**(5): 1612–17.

World Health Organization (1979) *Handbook for Reporting Results of Cancer Treatment*. Geneva: WHO, pp. 15–22.

Yeh CH, Chang CW, Chang PC (2005) Evaluating quality of life in children with cancer using children's self-reports and parent-proxy reports. *Nursing Research* **54**(5): 354–62.

Further reading

Anon. (1991) Development of a staging system for chemotherapy-induced stomatitis. Western Consortium for Cancer Nursing Research. *Cancer Nursing* **14**(1): 6–12.

Anon. (1998) Assessing stomatitis: refinement of the Western Consortium for Cancer Nursing Research (WCCNR) stomatitis staging system. *Canadian Oncology Nursing Journal* **8**(3): 160–5.

Barbosa TS, Gaviao MB (2008) Oral health-related quality of life in children: part III. Is there agreement between parents in rating their children's oral health-related quality of life? A systematic review. *International Journal of Dental Hygiene* **6**(2): 108–13.

Cremeens J, Eiser C, Blades M (2006) Factors influencing agreement between child self-report and parent on the Pediatric Quality of Life Inventory 4.0 (PedsQL) generic. *Health and Quality of Life Outcomes* **4**: 58.

Cruz LB, Ribeiro AS, Rech A, Rosa LG, Castro CG Jr, Brunetto AL (2007) Influence of low-energy laser in the prevention of oral mucositis in children with cancer receiving chemotherapy. *Pediatric Blood & Cancer* **48**(4): 435–40.

Filstrup SL, Briskie D, da Fonseca M, Lawrence L, Wandera A, Inglehart MR (2003) Early childhood caries and quality of life: child and parent perspectives. *Pediatric Dentistry* **25**(5): 431–40.

Ishii E, Yamada S, Higuchi S, Honjo T, Igarashi H, Kanemitsu S, Kai T, Ueda K (1989) Oral mucositis and salivary methotrexate concentration in intermediate-dose methotrexate therapy for children with acute lymphoblastic leukemia. *Medical and Pediatric Oncology* **17**(5): 429–32.

Lynn MR (1986) Determination and quantification of content validity. *Nursing Research* **35**(6): 382–5.

Olson K, Hanson J, Hamilton J, et al. (2004) Assessing the reliability and validity of the revised WCCNR stomatitis staging system for cancer therapy-induced stomatitis. *Canadian Oncology Nursing Journal* **14**(3): 168–74, 176–82.

Chapter 5

Facing the challenges of primary malignant brain tumours

Shanne McNamara

Primary malignant brain tumours are one of the most complex and devastating cancers because patients have a universally poor prognosis and, after initial treatments of surgery, radiotherapy and chemotherapy, further treatment options are limited (Uddin & Jarmi 2008). Therefore patients do not benefit from early detection of recurrence and their management is essentially palliative (Brada & Guerrero 1997). The diagnosis can be drastic for both the patient and their family because it can affect them physically, cognitively, psychologically and socially, and all of these problems are compounded by a poor prognosis. For healthcare professionals, the care and management is a challenge, in terms of determining the best treatment, assisting rehabilitation and ensuring continuing support (Guerrero 1998). It is argued that the care required is often directed by the patient and carers themselves, and is usually best managed outside the hospital setting. The main focus of care is to maximise the patient's quality of life (National Collaborating Centre for Cancer [NCCC] and the National Institute for Health and Clinical Excellence [NICE] 2006).

This chapter will outline the incidence, diagnosis, symptoms and treatment of primary malignant brain tumours. The specific problems experienced by the patients, such as physical dysfunction, communication difficulties, cognitive impairment and psychological distress, will be explored. The management of the complication of seizures will be discussed, along with the implications for patients' quality of life. Radiotherapy, chemotherapy and steroid therapy will be summarised in relation to survival, quality of life and side effects, with particular attention to the need for a multidisciplinary approach to care. Finally, palliative and end-of-life care needs will be explored.

Incidence

From a report by Cancer Research UK (2009a), the incidence of primary brain and other central nervous system tumours in the United Kingdom was 4555 new cases in 2005. Primary brain tumours occur in approximately 7 per 100 000 population, representing just

Perspectives on Cancer Care. Edited by Josephine (Tonks) N. Fawcett and Anne McQueen
© 2011 Blackwell Publishing Ltd

2% of all cancers (Cancer Research UK 2009a). They are the eighth most common cancer in people of working age and the fifth commonest cause of death in people under the age of 65 years. Primary malignant gliomas are most common, accounting for around 80% of all brain tumours (Levin et al. 2001). Gliomas occur in people of all ages, are the commonest type of solid tumours in children, and affect men more commonly than women (Cancer Research UK 2009a). There has been some suggestion that the incidence is increasing. At one time this was thought to be a result of more frequent diagnosis due to improved imaging techniques (Brada & Thomas 1995). However, Brandes (2003) reports that the incidence is definitely increasing. The majority of these cases will be high-grade gliomas, which have a poor prognosis despite improvements in treatment (Rampling et al. 2004; Krex et al. 2007).

Origins and classification

The brain substance consists of nerve cells called neurons and supportive tissue called glia. The glia comprises of three cell types; astrocytes, oligodendrocytes and ependymal cells (Hickey & Armstrong 1997). Most primary brain tumours arise from the supportive tissue and are classified according to their cell of origin and stage of development. They are referred to as gliomas. The World Health Organization (WHO) (Louis et al. 2007) classifies gliomas into four grades (See Table 5.1).

Aetiology

As with other cancers, it is believed that brain tumours result from one or more mutations in cellular DNA (Henderson 2006). The majority of brain tumours appear to arise randomly (NCCC & NICE 2006). However, a small proportion is associated with familial conditions such as neurofibromatosis, tuberous sclerosis and familial adenomatous polyposis (Schwartzbaum et al. 2006; Wen & Kesari 2008). These genetic predispositions are rare and are not discussed here in any further detail. Interestingly, brain tumours are more common among affluent groups, and less developed countries have a lower incidence (NCCC & NICE 2006). Exposure to radiation is known to be a cause of primary malignant brain tumours and other cancers, and has been reported in patients who were treated with radiation, for tinea capitis and acute lymphoblastic leukaemia (Salvati et al. 2008).

Chemical carcinogens also appear to be an influencing factor. Despite the lack of conclusive evidence, people in certain occupations, such as farmers, chemists, veterinar-

Table 5.1 World Health Organization glioma grading system

Low grade	Grade I	Pilocytic astrocytoma
Low grade	Grade II	Astrocytoma and oligodendroglioma
High grade	Grade III	Anaplastic astrocytoma and anaplastic oligodendroglioma
High grade	Grade IV	Glioblastoma

ians, workers in rubber factories and those exposed to magnetic fields, have been shown to have an increased risk of brain tumours (Brada & Thomas 1995). More recently, the use of mobile telephones has been associated with an increased risk of brain tumours. A meta-analysis by Khurana et al. (2009) has indicated that there is sufficient epidemiological evidence to suggest a link with prolonged mobile telephone usage and the development of a tumour.

There are known to be two genetic pathways for the formation of glioblastoma, WHO grade IV. Primary (de novo) glioblastoma accounts for the majority and occurs mainly in older people with a short clinical history. In others, secondary glioblastoma develops from pre-exisiting low-grade astrocytomas and mainly affects younger people (Benjamin et al. 2003). Unlike other cancers, glioblastomas rarely spread to other parts of the body but can metastasise to the spinal cord.

Clinical manifestations of primary malignant brain tumours

The presenting symptoms of primary malignant brain tumours relate to raised intracranial pressure and local or general brain dysfunction (NCCC & NICE 2006) (see Box 5.1).

Box 5.1 **The symptoms that patients with primary malignant brain tumours may experience**

- Headache.
- Nausea/vomiting.
- Seizures.
- Cognitive problems.
- Physical function.
- Personality changes.

Source: Uddin & Jarmi (2008)

Raised intracranial pressure

The signs and symptoms of raised intracranial pressure are headache, vomiting and papilloedema (Brada & Thomas 1995). Papilloedema is caused by an increase in cerebral spinal fluid pressure around the optic nerve, which impairs the outflow of venous blood. This results in oedema or swelling of the optic disc; unrelieved papilloedma usually leads to a slow and progressive visual deterioration (Wegman 1993). In some instances the raised intracranial pressure will be severe and will rapidly cause altered levels of consciousness as vital centres within the brain become compressed (NCCC & NICE 2006).

Local or general brain dysfunction

The specific, and often distressing, symptoms of primary malignant brain tumours depend on its location in the brain and can include seizures, visual disturbance, focal neurological

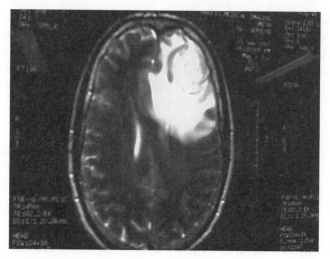

Figure 5.1 A computed tomography scan of a left frontal glioblastoma with surrounding oedema.

deficits, speech and understanding difficulties, cognitive decline, personality changes and memory and behavioural changes (NCCC & NICE 2006; Wen & Kesari 2008) (see Figure 5.1). There are wide variations in the abruptness of the onset of these symptoms, which usually varies with the histological grade and site of the tumour. As brain tumours are relatively rare, and may present with a wide range of symptoms, many patients will have had other diagnoses considered before finally arriving at the diagnosis of a brain tumour. This often increases anxiety and stress for the patient and their family and can only be exacerbated if there is a decline in cognitive function which may necessitate an increased need for psychological, psychiatric, social and physical support (NCCC & NICE 2006).

Prognosis

As discussed above, the majority of the presenting brain tumours will be high-grade gliomas, which have a poor prognosis despite improvements in treatment (Krex et al. 2007). The most important prognostic factors are:

- age;
- histology;
- presenting symptoms and degree of neurological deficit;
- performance status.

Table 5.2 Karnofsky rating scale for functional status

Rating %	Functional status
100	Normal, no complaints; no evidence of disease
90	Able to carry on normal activity, minor signs or symptoms of disease
80	Normal activity with effort, some signs or symptoms of disease
70	Cares for self, unable to carry on normal activity or to do active work
60	Requires occasional assistance, but is able to care for most personal needs
50	Requires considerable assistance and frequent medical care
40	Disabled, requires special care and assistance
30	Severely disabled, hospital admission is indicated although death not imminent
20	Very sick, hospital admission necessary, active supportive treatment necessary
10	Moribund, fatal processes progressing rapidly
0	Dead

Source: Karnofsky et al. (1948)

It is known that patients who are younger have a better prognosis for gliomas of all grades (Giles & Gonzales 2001); however, histology is the most important factor in prognosis (Uddin & Jarmi, 2008). Patients who have seizures at presentation have a better prognosis (Berger & Keles 1995). This is probably due to the fact that they are likely to be investigated sooner than a patient presenting with more subtle symptoms.

Survival in patients with high-grade gliomas decreases in line with performance status. That is, the poorer the performance status, the poorer the prognosis (Uddin & Jarmi 2008). Two scales are commonly used in neuro-oncology to measure performance status: the Karnofsky performance (KPS) rating scale (Karnofsky et al. 1948) (see Table 5.2) and the WHO performance status scale first published in 1979 (WHO 1979) (see Table 5.3). Additionally, the extent of surgical resection will help guide the clinician when estimating prognosis (Hentschel & Sawaya 2003).

Table 5.3 WHO performance status criteria

Grade	WHO status
0	Fully active, able to carry on all pre-disease performance without restriction
1	Restricted in physically strenuous activity but ambulatory and able to carry out work of a lighter or sedentary nature, e.g. light housework, office work
2	Ambulatory and capable of all self-care but unable to carry out any work activities. Up and about more than 50% of waking hours
3	Capable of only limited self-care, confined to bed or chair more than 50% of waking hours
4	Completely disabled. Cannot carry out any self-care. Totally confined to bed or chair
5	Dead

Source: WHO (1979)

Impact of diagnosis on the patient and their family

Many patients with primary malignant brain tumours will not have major neurological deficits. Consequently, when they are given the diagnosis it comes as a shock for the patient and their family (Guerrero 2005). However, as a direct result of the tumour or from side effects of treatment, patients with a brain tumour may experience symptoms that drastically affect their ability to function normally (Khalili 2007). They encounter many losses that may include the loss of communication, short-term memory, mobility, hair, strength and endurance, the ability to drive and independence (Khalili 2007). Indeed, Armstrong (2004) found that, because of ongoing symptoms, only 18% of patients returned to work. A number of conditions are commonly associated with the diagnosis and treatment of brain tumours including seizures, confusion, deep vein thrombosis and the effects of corticosteroids (Taillibert et al. 2004). Furthermore, many patients will suffer from depression, with various authors reporting an incidence between 35% and 93% (Pelletier et al. 2002; Litofsky et al. 2004; Mainio et al. 2005). Mainio et al. (2005) suggest that quality of life is adversely affected by depression, yet many patients are not treated with antidepressants (Litofsky et al. 2004). In turn, depression correlates closely with fatigue, emotional distress and existential distress (Pelletier et al. 2002). Pelletier et al. (2002) advise that a better understanding of emotional distress would result in effective intervention which would thereby improve quality of life. One of the most difficult issues for families is coping with the loss of the person before the diagnosis as a result of personality changes, cognitive decline, difficulties in communication and changes in body image (Guerrero 2002; Khalili 2007). Sherwood et al. (2004) suggest that coping with personality changes and changes in behaviour causes family anxiety because they do not know how to deal with these changes. Thus, optimal care of the patient, their family and/or carers will require input from many healthcare professionals, depending on their specific needs (NCCC & NICE 2006). Nurses have an important role in supporting the patient and their family through all stages of their illness (Khalili 2007), and it especially important that they plan future care with the interest of the patient at heart, thus avoiding stressful situations and crisis intervention (Guerrero 2002). The future place of care for the patient will be dependent on the needs of the individual and could include hospice, nursing home, rehabilitation centres and the patient's home (Guerrero 2002).

Diagnostic investigations

Neuro-imaging

The National Institute for Health and Clinical Excellence (NCCC & NICE 2006) guidance on improving outcomes for people with brain and other CNS tumours outlines the diagnostic process. Computed tomography (CT) scan and magnetic resonance imaging (MRI) scans are used to determine the diagnosis and are helpful for planning the surgical intervention. Other imaging techniques are not routinely required, but positron emission tomography (PET) scans or single photon emission computed tomography (SPECT) scans may be used in some cases. Functional MRI and the use of MR spectroscopy and diffusion tensor analysis may improve the diagnosis and provide preoperative information (NCCC & NICE 2006; Wen and Kesari 2008). However, whenever possible, it is best practice to obtain histological classification. Neuro-imaging continues to be necessary following treatments to assess the response to interventions or to identify progression (Cha 2006) (see Figure 5.1).

Histopathology

The histological appearance of a glioblastoma is of poorly differentiated astrocytic cells with brisk mitotic activity and atypical neuclei. There is also necrosis and microvascular proliferation (Louis et al. 2007). With growing research, molecular analysis will be increasingly used to characterise brain tumours and may provide more sensitive information about prognosis and expected therapeutic response (NCCC & NICE 2006).

Treatment

There should be a multidisciplinary approach to the treatment of patients with primary malignant brain tumours (NCCC & NICE 2006). The main aim of treatment is always to increase survival and maximise quality of life (NCCC & NICE 2006). Because the treatment for primary malignant brain tumours is often palliative, the benefits of treatment must be considered carefully, as the degree of toxicity may outweigh the survival benefit (Guerrero 2005).

Generally there are three treatments that are considered: surgery, radiotherapy and chemotherapy. Additionally many of the symptoms, identified above, are managed medically (Wen & Kesari 2008). For patients with glioblastoma, who have a good performance status, a surgical resection followed by radiotherapy plus concomitant and adjuvant chemotherapy is recommended (Stupp et al. 2005).

Surgery

Ideally, a sample of the tumour is required for histopathological grading. This can be obtained either by biopsy or surgical resection, and the choice will be dependent on the anatomical position of the tumour (NCCC & NICE 2006). There are several possible surgical procedures including sterotactic guided biopsy, neuro-radiologically guided biopsy, open biopsy, craniotomy and resection, 'awake' craniotomy, and craniotomy with the insertion of carmustine implants (biodegradable polymer discs containing the antineoplastic agent, carmustine) (NCCC & NICE 2006).

Biopsy

Stereotactic biopsy is performed when the tumour is located in a part of the brain that is critical and where attempt at resection would be unsafe (Wen & Kesari 2008). The biopsy will only determine the tumour's histological picture as a guide to non-surgical treatment.

Sometimes the risk associated with a biopsy is considered to be too high. In these situations treatment is based on the radiological diagnosis (NCCC & NICE 2006).

Craniotomy

Whenever possible a craniotomy and resection of the tumour is advantageous in terms of overall survival and improvement of symptoms. However, due to the infiltrative nature of high-grade gliomas, it is not possible to remove the tumour completely (NCCC & NICE 2006; Wen & Kesari 2008). When possible, maximal surgical resection should be completed as this will reduce the symptoms of the tumour (Wen & Kesari 2008). New technology such as intraoperative MRI, fluorescence-guided surgery and sonic wands has improved the safety and assisted in achieving a more complete resection (Wen & Kesari 2008).

Carmustine implants

Carmustine implants are recommended only when it has been possible to remove 90% of the tumour (NICE 2007). They can be used in newly diagnosed high-grade glioma and upon recurrence in glioblastoma.

Westphal et al. (2003) report on a phase III trial of the use of carmustine implants for newly diagnosed high-grade glioma at 38 centres in 14 countries (see Chapter 9). The results showed that the median survival was significantly longer in patients who received the implants compared to those receiving placebo (13.8 months versus 11.6 months; $P = 0.017$). A phase III, prospective, randomised, double blind, placebo-controlled trial was conducted on patients with tumour progression in 27 centres. The six-month survival rate increased from 47% to 60% ($P = 0.061$) with the use of carmustine implants (Brem et al. 1995). Carmustine implants should be considered for patients presenting on tumour progression who are eligible for re-resection.

In some centres carmustine implants are used at initial surgery and on tumour recurrence (Krzeminski et al. 2008). Other centres are combining the use of carmustine wafers followed by radiotherapy with concomitant and adjuvant chemotherapy with temozolomide (LaRocca & Mehdorn 2009), although this is not currently common practice in the United Kingdom. However, Spiegel et al. (2007), following a meta-analysis, concluded that the combination of carmustine implants and temozolomide may be more effective than single-agent chemotherapy.

Radiotherapy

Marie Curie was the first scientist to use radioisotopes to treat cancer. Radiotherapy damages the cell's DNA, thereby causing cell death, in particular when the cell is replicating (Faithfull 2006). It causes damage to both normal and abnormal cells, therefore it is important to minimise the dose affecting normal cells as much as possible. Advances in radiotherapy resulting in better delivery techniques, such as intensity modulated radiotherapy (IMRT) and conformal therapies, where the beams of radiation used in treatment are shaped to match the tumour, assist in this aim (Faithfull 2006). Patients with primary malignant brain tumours commonly receive external beam radiotherapy using high-energy X-rays. This type of radiotherapy is delivered using a linear accelerator (Plate 4).

To deliver radiotherapy to the brain it is necessary that a beam-directed shell to fit the patient is made. Such shells are commonly made from thermoplastic (see Plate 5). The treatment is usually planned using a CT simulator (see Plate 6). The dose is measured in grays (Gy), as the amount of energy absorbed per unit mass of tissue (Faithfull 2006).

Overexposure to X-rays is unsafe; therefore the therapy radiographers, other healthcare professionals and relatives are not allowed into the treatment room. The treatment room will either have heavy lead doors, or, more likely, a maze corridor. The patient is observed throughout the treatment via a monitor.

Brachytherapy, a form of cancer treatment using localised radiotherapy, is not considered for use in newly diagnosed glioblastoma because its value has not been established in a randomised clinical trial (Salcman 2001). Some small-scale studies have been undertaken in the use of brachytherapy in recurrent malignant glioma, which suggest it is safe to use and has some survival benefit for patients with a good performance status (Chan et al. 2005; Fabrini et al. 2009).

Radiotherapy is probably the most effective treatment for malignant gliomas, doubling the length of survival to a median of 9–12 months (Stupp et al. 2005). The type of radiotherapy most commonly used for malignant gliomas is external beam radiotherapy. A radical course of 60 Gy in 30 fractions is usually given Monday to Friday for six weeks. When patients are less well, frail and elderly, or their performance status is poor, a palliative course of radiotherapy is considered. This regime is 30 Gy in six fractions frequently delivered over two weeks on alternate days (Whittle et al. 2002). Some oncology centres may have their own radiotherapy regimes for the palliative course of treatment. It is therefore always advisable to check before informing individual patients of the treatment plan.

Guerrero (2005) suggests that many of the treatments are disruptive to daily life as radiotherapy regimes can last up to six weeks and entail visits to the hospital on a daily basis. Travelling can be tiring and difficult for patients (Faithfull 2006), and especially so for patients with primary malignant brain tumours because they can no longer drive (DVLA 2009). Understandably, patients can find the effects of treatment upsetting as the side effects include alopecia, skin reactions, otitis, fatigue, somnolence, nausea and vomiting. Patients generally feel vulnerable, have low self-esteem and feel out of control (Guerrero 2005; Taillibert & Delattre 2005). Therefore, it is important that patients understand the practicalities and consequences of treatment and that staff are sensitive to their psychological needs.

Radiotherapy reactions

Patients will experience some reactions to radiotherapy. These reactions are commonly divided into early acute, early delayed and late reactions (Brada & Thomas 1995; Karim 1995). Early acute reactions may occur during the course of treatment and include fatigue, skin reactions and hair loss (Karim 1995). Early delayed reaction is usually referred to as somnolence syndrome (Shenouda et al. 1997; Faithfull & Brada 1998). The effect of radiotherapy is insidious in nature and late delayed reactions result in necrosis and demyelination, two to three years after treatment, in a small percentage of patients (Brada & Thomas 1995; Karim 1995). Patients with glioblastoma are unlikely to live this long; however, it is an important factor in the careful planning of treatment, especially for children and adults with curable tumours (Brada & Thomas 1995). The recent addition of temozolomide chemotherapy has led to a phenomenon known as pseudo-progression. Progressive and enhancing lesions are seen on scans following treatment which are not due to tumour progression but are treatment related (Brandsma et al. 2008). This can occur in around 50% of patients, who may require corticosteroids or further surgery (Brandsma et al. 2008; Taal et al. 2008).

Skin care

Most patients will experience some reaction of the skin due to radiotherapy (Naylor 2006). This will vary from person to person, ranging from mild erythema or dry desquamation to moist desquamation (Guerrero 2005). A particular affected area is behind the ear, especially when patients wear glasses (Guerrero 2005). Wells et al. (2004) suggest that washing the area with mild soap and water is sufficient as there is no symptomatic benefit in applying cream. However some patients find the use of aqueous cream beneficial. Each radiotherapy centre will have a policy on skin care and the reader is advised to check before making suggestions to patients. Necrosis of the skin is now rarely seen, because of improved delivery techniques (Naylor 2006).

Somnolence syndrome following radiotherapy

Fatigue and somnolence syndrome have been reported in the literature as being a problem for patients who undergo cranial irradiation (Shenouda et al. 1997; Faithfull & Brada 1998). Somnolence has been described as causing fatigue, lethargy, an overwhelming feeling of exhaustion, fever, anorexia, irritability, slowing of mental processes, seizures, transient worsening of disease symptoms such as limb weakness, headaches and nausea and has been linked to anxiety and depression. Fatigue is also well documented as being a problem for patients with malignant disease following radiotherapy and chemotherapy. Other studies into fatigue in patients with cancer have described deteriorating effects on quality of life, levels of energy, motivation, sleep patterns, cognition and social functioning (Stone et al. 2001). Despite increasing work into both fatigue and somnolence, there is no known cause, and have been limited attempts at effective assessment and intervention (see Chapter 8). Catt et al. (2008) recommend informing patients that this syndrome can occur in as many as 80% of cases.

When considering the syndrome of somnolence, many studies can be criticised for their use of patients with wide-ranging diagnosis, demographic factors and differing treatment regimes, and for ignoring other factors which might be responsible for the severity and frequency of somnolence. It has been speculated that somnolence syndrome may be due to demyelination, and the severity may depend on the type of tumour, its location within the brain, the intensity and type of radiotherapy delivered and the age of the patient.

There is debate in the literature as to when somnolence is most likely to occur, with Faithfull and Brada (1998) finding two instances of between 11 and 21 days post-radiotherapy and another phase at 31 and 33 days, and Shenouda et al. (1997) reporting somnolence occurring at 47 and 67 days. This two-stage pattern puts the theory of demyelination into question. Patients should be informed that somnolence syndrome is a possibility, because they may fear that the symptoms are suggestive of recurrence. The reintroduction of corticosteroids is indicated for these patients (Grant 2004).

Chemo-radiation

Clinical trials have shown that some chemotherapeutic drugs, molecular and antiangio-genic agents may enhance the effect of radiotherapy. As a consequence, patients who have had a craniotomy and resection now receive temozolomide chemotherapy, broadly referred to as chemo-radiation.

A randomised controlled trial performed by the European Organisation for Research and Treatment of Cancer (EORTC) and National Cancer Institute of Canada (NCIC) has shown that the combination of concomitant temozolomide with radical radiotherapy followed by a six-month adjuvant or maintenance phase prolongs survival of newly diagnosed patients with glioblastoma (Stupp et al. 2005). Prior to this treatment regime, the standard treatment for glioblastoma was surgical resection if possible, followed by radiotherapy with a median survival of around 9–12 months and a two-year survival of just 9% of patients. The results of this trial demonstrate a two-year survival of 26% (Stupp et al. 2005).

During this trial the tumour specimens were examined for *O*6-methylguanine-DNA methyltransferase (MGMT), and this marker was found to be an important prognostic indicator (Hegi et al. 2005). Tumours which contain methylated MGMT are unable to repair the chemotherapy-induced DNA damage, resulting in better overall survival for this group of patients (Stupp et al. 2006). Some centres in the United Kingdom are routinely testing for this marker, but at present the results are not used to influence management.

Generally, patients in the United Kingdom who receive chemo-radiation treatment have not had carmustine implants at surgery. As mentioned earlier, this practice may change in the future as there are some interesting reports of their combined use, thereby improving the prognosis of patients with glioblastoma (Spiegel et al. 2007). Nevertheless, following radiotherapy, with or without chemotherapy, most tumours recur in the same location (Wen & Kesari 2008).

Stereotactic radiotherapy or radiosurgery

Stereotactic radiotherapy is a type of radiotherapy delivered by a linear accelerator in daily fractions. Radiosurgery is delivered in a single fraction (Cancer Research UK 2009b). It requires the fitting of a special head frame. It is a very accurate conformal technique using a three-dimensional coordinate system to precisely target the tumour (Tsao et al. 2005). However, stereotactic radiotherapy or radiosurgery are rarely used for the initial treatment of high-grade gliomas because of their infiltrative nature. It is best used for small, well-defined round tumours such as metastases or acoustic neuromas (Cancer Research UK 2009b). Biswas et al. (2009) report that radiosurgery is a well-tolerated treatment when used as a boost or on recurrence. Nevertheless, Biswas et al. (2009) recommend that further clinical trials need to be carried out, especially since the advent of temozolomide, which would be the preferred choice of treatment with external beam radiotherapy.

Chemotherapy

Chemotherapy is the administration of cytotoxic drugs to kill malignant cells. Cytoxic drugs destroy all dividing cells, not just malignant cells. Therefore, there are associated toxicities, especially bone marrow depression, alopecia, mucositis and infertility (Coward & Coley 2006). The difficulty in treating malignant brain tumours is the inability for many drugs to cross the blood–brain barrier (Brada & Thomas 1995). If surgery is not possible, chemotherapy is the treatment of choice at relapse (NCCC & NICE 2006).

As already mentioned previously, temozolomide is the first choice of chemotherapy for patients newly diagnosed with glioblastoma. It is administered for the duration of radiotherapy and continued for 5 days in every 28 in the adjuvant phase, usually for six months (Stupp et al. 2005). Some authors recommend the long-term use of temozolomide and report that some patients have continued to take it for several years without any serious side effects (Khasraw et al. 2009). However, in general, chemotherapy is kept in reserve for patients presenting with tumour recurrence, and mostly only offers palliation (Sathornsumetee & Rich 2008; Wick et al. 2009). Previously the most common chemotherapy regime in the treatment of high-grade gliomas was a combination of three agents: procarbazine, lomustine (CCNU) and vincristine (PCV); this is still used in many centres (Schmidt et al. 2006). In a phase II study comparing temozolomide with procarbazine at first relapse, patients receiving temozolomide had a better outcome in survival and quality of life (Yung et al. 2000). Unfortunately there has been no comparison with the PCV regime.

With increasing knowledge of the molecular abnormalities of glioblastoma there is increasing interest in molecular target therapies. These drugs have the potential to increase the efficacy of existing chemotherapeutic agents. However, to date they have not demonstrated any benefit but warrant further clinical trials (Sathornsumetee & Rich 2008).

Medical management

Medications

Anticonvulsant medication

Many patients with primary malignant brain tumours will have seizures. The incidence ranges between 35% to 70% depending on the type of tumour and its location (Campbell 2006; NCCC & NICE 2006). The likelihood of developing seizures is related both to the site and the type of tumour (NCCC & NICE 2006). Most commonly, seizures are partial and secondary generalised, and prove difficult to manage. Seizures can have major social implications, including loss of independence, social isolation and driving restrictions (Campbell 2006). Patients with seizures should be managed with anticonvulsants, the choice of which should be carefully selected if treatment may at some point involve chemotherapy. Some anticonvulsant agents increase the metabolism of certain chemotherapeutic agents and reduce the efficacy of corticosteroids (Campbell 2006; Wen & Kesari 2008). Additionally, Taillibert and Delattre (2005) state that cognitive impairment can be exacerbated with the use of anticonvulsants.

Because patients with malignant gliomas are at a greater risk of developing deep vein thrombosis, the choice of anticonvulsant should be one that does not interact with anticoagulant medication (Campbell 2006). Many anticonvulsants cause weight gain, which can cause additional distress to the patient whose body image is already vulnerable (Campbell 2006). Body image is discussed in more detail later in this chapter. Although anticonvulsant prophylaxis has been under discussion for some time, there is an increasing belief that there is no benefit in prescribing prophylactic anticonvulsants for such patients, as the side effects outweigh the risk of having a seizure (Glantz et al. 2000; Taillibert & Delattre 2005).

Corticosteroids

Patients with high-grade glioma frequently develop raised intracranial pressure at some point during the course of their illness, and corticosteroids remain the most effective treatment (NCCC & NICE 2006; Wen & Kesari 2008). Unfortunately, corticosteriods have many side effects including gastric irritation, obesity, psychosis, myopathy, stress fracture, adrenal suppression, immunosuppression and the onset of diabetes mellitus, as listed in the *British National Formulary* (British Medical Association 2008). It is therefore recommended that patients are made aware of these side effects and that they carry a steroid treatment card (BMA 2008). Dexamethasone is the corticosteroid of choice and large doses, usually up to 16 mg, can be administered. Once the patient's condition has stabilised the dose should then be titrated against symptoms and discontinued where possible. Due to the risk of gastric irritation it is suggested that a H2 antagonist is prescribed prophylactically (McNamara & Kilbride 1999).

Anticoagulation therapy

Patients are at a greater risk of developing a deep vein thrombosis when they are diagnosed with a malignant glioma, with an incidence of 20% to 30% (Wen & Kesari 2008). It is known that there are angiogenic factors which increase the risk in patients with malignant gliomas (Junck 2004). Some clinicians recommend prophylaxis with low molecular-weight heparin, as the risk of intratumoral haemorrhage is low (Taillibert & Delattre 2005; Wen & Kesari 2008). Subcutaneous heparin or oral warfarin is the choice for long-term use. A vena cava filter can be fitted for patients who have pulmonary complications (Junck 2004).

Quality of life

The emotional impact of a brain tumour diagnosis can, in some patients, lead to depression, which may be difficult to diagnose due to tumour-induced cognitive and behavioural changes (Junck 2004). Pelletier et al. (2002) discuss aspects of quality of life while considering depression, fatigue, emotional distress and existential issues. As might be anticipated, patients who have had depressive illness before a diagnosis of a brain tumour are more likely to have depression following the diagnosis (Kilbride et al. 2007). Various other aspects need to be considered, including behavioural changes, cognitive dysfunction, anxiety and depression, and fatigue (Pelletier et al. 2002; Pangilinan et al. 2007). For example, some patients with brain tumours will become disinhibited, suffer from lability, and on occasions become aggressive (Pelletier et al. 2002). These symptoms are associated with neurological damage and associated treatments (Pangilinan et al. 2007). It is suggested that addressing the needs of the patient and helping them cope with their illness will improve quality of life (Pelletier et al. 2002; Pangilinan et al. 2007). However, depression is often under-diagnosed and patients fail to receive appropriate treatment with antidepressants and psychiatric and psychological support (Litofsky et al. 2004; Pangilinan et al. 2007; Wen & Kesari 2008). As a result of common alternative explanations for depressive symptoms, depression is frequently missed in this group of patients (Pangilinan et al. 2007). Pangilinan et al. (2007) list the symptoms of depression and alternative reasons for these symptoms (see Table 5.4), explaining why depression is often missed in patients with brain tumours. Treatment of depression will include medication, and serotonin reuptake inhibitors (SSRIs) are

Table 5.4 Depression experienced in the presence of brain tumour

Symptoms of depression	Other reasons for these symptoms
Increased levels of fatigue	Following radiotherapy Due to anticonvulsants Insomnia due to corticosteroids Myopathy due to steroids Physical dysfunction
Decreased concentration	Cognitive decline Poor memory Effects of anticonvulsants Following radiotherapy
Weight changes	Weight gain due to corticosteroids and anticonvulsants Weight loss due to poor memory and lack of motivation Weight loss due to side effects of oncological treatments
Insomnia	Due to corticosteroids
Psychomotor slowing	Due to anticonvulsants Due to tumour
Decreased motivation	Due to tumour effects Due to fatigue following treatment Due to fatigue with anticonvulsants

commonly recommended along with psychotherapy, family training and counselling (Pangilinan et al. 2007).

Anxiety has been reported by Kilbride et al. (2007), especially in patients who are waiting for radiotherapy following surgery and their diagnosis. The provision of information in an attempt to reduce levels of anxiety is recommended (Kilbride et al. 2007). Information can empower patients and help them gain control, which may be of psychological benefit. However, providing information and communicating with patients with brain tumours can be difficult due to cognitive impairment, dysphasia and loss of insight into their condition (Guerrero 2005).

Reactions to receiving news of a serious diagnosis are unpredictable and complex and can include anger, fear, loneliness and guilt (Lakasing 2007; McNamara 2008). Khalili (2007) describes how patients with primary malignant brain tumours suffer feelings of hopelessness. This diagnosis includes many losses that have already been described; nevertheless, some patients manage to conquer their fears and accept the diagnosis and poor prognosis (O'Kelly and O'Kelly 2006).

Other aspects affecting quality of life include loss of role and social interaction (Khalili 2007). In part hindering the return to work and social interaction is the driving restriction imposed on patients following their diagnosis. The length of time off driving is dependent on several factors: grade of the tumour and its position, whether the patient has seizures, and whether surgery has been performed. Patients diagnosed with a brain tumour are advised to notify the DVLA by writing to the Medical Adviser, Driver and Vehicle Licensing Agency, Swansea, SA99 1DL (further information can be found at www.dvla.org.uk).

Body image

In the introduction to this chapter it was acknowledged that brain tumours could affect patients physically, cognitively, psychologically and socially. This implies wide and varied reactions to such a diagnosis. Individuals will of course be affected differently according to the site and nature of the tumour and how they individually respond to such suffering and anguish. Physical, cognitive, psychological or social changes, affecting one's appearance, behaviour or functioning, inevitably have an impact on one's body image. Grogan (1999) recognised that body image embraces perceptions, thoughts and feelings about one's body. Thus changes to the image one has of oneself, for example, as an active, competent, healthy individual, can be threatened from the point of any cancer diagnosis, since cancer and its treatments can cause significant alteration to the way one views, thinks and feels about oneself as an individual.

This is particularly relevant to patients with malignant brain tumours because they can experience many body changes such as hemiparesis, dysphasia, mobility problems and/or alopecia following surgery, as well as weight gain due to corticosteroid therapy and anticonvulsants. While some bodily changes may be temporary, others will be permanent and will necessitate ongoing adjustment physically and emotionally (Guerrero 2002; White 2002). Alopecia, for example, is a significant concern for many patients with cancer (Batchelor 2006); for patients receiving radiotherapy to the brain this alopecia may be permanent.

Individuals experiencing altered body image have not only to cope with and adjust to the change, but they will also experience a sense of loss or grief. Furthermore, the emotional impact of sometimes sudden changes to one's sense of self can have significant psychological and social consequences. Embarrassment, lowered self-confidence and lowered self-esteem can adversely affect social interactions and may lead to social withdrawal (Newell 1999; Guerrero 2002).

Nurses have an important role in assessing the impact of changes to body image and how individuals adjust to them. Individuals will use their own coping strategies. Problem-focused and emotion-focused strategies have their place (Lazarus & Folkman 1984). Also, some patients are driven to seek out information and think through their situation, while others prefer to adopt avoidant strategies as a means of coping. Social support has a significant contribution to a person's adaptation to their disease, treatment and the concomitant changes to their body image (Price 1990). Health professionals, as well as the patient's family and friends, have an important role in supporting the patient by accepting their bodily changes and adopting a positive, hopeful attitude.

Palliative care

NCCC and NICE (2006) recommend that all patients with primary malignant brain tumours have access to specialist palliative care services (see Chapter 12). Palliative care is described by the World Health Organization (2002) as:

> A support system which addresses the individual needs to enable patients to cope with disease impairments and live actively until death.

> www.who.int

It is expected that, as patients enter the final stage of the disease, it will result in yet further neurological and cognitive deficits, personality changes, epilepsy, side effects of medication, and/or fatigue, and anxiety and depression. In the palliative phase, patients with primary malignant brain tumours frequently experience the symptoms of raised intracranial pressure, which is usually managed with corticosteroids (McNamara & Kilbride, 1999; Taillibert & Delattre 2005). However, the use of corticosteroids is based on clinical experience, as there is a lack of clinical trials on their effect and use (Junck 2004).

The management of seizures may present a problem. Lakasing (2007) recommends the use of rectal and subcutaneous administration of medications for patients who experience seizures and are unable to swallow during the last stage of their disease. Relatives often become distressed and worried when patients are unable to swallow. It is therefore important that time is taken to explain to them that the patient is not in any discomfort. Thirst is not a problem at the end of a patient's life because sodium and fluid are lost proportionately (Bavin 2007). It has been suggested that artificial rehydration may cause increased peritumoral, cerebral and peripheral oedema

(Bavin 2007). The benefits of artificial rehydration are anecdotal; detrimental effects may include increased gastric and pulmonary secretions leading to nausea, vomiting and congestion. However, some are of the opinion that hydration can increase alertness and wellbeing, thereby giving a psychological lift and hope for the patient and relatives (Bavin 2007).

A multidisciplinary approach

It is recommended by the NCCC and NICE (2006) that a specialist multidisciplinary team manages patients with malignant brain tumours. This should ensure that patients are diagnosed correctly and receive the most appropriate care and interventions. Patients will therefore come into contact with many healthcare professionals depending on their specific needs. In considering this factor, combined with their poor prognosis, it is crucial that their care is streamlined and that the patient and their carers understand the individual roles of other healthcare professionals and who should be their first point of contact (Park 2007).

The future

The progress in the treatment of primary malignant brain tumours in the last 10 years has been encouraging, with improved outcome in terms of survival and quality of life, alongside the introduction of temozolomide and carmustine implants (Dunn & Black 2003; Stupp et al. 2005). It has been known for some time that molecular testing of the tumour samples in the pathology laboratory may help identify patients most likely to respond to individual treatment (NCCC & NICE 2006; Stupp et al. 2006). For example, when examining $O6$-methylguanine-DNA methyltransferase (MGMT) in the tumour sample, Hegi et al. (2005) identified that when the MGMT promoter is methylated the prognosis of this patient is likely to be better than if the gene is unmethylated. Other molecular markers, for example, the loss of chromosome 10, mutation or loss of the *TP53* gene and epidermal growth factor receptor, are also thought to have an influence on response to treatment (Wen & Kesari 2008). It has been known for some time that in patients with oligodendroglioma a loss of heterozygosity in a tumour suppressor gene on chromosomal arms 1p and 19q indicates a better response to treatment (Rampling et al. 2004).

As already discussed, the use of carmustine implants and their combined use with temozolomide (Spiegel et al. 2007; Krzeminski et al. 2008; LaRocca and Mehdorn, 2009) may be a more common occurrence in the future.

Nevertheless, this diagnosis remains complex and devastating for the patient and their families. It is an aspiration of the author that the overall management of patients with primary malignant brain tumours will continue to improve and all aspects of their ongoing care should concentrate on maintaining quality of life.

References

Armstrong TS (2004) Introduction to brain tumour series. *Seminars in Oncology Nursing* **20**(4): 221–3.

Batchelor D (2006) Alopecia. In: Kearney NE, Richardson A (eds) *Nursing Patients with Cancer: Principles and Practice*. Edinburgh: Elsevier/Churchill Livingstone.

Bavin L (2007) Artificial rehydration in the last days of life: is it beneficial? *International Journal of Palliative Nursing* **13**(9): 445–9.

Benjamin R, Capparella J, Brown A (2003) Classificatio, of glioblastoma multiforme in adults by molecular genetics. *Cancer Journal* **9**(2): 82–90.

Berger MS, Keles E (1995) Epilepsy associated with brain tumours. In: Kaye AH, Laws ER (eds) *Brain Tumours*. Hong Kong: Churchill Livingstone.

Biswas T, Okunieff P, Schell MC, et al. (2009) Stereotactic radiosurgery for glioblastoma: retrospective analysis. *Radiation Oncology* **4**: 11.

Brada M, Guerrero D (1997) One model of follow-up care. In: Davies E, Hopkins A (eds) *Improving Care for Patients with Malignant Cerebral Glioma*. London: RCP Publications.

Brada M, Thomas DGT (1995) Tumours of the brain and spinal cord in adults. In: Peckham M, Pinedo HM, Verones U (eds) *Oxford Textbook of Oncology 2*, Sections 8–20 and Index. Oxford: Oxford Medical Publications.

Brandes AA (2003) State-of-the-art treatment of high-grade brain tumors. *Seminars in Oncology* **30** (suppl 19): 4–9.

Brandsma D, Stalpers L, Taal W, Sminia P, Van den Bent MJ (2008) Clinical features, mechanisms, and management of pseudoprogression in malignant gliomas. *Lancet Oncology* **9**(5): 453–61.

Brem H, Piantadosi S, Burger PC, et al. (1995) Placebo-controlled trial of safety and efficacy of intraoperative controlled delivery by biodegradable polymers of chemotherapy for recurrent gliomas. *Lancet* **345**: 1008–12.

British Medical Association (BMA) (2008) *British National Formulary*. BMJ Group & RPS Publishing, pp. 380–2.

Campbell J (2006) Brain tumour related epilepsy: The experience of a nurse-led seizure clinic in Scotland. *British Journal of Neuroscience Nursing* **1**(5): 218–24.

Cancer Research UK (2009a) UK Brain and Central Nervous System Cancer incidence statistics. http://info.cancerresearchuk.org/cancerstats/types/brain/incidence/ (accessed 8 September 2009).

Cancer Research UK (2009b) Cancer Help UK. *Cancer treatments: Radiotherapy* http://www.cancerhelp.org.uk/help/default.asp?page=16651 (accessed 8 September 2009).

Catt S, Chalmers A, Fallowfield L (2008) Psychosocial and supportive-care needs in high-grade glioma. *Lancet Oncology* **9**(9): 884–91.

Cha S (2006) Update on brain tumour imaging: from anatomy to physiology. *AJNR American Journal of Neuroradiology* **27**: 475–87.

Chan TA, Weingart JD, Parisi M, et al. (2005) Treatment of recurrent glioblastoma with GliaSite brachytherapy. *International Journal of Radiation, Oncology, Biology and Physics* **62**(4): 1133–9.

Coward M, Coley HM (2006) Chemotherapy. In: Kearney N, Richardson A (eds) *Nursing Patients with Cancer: Principles and Practice*. Edinburgh: Elsevier/Churchill Livingstone.

Driver and Vehicle Licensing Agency (DVLA) (2009) http://www.dvla.gov.uk/medical.aspx.

Dunn IF, Black PM (2003) The neurosurgeon as local oncologist: cellular and molecular neurosurgery in malignant glioma therapy. *Neurosurgery* **52**: 1411–24.

Fabrini MG, Perrone F, De Franco L, Pasqualetti F, Grespi S, Vannozzi R, Cionini L (2009) Perioperative high-dose-rate brachytherapy in the treatment of recurrent malignant gliomas. *Strahlentherapie und Onkologie* **185**(8): 524–9.

Faithfull S (2006) Radiotherapy. In: Kearney N, Richardson A (eds) *Nursing Patients with Cancer: Principles and Practice.* Edinburgh: Elsevier/Churchill Livingstone.

Faithfull S, Brada M (1998) Somnolence syndrome in adults following cranial irradiation for primary brain tumours. *Clinical Oncology* **10**(4): 250–4.

Giles GG, Gonzales MF (2001) Epidemiology of brain tumours and factors in prognosis. In: Kaye AH, Law ER (eds) *Brain Tumours: An Encyclopedic Approach*, 2nd edn. Edinburgh: Churchill Livingstone.

Glantz MJ, Cole BF, Forsyth PA, et al. (2000) Practice parameter: anticonvulsant prophylaxis in patients with newly diagnosed brain tumours: Report of the Quality Standards Subcommittee of the American Academy of Neurology. *Neurology* **54**: 1886–93.

Grant R (2004) Overview: Brain tumour diagnosis and management. Royal College of Physicians Guidelines. *Journal of Neurology Neurosurgery and Psychiatry* **75**: ii18–23.

Grogan S (1999) *Body Image*. London: Routledge.

Guerrero D (1998) Caring for patients with central nervous system metastases. *Nursing Times* **99** (08): 30–4.

Guerrero D (2002) Neuro-oncology: a clinical nurse specialist perspective. *International Journal of Palliative Nursing* **8**(1): 28–9.

Guerrero D (2005) Understanding the side effects of cranial irradiation and informing patients and carers. *British Journal of Neuroscience Nursing* **1**(3): 118–21.

Hegi ME, Diserens AC, Gorlia T, et al. (2005) MGMT gene silencing and benefit from temozolomide in glioblastoma. *New England Journal of Medicine* **352**(10): 997–1003.

Henderson JW (2006) Treatment of glioblastoma multiforme: a new standard. *Archives of Neurology* **63**: 337–41.

Hentschel SJ, Sawaya R (2003) Optimizing outcomes with maximal surgical resection of malignant gliomas. *Cancer Control: Journal of the Moffitt Cancer Center* **10**(2) (http://www.medscape.com/viewarticle/452004).

Hickey JV, Armstrong T (1997) Brain tumours. In: *The Clinical Practice of Neurological and Neurosurgical Nursing*, 4th edn. Philadelphia: Lippincott Williams & Wilkins.

Junck L (2004) Supportive management in neuron-oncology: opportunities for patient care, teaching and research. *Current Opinion in Neurology* **17**: 649–53.

Karim ABMF (1995) Radiotherapy and radiosurgery for brain tumours. In: Kaye AH, Laws ER (eds) *Neuro-oncology*. Amsterdam: Elsevier.

Karnofsky DA, Ableman WH, Craver LF, Burchenal JH (1948) The use of nitrogen mustards in the palliative treatment of carcinoma. *Cancer* **56**: 634–56.

Khalili Y (2007) Ongoing transitions: The impact of a malignant brain tumour on patient and family. *Axone* **28**(3): 5–13.

Khasraw M, Bell D, Wheeler H (2009) Long-term use of temozolomide: could you use temozolomide safely for life in gliomas? *Journal of Clinical Neuroscience* **16**(6): 854–5.

Khurana VG, Teo C, Kundi M, Hardell L, Carlsberg M (2009) Cell phones and brain tumours: a review including the long-term epidemiologic data. *Surgical Neurology* **72** (3): 205–14.

Kilbride L, Smith G, Grant R (2007) The frequency and cause of anxiety and depression amongst patients with malignant brain tumours between surgery and radiotherapy. *Journal of Neuro-oncology* **84**: 297–304.

Krex D, Klink B, Hartmann C, et al. (2007) Long-term survival with glioblastoma multiforme. *Brain* **130**: 2596–606.

Krzeminski JP, Piquer J, Riesgo P (2008) Repeated implantation of interstitial chemotherapy to treat malignant gliomas. *Neurosurgery Quarterly* **18**(4): 286–9.

Lakasing E (2007) Palliative care in primary care. *Geriatric Medicine* **37**(11): 20–5.

LaRocca RV, Mehdorn HM (2009) Localised BCNU chemotherapy and the multimodal management of malignant glioma. *Current Medical Research and Opinion* **25**(1): 149–60.

Lazarus RS, Folkman S (1984) *Stress: Appraisal and Coping.* New York: Springer.

Levin VA, Leibel SA, Gutin PH (2001) Neoplasms of the central nervous system. In: DeVita VT Jr, Hellman S, Rosenberg SA (eds) *Cancer: Principles and Practice of Oncology*, 6th edn. Philadelphia: Lippincott Williams & Wilkins, pp. 2100–60.

Litofsky NS, Farace E, Anderson F Jr, Meyers CA, Huang W, Laws ER Jr (2004) Depression in patients with high grade glioma: results of the Glioma Outcomes Project. *Neurosurgery* **54**: 358–66.

Louis DN, Ohgaki H, Wiestler OD, Cavenee WK (eds) (2007) *WHO Classification of Ttumours of the Central Nervous System.* Lyon: WHO Press.

Mainio A, Hakko H, Niemela A, Koivukangas J, Rasanen P (2005) Depression and functional outcome in patients with brain tumours: a population based 1-year follow-up study. *Journal of Neurosurgery* **103**: 841–7.

McNamara S (2008) An overview of palliative care for patients with brain tumours: an interprofessional approach. *British Journal of Neuroscience Nurses* **4**(9): 435–7.

McNamara S, Kilbride L (1999) Treating primary brain tumours with dexamethasone. *Nursing Times* **95**(47): 54–7.

National Collaborating Centre for Cancer (NCCC) and the National Institute for Health and Clinical Excellence (NICE) (2006) *Service guidance for improving outcomes in brain and other CNS cancers – the manual.* London: NCCC & NICE.

National Institute for Health and Clinical Excellence (NICE) (2007) Carmustine implants and temozolomide for the treatment of newly diagnosed high-grade glioma. www.nice.org.uk/TA121

Naylor WA (2006) Skin and wound care. In: Kearney N, Richardson A (eds) *Nursing Patients with Cancer: Principles and Practice.* Edinburgh: Elsevier/Churchill Livingstone.

Newell RJ (1999) Altered body image: a fear-avoidance model of psycho-social difficulties following disfigurement. *Journal of Advanced Nursing* **30**: 1230–8.

O'Kelly E, O'Kelly C (2006) *Chasing Daylight: how my forthcoming death transformed my life.* New York: McGraw-Hill.

Pangilinan PH, Kelly BM, Pangilinan JM (2007) Depression in the patient with brain cancer. *Community Oncology* **4**(9): 533–7.

Park L (2007) The multidisciplinary approach to care. *Mims Advances.* Medical Imprint. Haymarket. 6–8.

Pelletier G, Verhoef MJ, Khatri N, Hagen N (2002) Quality of life in brain tumour patients: the relative contributions of depression, fatigue, emotional distress and existential issues. *Journal of Neurooncology* **57**: 41–9.

Price B (1990) A model for body image care. *Journal of Advanced Nursing* **15**: 585–93.

Rampling R, James A, Papanastassiou V (2004) The present and future management of malignant brain tumours: surgery, radiotherapy, chemotherapy. *Journal of Neurology, Neurosurgery and Psychiatry* **75**: 24–30.

Salcman M (2001) Glioblastoma multiforme and anaplastic astrocytoma. In: Kaye AH, Laws E.R. Jr. (2001) *Brain Tumours*, 2nd edn. Edinburgh: Churchill Livingstone.

Salvati M, D'Elia A, Melone GA, et al. (2008) Radio-induced gliomas: 20 years experience and critical review of on pathology. *Journal of Neurooncology* **89**(2): 169–77.

Sathornsumetee S, Rich JN (2008) Designer therapies for glioblastoma multiforme. *Annals of the New York Academy of Sciences* **1142**: 108–32.

Schmidt F, Fischer J, Herrlinger U, Dietz K, Dichgans J, Weller M (2006) PCV chemotherapy for recurrent glioblastoma. *Neurology* **66**(4): 587–9.

Schwartzbaum JA, Fisher JL, Aldape KD, Wrensch M (2006) Epidemiology and molecular pathways of glioma. *National Clinical Practice Neurology* **2**(9): 494–503.

Shenouda G, Souhami L, Podgorsak EB, et al. (1997) Radiosurgery and accelerated radiotherapy for patients with glioblastoma. *Canadian Journal of Neurological Sciences* **24**(2): 110–15.

Sherwood PR, Given BA, Doorenbos AZ, Given CW (2004) Forgotten voices: lessons from bereaved caregivers of persons with a brain tumour. *International Journal of Palliative Nursing* **10**(2): 67–75.

Spiegel BM, Esrailian E, Laine L, Chamberlain MC (2007) Clinical impact of adjuvant chemotherapy in glioblastoma multiforme: a meta-analysis. *CNS Drugs* **21**(9): 775–87.

Stone P, Richardson A, A'Herm R, Hardy J (2001) Fatigue in patients with cancer of the breast or prostate undergoing radical radiotherapy. *Journal of Pain & Symptom Management* **22**(6): 1007–15.

Stupp R, Mason WP, van den Bent MJ, et al.; European Organisation for Research and Treatment of Cancer Brain Tumor and Radiotherapy Groups; National Cancer Institute of Canada Clinical Trials Group (2005) Radiotherapy plus concomitant and adjuvant temozolomide for glioblastoma. *New England Journal of Medicine* **352**: 987–96.

Stupp R, Hegi ME, van den Bent MJ, et al., on behalf of the European Organisation for Research and Treatment of Cancer Brain Tumor and Radiotherapy Groups and the National Cancer Institute of Canada Clinical Trials Group (2006) Changing Paradigms: An update on the multidisciplinary management of malignant glioma. *Oncologist* **11**(2): 165–80.

Taillibert S, Delattre JY (2005) Palliative care in patients with brain metastases. *Current Opinion in Oncology* **17**(6): 558–92.

Taillibert S, Laigle-Donadey F, Sanson M (2004) Palliative care in patients with primary brain tumours. *Current Opinion in Oncology* **16**: 587–92.

Taal W, Brandsma D, de Bruin HG, et al. (2008) Incidence of early pseudo-progression in a cohort of malignant glioma patients treated with chemoirradiation with temozolomide. *Cancer* **113**(2): 405–10.

Tsao MN, Metha MP, Whelan TJ, et al. (2005) The American Society for Therapeutic Radiology and Oncology (ASTRO) Evidence-based review of the role of radiosurgery for malignant glioma. *International Journal Radiation Oncology Biology Physics* **63**: 147–55.

Uddin ABM, Jarmi T (2008) Glioblastoma Multiforme. Available at: http://emedicine.medscape.com/article/1156220-overview (accessed 18 May 2009)

Wegman JA (1993) Central nervous system cancers. In: Groenwald SL, Frogge MF, Goodman M, Yarbro CH (eds) *Cancer Nursing: Principles and Practice*. Boston, MA: Jones & Bartlett.

Wells M, Macmillan M, MacBride S, et al. (2004) Does aqueous or suralfate cream affect the severity of erythematous radiation skin reactions? *Radiation and Oncology* **73**(2): 153–62.

Wen PY, Kesari MD (2008) Malignant gliomas in adults. *New England Journal of Medicine* **359**: 492–507.

Westphal M, Hilt DC, Bortey E, et al. (2003) A phase 3 trial of local chemotherapy with biodegradable carmustine (BCNU) wafers (Gliadel wafers) in patients with primary malignant glioma. *Neuro-oncology* **5**: 79–88.

White CA (2002) Body images in oncology. In: Cash TF, Pruzinsky T (eds) *Body Image: A Handbook of Theory, Research and Clinical Practice*. New York: Guilford Press.

Whittle IR, Basu N, Grant R, Walker M, Gregor A (2002) Management of patients aged > 60 years with malignant glioma: good clinical status and radiotherapy determine outcome. *British Journal of Neurosurgery* **16**(4): 343–7.

Wick A, Pascher C, Wick W, et al. (2009) Rechallenge with temozolomide in patients with recurrent gliomas. *Journal of Neurology* **256**(5): 734–41.

World Health Organization (1979) *WHO handbook for representing results of cancer treatments.* Geneva: WHO.

World Health Organization (2002) WHO definition of palliative care. www.who.int/cancer/palliaitve/definition/en.

Yung WKA, Albright RE, Olson J, et al. (2000) A phase II study of temozolomide vs. procarbazine in patients with glioblastoma multiforme at first relapse. *British Journal of Cancer* **83**(5): 588–93.

Chapter 6

Cancer and the surgeon

Ashley Brown

When an individual is diagnosed with cancer they and their family are anxious and fearful – fearing the worst yet hoping for the best outcome. One of the many initial thoughts is 'can I get rid of this?' or 'is it possible for me to be cured of this cancer?' When possible, surgery to completely remove a tumour generally results in the best outcome, although some cancers may respond better to other forms of treatment. Usually the best results are when surgery is combined with other forms of treatment. To date the surgeon has been pre-eminent in cancer treatment, with the aim of removing the cancerous tissue. However, the role of the surgeon is changing with the advent of new regimes in chemotherapy and in radiotherapy. Until recently, the inclusion of these two treatment modalities into most of the common cancers had been peripheral, but with the advent of new anticancer agents, this is no longer the case. Surgery itself, though, has many exciting new developments to consider in its role in optimal cancer treatments, including minimally invasive techniques, micro and non-invasive and even robotic methods. This chapter will provide a flavour of the cancer surgeon's perspective of their work in this area, and will focus on the events and experiences that may be encountered by a patient from their initial diagnosis, and the possible surgical treatment.

Becoming a cancer surgeon

For those doctors who choose to follow a career pathway as a cancer surgeon, their work can be emotionally and technically challenging but also immensely satisfying. Towards the end of training to become a surgeon, they can elect to become a specialist in cancer surgery. He or she will need to spend time in a specialised cancer unit, and this final period of training may take several years before the trainee becomes a consultant. Whether the surgeon likes it or not, he or she will have to share some of the emotional burden of the disease with patients and relatives. Patients will often attribute success or failure of cancer treatment to the skill (or otherwise) of the surgical team, not perhaps fully appreciating that clinical staging is a far better discriminator as to future disease behaviour. For all that, the best reward is to see a patient who is disease-free at five or ten years after treatment.

Perspectives on Cancer Care.   Edited by Josephine (Tonks) N. Fawcett and Anne McQueen
© 2011 Blackwell Publishing Ltd

Surgery as a treatment regime for cancer

Until the recent past, surgery was the only option for the treatment of most cancers. In the last few decades, however, two other modalities have been increasingly used: radiotherapy and chemotherapy. Within 'chemotherapy' it may be best to include treatment with monoclonal antibodies. Non-surgical treatments have an immediate appeal to patients. There is no cutting, no inpatient recovery and none of the risks associated with surgery. However, neither of these other modalities is risk-free, and patients have other real fears of such treatments. Chemotherapy can be particularly toxic to all systems of the body and, instead of the 'short sharp knock' from surgery, chemotherapy treatment and its side effects can be drawn out over many months. Its complications, such as neuropathy associated with the taxane class of chemotherapeutic agents, can persist for a lifetime (Hagiwara & Sunada 2004). Most chemotherapeutic agents are both cardiotoxic and nephrotoxic, and since the largest proportion of the 'cancer population' is elderly, often already experiencing cardiac problems, then clearly many patients may not be suitable for at least some forms of chemotherapy. Radiotherapy also has its share of long-term complications, for example, the haemorrhagic proctitis that can occur after radiotherapy for prostate cancer (Donner 1998). It has been stated, by some who have a self-awarded crystal ball with which to look into the future, that the role of the surgeon in times to come in cancer treatment will be merely that of a diagnostic technician, and even that may be at the tip of a biopsy needle! (Sikora 2008). This may be so, but possibly is not yet just round the temporal corner.

Principles of cancer surgery

The foremost principle of cancer surgery is quite simple. The tumour should be completely removed in a way in which the possibility of local or distant recurrence is put to the minimum. This can at times be a daunting task for the surgeon and, depending on the stage of cancer development, may not be a realistic option for the patient. The possible surgical options in relation to cancer can be viewed in three distinct situations: when surgery is potentially curative, surgery for disease recurrence and palliative surgery.

The surgeon and potentially curative surgery

All the staff in a cancer service hope to receive patients who have a chance of cure, i.e. their disease process has not reached an advanced and incurable stage. Although removal of a tumour may seem straightforward, this may be a daunting and challenging proposition for patient and surgeon. In some types of cancer, radical removal is less of a challenge but in others, such as a cancer of the oesophagus, the operation is of great magnitude.

One of the many advantages of modern scanning, whether it is ultrasound, computed tomography (CT), magnetic resonance imaging (MRI) or positron emission tomography (PET), is that the imaging process will detect secondary disease in a way which, 20 years ago, would have been quite impossible. This is immensely valuable in that it shows the extent of the disease and enables assessment of the most appropriate surgical procedure.

Clearly radical surgery is not indicated if, on modern imaging techniques, the evidence is that there is no chance of a cure.

While radical or curative surgery may be thought of as routine for the surgeon, any surgery is traumatic for the patient, both physically and emotionally. On the patient's side the operating day may well be a terrifying ordeal, despite all the advances in surgery, anaesthesia and pain relief. Many questions will occur to the patient, and worries will surface as the operating time draws near, such as will they survive the operation? Operative deaths are now extremely rare. However, in some types of surgery, for example, for oesophago-gastric cancer, there is a very real mortality from associated complications. In the United Kingdom (UK), for oesophageal tumours, the national 30-day mortality approaches 10–15% (Crofts 2000). However, the issue of operative morbidity is very real. Will the patient feel mutilated by the cancer surgery? That may well be so in the case of a permanent stoma. Will bodily functions be reasonably normal? A permanent ileostomy, urostomy or colostomy will ensure that there is no return to 'normality'. The critical question is always the hope for, and chance of, a cure. An idea of probability might help, but statistics are never that reassuring to the individual patient. What about work? A well-known female politician once said that the hallmark of good treatment is the return to work and starting to pay income tax once more. Cynical maybe, but work forms an important part of most people's lives and is not just related to money. It is well known that a person withdrawn from work, for whatever reason, is more prone to mental and physical disorders (Williams 2008), and reassurance about a return to work is important. If employment is out of the question, an unusual state of affairs, then it should be possible to outline positive aspects of the outcome, especially in regard to family relationships and pursuit of other, perhaps new, interests.

The surgeon and cancer recurrence

In this situation, the patient will look to the medical staff to see if the situation can be retrieved and the patient set on the road to cure again. Often, sadly, this is not the case and the old phrase that 'you have only one bite of the cherry' is applicable to surgical endeavours in the treatment of cancer. Re-looks and re-attempts are fraught with difficulty for the surgeon and danger for the patient. However, despite this, in many instances, repeat operation does hold some chance of success. In managing all patients with recurrent disease, the surgeon must temper enthusiasm for 'doing something' in the knowledge that it is easy to make a patient worse by intemperate and badly thought-out 're-look' surgery. The multidisciplinary team is an invaluable resource for discussing these problems and pursing the best possible solutions.

The surgeon and palliation

The patient and relatives in this situation will hope against hope that the surgeon has some 'fix' for the problem. An example would be small bowel obstruction seen in carcinomatosis peritonei, which is often seen in advanced cancer of the ovary or pancreas. Radiography will show gross bowel obstruction, so why should the surgeon be reluctant to reoperate? From the wealth of the cancer surgeon's knowledge and experience, it is unlikely there will be just a simple kink or band causing the obstruction. Instead there may be a myriad of obstructing nodules of cancer which in practical terms are neither excisable nor indeed 'by-passable'. If surgery is attempted the patient may well be made worse and may also have to endure the potential burden of a fistula or even peritonitis. The surgical teaching here is quite simple: proceed with great caution. Injudicious surgery in this case may well hasten the patient's disease process. Having aired this necessary caution, there will be some patients whose life can be improved by further surgery and the proposition will be discussed, as indicated, at the appropriate multidisciplinary meeting, where the best decision for each individual patient will be made.

The surgeon and the patient newly diagnosed with cancer

When a patient is first diagnosed with cancer they are apprehensive and frightened; their family may be even more so. The fear experienced is, to a large extent, fear of the unknown and the uncertain. Clearly the eventual outcome cannot be given to the patient as nobody will know that, but it is always possible and important to keep the patient informed about the procedures and possibilities along the way. An outline of the disease process and the possible lines of treatment can easily be given, and during this process the patient will get to know those people responsible for their treatment and care. Patients can accept the most awful news and accommodate to it, given time. Patients like a familiar face when they are in surroundings which are strange and sometimes, because of its association with such a diagnosis, perceived as hostile. This initial period represents a golden opportunity for the doctors and the nurses to gain the patient's trust and confidence before any treatment starts.

Referral of the patient

When a patient with cancer is initially referred to the surgeon this can carry with it a sense of optimism, suggesting that surgical removal of the tumour will take away the disease. It is not always as simple as this; but generally, when surgery is the initial treatment of choice, the prognosis for a patient is likely to be more favourable. If a patient's diagnosis is deemed to be without hope of cure, or when only palliation can be offered, then the surgeon may not be the appropriate referral. However, even in such circumstances palliative surgery can relieve distressing symptoms and offer a significant improvement to the patient's psychological wellbeing and quality of life. The fact that the patient is being 'sent to the surgeon' implies that there is at least a ray of sunshine in this rather bleak, forbidding and terse diagnosis.

The patient may find themselves in front of the surgeon by different paths including, first, from the general practitioner (GP). However, the days may well be gone when a GP could select the surgeon of their choice to investigate the patient and continue the treatment. It is now driven by the National Health Service computer system which rather works on the principle that the more quickly the referral is made the better the potential outcome for the patient (NHS 2004). Without a doubt this must be of benefit in early-stage cancer, but it has to be remembered that, for many tumours, symptoms may only occur after a cancerous tumour has been in existence for many months or years when, arguably, speed may not be the critical factor. It is also a sad reality that, for some cancer sufferers, their symptoms just do not appear on the 'cancer symptom radar'.

Referral may also come from within the hospital itself, when either an inpatient, admitted for other reasons to another medical or surgical department, may be found to have symptoms or signs of a cancer or the patient may have presented at the emergency department with symptoms suggestive of cancer more appropriate to another hospital directorate. In both circumstances the patient will be referred to the oncologists and surgeons by the intra-hospital mechanisms.

For many individuals, however, the referral will come from a cancer screening service. The NHS runs several cancer screening services for the 'well population'. Examples include breast, colorectal, gynaecological and prostate cancer screening. These often involve blood tests, endoscopy or radiology. Although rather resource consuming, a positive result places the patient on to a 'fast track' into well-laid-out pathways of investigation and treatment.

In the not too distant future, cancer screening is likely to be carried out with a simple blood test for genetic markers, to identify at least some of the more common cancers (Lonwagie et al. 2009). This will have tremendous repercussions on modes of referral. The test will probably be performed on 'well' patients, outside the hospital setting. Such tests will be relatively inexpensive and will, if positive, be followed by further survey and scrutiny in a diagnostic unit (Bosch et al. 2009). It is possible therefore that such screening will identify patients at an early stage of cancer progression, with obvious advantages to the patient population. This notion of an all-embracing cancer screening test has a superficial appeal but is fraught with practical drawbacks. What about the pre-malignant bowel polyp? What about pre-malignant breast changes? A negative test may well breed a false sense of security.

The multidisciplinary team

Caring for a patient with cancer is complex and requires input from a variety of specialists, working together towards the same aim or outcome for the patient. In this respect, interdisciplinary communication and decision making is of key importance. Each site-specific cancer has its own multidisciplinary team (e.g. breast, upper gastrointestinal (GI), lower GI, urology, chest, etc.). These teams have a constitution which varies between hospitals and also according to the site of the cancer. A typical multidisciplinary team might be constituted as follows:

- Chair – usually a clinician but could be a clinical nurse specialist
- Pathologist
- Surgeon
- Physician
- Endoscopist
- Imaging consultant
- Oncologist
- Radiotherapist

- Palliative care physician
- Clinical nurse specialist
- Stoma care nurse – as necessary
- A member of the nutrition team
- Clinical trials' nurse
- A representative of an outside organization such as Macmillan Cancer Support
- Ward/operating theatre staff
- Administrative coordinator.

The multidisciplinary team for any one site-specific cancer is likely to meet weekly to discuss the care decisions and management of patients at various stages of the treatment process (i.e. pre-admission, pre-treatment, post-treatment) or at any point where a problem in management and clinical decision making has arisen. Individual members of the multidisciplinary team may voice their opinions, no more than that, but these opinions form the basis of the eventual decision that is vital for the patient through their cancer journey.

Preparing for cancer surgery

The times are gone when a diagnosis of cancer was just followed shortly afterwards by the operating theatre. Nowadays a cancer is graded and staged to show its size, disposition and any evidence of local or distant spread. Once the grading and, particularly, staging classification is complete, then a treatment plan is formulated. The Tumour, Node, Metastases (TNM) staging classification of tumours respectively refers to the size and invasion of the tumour (T), the lymph node status (N) and the presence of metastases (M). To illustrate the significance of TNM staging and assuming the patient is of average fitness, below are four results for patients who have been 'staged' for rectal cancer.

T1, N0, M0   This patient will need an endoscopic procedure via the anus which will not involve opening the abdomen.

T2, N0, M0   This patient will need an anterior resection.

T3, N1, M0   This patient will need a long course of preoperative chemo-radiotherapy followed by an anterior resection of the bowel.

T3, N1, M1   This patient will need no primary attempt at curative surgery and will need further investigation to see if the metastasis is removable. Further discussion within the MDT is necessary.

From this simplified set of treatments according to the TNM classification, it should be evident that staging has a very real effect upon the treatment plan produced for each individual patient. The most valuable discriminator in terms of outcome in cancer surgery is, indeed, the staging. Clearly a T1, N0, M0 tumour should do better than a T3, N1, M1 tumour. However, many other factors merit consideration. Co-morbidity is very important and is usually summarised in the commonly used American Society of Anesthesiologists (ASA) grade to assess the patient's fitness for anaesthesia and surgery prior to an operation; this is normally carried out by the anaesthetist (Sackland 1941). A patient with diabetes mellitus whose medical history includes both myocardial infarction and a cerebrovascular accident (ASA grade III) is surely going to fare differently from the non-diabetic and complication-free individual (ASA grade I). As discussed, some elderly patients may have to be excluded from chemotherapy, because of the cardiotoxic and nephrotoxic effects of some chemotherapeutic agents. It is most unusual, however, for a patient to be excluded from a surgical operation. This rather implies that, in these circumstances, surgery may be the default in terms of therapy for cancer. It is hardly surprising, therefore, that most visceral operations for cancer have a well-defined 30-day mortality. In-hospital mortality, as audited, is defined as death within 30 days following intervention; however, Visser et al. (2009) suggest that this does not represent true risk and that perhaps a 90-day mortality would provide a better estimation of risk when counselling patients.

Recovering from cancer surgery

Recovery from major cancer surgery, in particular, varies according to many factors, especially the ASA grading. Most importantly, the operation should have 'gone well'. A technically 'difficult' operation that might substantially overrun the usual time span allotted for the procedure casts a potential cloud over the likelihood of a smooth recovery. The surgical team will know if an operation has proved difficult and will be extra vigilant for postoperative problems. In addition, modern facilities in the form of the high dependency unit (HDU) and intensive therapy unit (ITU) are vital in the part they play in optimal recovery. Without these two vital components of 'critical care', many surgeons would be very reluctant to embark upon surgical treatment for a major visceral cancer. As indicated, surgery is not without risks, not only during surgery and anaesthesia but in the postoperative period; especially the immediate postoperative period.

Complications can sometimes present themselves at the most inauspicious moment: in the early hours of the morning or at the weekend when the patient's specialist staff are not on hand and when fewer staff are available. Surgical complications are often not foreseen and are often not associated with poor surgery or poor decision making (Atkins et al. 2004). Even in the best of circumstances, the anastomosis that leaks, the wound which dehisces or becomes infected, the sudden pulmonary embolism are all complications that are familiar to surgeons and surgical nursing staff. That is not to say that any one should be accepting of, or tolerant towards, any complication. In a foreseeable complication such as pulmonary embolism, active prophylaxis should be evident. Once the complication has occurred, then it will need to be confirmed and treated in the most efficient and expeditious way.

Careful audit will reveal the surgeon more prone to complications and who might require further training, but even this statement needs a qualifier. One particular surgeon may have a seemingly higher complication rate than others. However, this individual may be the person who takes most of the more 'difficult' cases which other colleagues may have eschewed. Reference has already been made to oesophagectomy for oesophageal cancer (known as the Ivor-Lewis procedure), which has a complication rate of 50–70%. However, this is the most invasive operation generally performed for visceral cancer, and other procedures in other parts of the body will not be expected to be attended by such a fearsome morbidity rate.

Follow-up

A member of the administrative staff in the NHS nowadays might argue that surgeons should be operating and seeing new patients and not continuing to be involved with the follow-up of existing patients. This has a ring of plausibility about it, but for cancer work and care, it may be incorrect (Waghorn et al. 1995). Examine the following scenario. The situation is one where a patient has had a total cystectomy for bladder cancer, or another who has had an anterior resection for rectal cancer. For such patients there can be the risk of certain mechanical problems in their surgical recovery. However, these problems can often be resolved with advice, information and even instruction, confidently given by the expert surgeon and the appropriate clinical nurse specialist, but are unlikely to be resolved as effectively by less specialised personnel. A lack of confidence in those caring for them in the surgical recovery period is a major concern for the postoperative patient in the first few months after cancer surgery, threatening their sense of self-worth and self-efficacy at a critical time on the cancer journey.

In addition to supportive advice for the patient, there are two other major reasons for closely monitoring the patient who has undergone cancer surgery. First, there is the possibility of recurrent disease or, indeed, a new primary cancer. Second, the surgical staff have to know how their patients are progressing. Without this they have no opportunity of knowing their cancer surgery outcomes and how these might compare with those of other units, both at home and overseas. Under the umbrella of audit, these facts are vital, particularly to those analysing the circumstances where things have not progressed as smoothly as hoped for or anticipated or, equally, when outcomes have been particularly, and even unexpectedly, good.

Palliative care

The patient referred to the palliative care team is not a surgical failure. Clearly, and by definition, if the patient with cancer finds they have been referred to the palliative care consultant and team, then the disease is regarded as now being beyond cure. However, this by no means implies that the patient is not in a position to be helped. Often the patient is referred to palliative care by the surgeons, as they are often the people most likely to know the facts about disease progression or recurrence and who are in day-to-day contact with the patient. The benefits of a good liaison between the palliative care team and the surgeons cannot be overstated. The palliative care team is likely to know much more about facilities for home and hospice care than the surgeons, and so their involvement is vital once the Rubicon has been crossed and the patient can no longer be deemed amenable to curative means. The palliative care team will also have the specific expertise in the management of cancer pain (see Chapter 7) and will have a close working relationship with other pain-relieving services.

The surgeon and the clinical nurse specialist

The role of the clinical nurse specialist has been mentioned and is pivotal in the way the NHS cancer service is run. This person assumes a central role, much appreciated by patients, surgeons and other surgical staff alike. The clinical nurse specialist post came about with the implementation of the *Calman Hine Report* (DH 1995). At the same time, the concept of the multidisciplinary team was being implemented, and gave a completely new direction to the way in which cancer services were run in the UK (see Chapter 1). Valued aspects of the clinical nurse specialist's role, from the perspective of the cancer surgeon, are discussed below.

Friend and advocate to the patient

It is important for the patient with cancer to have a friend and advocate through their treatment trajectory. Although the key decisions about treatment options and their alternatives for the patient are made by the multidisciplinary team, one of the shortcomings is that the single most important person in the discussion is absent: the patient. Accordingly, when the patient is being discussed at the multidisciplinary team meetings, the clinical nurse specialist can view the suggestions and therapeutic options from the perspective of the patient and family. This is particularly to the purpose as they may be the only person present who has spent sufficient time with the patient and family to appreciate their hopes, fears and expectations of treatment options and, indeed, the suitability of the patient for some of the more aggressive forms of cancer therapy.

Advocate for the hospital

In a reciprocal fashion, the clinical nurse specialist is the hospital's advocate to the patient. The following serves to illustrate this. At the multidisciplinary team meeting, the needs of a patient who has a newly diagnosed distal, large bowel cancer, with a degree of local spread, has been fully discussed. The patient is coming to the surgeon's clinic to hear the news of confirmation of diagnosis and treatment plans. The surgeon is unlikely to have sufficient time in a busy clinic to elaborate on the decisions in a way that the patient needs and deserves. It falls to the clinical nurse specialist to do so, explaining and often re-explaining the necessary facts: the diagnosis, the degree of advancement, the need for surgery which will probably involve at least a temporary stoma, as well as the need for a long course of preoperative chemotherapy and radiotherapy. The clinical nurse specialist must also respond to the patient's need to know the outlook for the future. All this news will, more often than not, make this one of the worst days in the life of the patient. The clinical nurse specialist will probably see the patient several times, to discuss all these facts more fully and to examine their various connotations and implications; for example, for the male patient, the possibility of postoperative impotence will need to be addressed. Great tact and patience are necessary and, above all, time. Time to spend with the patient, and excellent communication skills, are paramount.

A familiar presence

The clinical nurse specialist and the surgeon are the familiar faces, mentioned earlier, when the patient comes to be admitted. The friendly and confident clinical nurse specialist plays a vital part in preoperative preparation. The clinical nurse specialist will be expected to field all sorts of technical, procedural and emotional questions such as those concerning the operation, consequences in terms of altered body image, chemotherapy and radio-therapy, the chances of cure, postoperative treatment with further chemotherapy, as well as the ever-lurking question of a possible familial trait (see Chapter 2). Many clinical nurse specialists run their own cancer follow-up clinics (Moore et al. 2006) in association with surgical clinics, and patients find it reassuring to know that the familiar face will be there on a long-term basis, to answer their concerns.

Facilitating research

It was a clear tenet of the *Calman Hine Report* (DH 1995) that, as far as possible, all patients might be incorporated into a clinical trial (see Chapter 9). Most hospitals will have a clinical trials nurse, but the delicate question may first be broached by the clinical nurse specialist. In colorectal cancer, for example, where the national cure rate hovers stubbornly at only 50%, research is vital and larger numbers of patients need to be recruited into national trials.

Understanding the genetic basis of cancer

The clinical nurse specialist will need a working knowledge of the genetics of his or her site-specific cancers (see Chapter 2). The clinical nurse specialist may run a screening family history clinic for those who could be at risk of inherited disease. Those people whom the clinical nurse specialist regards as meriting further genetic enquiry will be passed on to a regional genetic service. The science of genetics, as well a working knowledge of statistical risk of disease, is not for the mathematically faint-hearted!

Follow-up care after discharge

The patient who is concerned that all is not well following discharge after surgery has a whole range of possible contacts. The GP, NHS Direct/24 or the local emergency department are just some of the options. A good clinical nurse specialist service will have a ready answer for the patient who telephones during office hours. According to what the patient says, the response instigated by the clinical nurse specialist may vary from a word of telephone advice, a booking into the next clinic or immediate admission back into the hospital.

The joys and heartaches of a cancer surgeon

Surgery is basically a process of trying to do some good by using instruments within the patient's body. It seems conspicuously obvious that this is likely to carry risk and, however small that risk, it is inevitable that sometimes things will go wrong. It is vital that the patient understands this before the surgery. In complaints and litigation, a common theme is 'nobody ever told us this'. Clearly this notion has implications for the way in which consent is obtained, and illustrates the importance of involving the patient and family with information about possible outcomes – both good and bad. All experienced cancer surgeons carry in their consciousness, somewhere, a small cemetery of patients who succumbed after their operations. The cemetery is of bitterness and regret where the surgeon seeks a reason for such outcomes. Adjacent to this cemetery will be a list of living patients in whom the surgeon can say 'if only': if only the operation had been undertaken differently or if intraoperative or postoperative decisions had been different. The patient survived, but might have survived better if clinical decision making had been different. William Shakespeare in *Julius Caesar* expressed it thus: 'The evil that men do lives after them; the good is oft interred with their bones' (Act III, Scene II). This can be applied to surgical staff too!

Despite heartaches experienced, one of the supreme joys for a surgeon is to see the patient 10 or 20 years after surgical treatment who is well and disease-free.

Changing surgical techniques: past, present and future

As recently as 25 years ago, open cancer surgery had arrived at a level of refinement that seemed likely not to change much in the future. Then came the advent of laparoscopic surgery in the late 1980s (Way 1990). Initially laparoscopic techniques were introduced by gynaecologists and then surgery for gallbladder removal became largely laparoscopic. Much visceral cancer surgery is now performed with such minimally invasive methods. The principle of the surgical excision of cancer has not changed radically. What has changed is the conversion to very small incisions and the use of 'tools' by the surgeon which are manipulated, not primarily with the help of the direct vision of the surgeon's eyes, but by the use of microchip cameras connected to high-definition television screens. Will cancer survival statistics be improved? Possibly not. Will the complication rates go down? Perhaps so. Infective complications, especially with methicillin-resistant *Staphylococcus aureus* (MRSA) are less common after laparoscopic surgery (Siddiqui & Khan 2006). Incisional hernia is also less common than after open surgery (Anderson et al. 2008).

These advances in the surgical approach, made possible by technical advances leading to improved and precise instrumentation and the use of miniature cameras, have been fuelled by increasing patient demand. On reflection it is not a total surprise that, given a choice, most people will choose a few minor incisions as opposed to a 12-inch wound, especially if it means a shorter time as an inpatient in hospital. On the horizon is the prospect of abdominal surgery without any abdominal incision, by means of natural orifice surgery. In natural orifice surgery, the laparoscopic instruments are introduced via the vagina or, in men, via a transoral gastroscope placed in the stomach (Baron 2007). Many would say this is not only unwise but technically verging on the impossible. The same words would have been used 25 years ago regarding laparoscopic surgery, so it may be prudent simply to conclude that currently we do not know the place that natural orifice surgery will occupy in the future. In addition, advances have been made to improve the patient's surgical journey in the form of multimodal strategies whereby the stress of surgery itself can be reduced, recovery enhanced and the patient enabled to return to normal function as soon as possible (Kehlet & Wilmore 2002).

Monitoring progress in cancer surgery

It is important that data are recorded and monitored to facilitate progress. Audit allows one to look to the past, which is unalterable. It allows us to assess the present performance and also allows redirection or rerouting, if it would seem advisable, for the future. In cancer services, a few, relatively simple data should be easy to gather, such as the numbers of patients treated, the staging of the cancers, the types of surgical technique, the 30-day mortality and five-year disease-free survival. Clearly the latter measurement has to be the most troublesome to gather. A surgeon needs to be in post for five years to fulfil this most simple of parameters. For many cancers, five-year survival is not appropriate in its use as a point at which the patient may be said to be cured. It may hold true for most gastrointestinal cancers but will not be so useful in breast cancer or malignant melanoma, as both have a fickle reputation as to the time to recurrence. Audit, however, is vital if used constructively in reshaping and redefining roles and practices.

Conclusion

Surgery remains the mainstay of the treatment of many forms of cancer. Radiotherapy and chemotherapy are often still second-line treatments, although this may change in the future. The surgery is often difficult and challenging, but nonetheless the reward is seeing a patient pulled back from a certain and perhaps premature death. The fact that many successfully treated patients return to their normal, day-to-day activities may be a tribute to the surgery but is also testament to their own bravery and fortitude.

References

Anderson LP, Klein M, Gogenu I, Rosenburg J (2008) *Surgical Endoscopy* **22**: 2026–9.

Atkins BZ, Shah AS, Hutcheson K, et al. (2004) Reducing hospital mortality following oesophagectomy. *Annals of Thoracic Surgery* **78**(4): 1170–6.

Baron TH (2007) Natural orifice transluminal endoscopic surgery. *British Journal of Surgery* **94**(1): 1–3.

Bosch X, Aibar J, Capell S, Coca A, López-Soto A (2009) Quick diagnosis units: a potentially useful alternative to conventional hospitalisation. *Medical Journal of Australia* **191**(9): 496–8.

Crofts TJ (2000) Ivor-Lewis oesophagectomy for middle and lower third oesophageal lesions – how do we do it. *Journal of the Royal College of Surgeons (Edinburgh)* **45**(5): 296–303.

Department of Health (1995) *A Policy Framework for Commissioning Cancer Services: A report by the Expert Advisory Group on Cancer to the Chief Medical Officers of England and Wales (Calman Hine Report)*. London: DH.

Donner CS (1998) Pathophysiology and therapy of chronic radiation induced injury to the colon. *Digestive Diseases* **85**(16): 253–61.

Hagiwara H, Sunada Y (2004) Mechanisms of taxane neurotoxicity. *Breast Cancer* **11**(1): 82–4.

Kehlet H, Wilmore DW (2002) Multimodal strategies to improve surgical outcome. *American Journal of Surgery* **183**(6): 630–41.

Lonwagie J, Pommerian W, Brichard G, et al. (2009) A plasma-based colorectal cancer screening assay using DNA methylation markers – first results of multicentre studies. *European Journal of Cancer Supplements* **7**(3): 9.

Moore S, Wells M, Plant H, Fuller F, Wright M, Corner J (2006) Nurse specialist led follow-up in lung cancer: the experience of developing and delivering a new model of care. *European Journal of Oncology Nursing* **10**(5): 364–77.

National Heath Service (2004) *An introduction to electronic booking, choice of hospital and appointment* (www.chooseandbook.nhs.uk).

Sackland M (1941) Grading for surgical procedures. *Anesthesiology* **2**: 281–4.

Siddiqui K, Khan AFA (2006) Comparison of frequency of wound infection: open vs laparoscopic cholecystectomy. *Journal of Ayub Medical College* **18**(3): 21–4.

Sikora K (2008) *Personal address to AGM.*, Association of Surgeons, Bournemouth, UK.

Visser BC, Keegan H, Martin M, Wren SM (2009) Death after colectomy: it's later than we think. *Archives of Surgery* **144**(11): 1021–7.

Waghorn A, Thompson J, McKee M (1995) Routine surgical follow-up: do surgeons agree? *BMJ* **11**(7016): 1344–5.

Way LW (1990) Changing therapy for gallstone disease. *New England Journal of Medicine* **323**(18): 1273–4.

Williams N (2008) *Health: unemployment and employment: the link between health and work.* London: Department of Work and Pensions (www.facoccmed.ac.uk/library/docs/comppnw3.ppt).

Chapter 7

Cancer pain

Papiya B. Russell and Anil Tandon

Pain is often one of the first symptoms people think of when they hear the word 'cancer', and many people believe that pain is an inevitable part of having cancer (Cleeland 1984; Levin & Cleeland 1985; Thomason et al. 1998). Thoughts of both 'cancer' and 'pain' can cause profound fear for both patients and their family members. Patients fear what may lie ahead and family members may fear that they will helplessly watch the suffering of their loved one. Those who have cared for patients with cancer are familiar with the worries people have about suffering pain and appreciate that these issues need to be addressed, as well as treating the pain.

While some fears may be based on a 'fear of the unknown' and some misapprehensions, concerns about pain are not without some basis. It is estimated that about 70% of patients with advanced cancer experience pain (Portenoy 1989), and for some this can be severe. When pain is not taken seriously, or is under-recognised or under-treated, patients can suffer great distress and this will affect their physical activity, psychological state and quality of life (Zaza & Baine 2002; Al-Atiyyat 2008).

Fortunately, improvements have been made over the years and the skilful use of medications is now able to alleviate pain and provide comfort to patients throughout their cancer journey. However, despite the advances made in managing and understanding cancer pain, there still remain many fears amongst patients and carers which can create barriers to good pain control. These include the unwanted side effects of pain-relieving drugs, such as sedation, confusion, tolerance or addiction (Paice et al. 1998; Al-Atiyyat 2008) and fear that analgesia might mask the signs of cancer progression and delay possible further treatment. Patients may simply worry about not being a 'good patient' should they complain of pain (Al-Atiyyat 2008). Informal carers of patients with cancer may also worry about being responsible for pain medication and the need to balance their wish for their loved one to be comfortable with, often unfounded, fears of overmedication, causing side effects or even encouraging addiction or hastening death (Vallerand et al. 2007). Unfortunately some of these misconceptions and lack of understanding are still shared by many healthcare professionals, due to inexperience or deficiencies in education (Jacobsen et al. 2007).

Notwithstanding this, our understanding of cancer pain has improved greatly over recent years, and when this knowledge is coupled with availability of a wider variety of

Perspectives on Cancer Care.   Edited by Josephine (Tonks) N. Fawcett and Anne McQueen
© 2011 Blackwell Publishing Ltd

effective analgesics, it is estimated that approximately 88% of cancer pain should be controllable using basic principles, such as the World Health Organization (WHO) ladder (Ventafridda et al. 1987; Zech et al. 1995).

This chapter will focus on the management of cancer pain and begin with exploring the concept of 'total pain' first propounded by Dame Cicely Saunders (Saunders 1966: 139; Saunders 1996) and demonstrate how such a concept has facilitated further understanding of the holistic nature of the pain experience. Methods of assessing pain and the use of the all-important WHO ladder in the management of pain will be discussed. Particular emphasis is given to the understanding and use of opioid analgesics, so often central to optimal pain relief in cancer-related pain. Neuropathic pain will also be given attention because of its significance in some patients with cancer, and the particular medications used in alleviating this type of pain. Use of adjuvant analgesics and the place of radiotherapy, chemotherapy and complementary therapy will also be briefly considered in the relief of pain.

The concept of total pain

Although not commonly referred to outside of palliative care services, total pain is an important concept, as it embraces the whole person, creating a picture of how the pain impacts on the living experience of the individual. Dame Cicely Saunders, considered to be the founder of modern hospice care, used this concept to describe how pain is not just experienced as a physical sensation; it is also experienced as emotional, spiritual and social sensations, affecting all aspects of a patient's life and impacting deeply on their sense of personhood; Saunders quotes the poignant words of a patient, 'all of me is wrong' (Saunders 1964; Clark 1999). The concept is depicted in Figure 7.1.

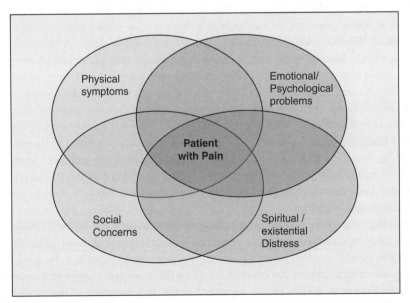

Figure 7.1   A depiction of the overlapping dimensions of total pain (based on Cicely Saunders' 'concept of total pain'; Saunders 1964).

These overlapping dimensions which may affect patients with cancer pain intuitively feel understandable to many healthcare professionals working in palliative care. If the perception of acute pain has developed as a protective function, a 'warning system that something is wrong' (Millan 1999; Woolf & Mannion 1999), then it is not surprising that the warning, the pain, also stimulates emotions such as anxiety and even alarm.

The experience and perception of pain

The original view of pain as a physical sensation, which mapped pain to tissue injury, was described in the 17th century by the philosopher René Descartes, who suggested that there was discrete connection from the origin of the pain in the body to the brain when he wrote: 'Fast moving particles of fire . . . the disturbance passes along the nerve filament until it reaches the brain' (Descartes 1664 cited in Colvin & Lambert 2008: 1). The brain, having detected the source of pain, could then initiate movement to remove the affected part of the body from the source of the tissue damage. However, this is too simplistic a notion and it is now known that many areas of the brain have an interconnected part to play in the detection and expression of pain, particularly in persistent or chronic pain.

Pain pathways

It is now well understood that the body's pain detection system starts with pain receptors, called nociceptors. These detect painful stimuli and transmit this signal, including the 'strength' of the signal, along pain nerves (neurons) to the central nervous system (CNS), which comprises the spinal cord and brain. The afferent neuron enters the CNS and meets the next neuron at the dorsal horn of the spinal cord, which is an important site where many opioids exert their effect (Kline & Wiley 2008). The second (central) neuron carries the signal to that part of the brain which maps the signal to where it is being generated in the body and records how strong the impulse is (Fine et al. 2004). All this takes milliseconds. This is 'nociceptive pain', which is detected within a normal nervous system and is how most types of pain are detected. Areas such as the limbic system and amygdala are involved with emotion and memory (Amunts et al. 2005; Carrasquillo & Gereau 2007). Painful information is fed into such centres, which then modify the pain sensation, perhaps based on our previous memories, experiences and emotions. When someone has cancer, which is usually a new experience for their body, the appearance of or an increase in pain detected through the amygdala and limbic system could easily cause fear or panic in a brain 'holding' fears about cancer. Thus, the pain pathways are interconnected, and also connect to the amygdala and limbic systems, which modulate the experience of pain, allowing the incorporation of memories and emotions.

Just as importantly, we now know that changes in neural pathways in the CNS can occur in *response* to repeated pain or its environmental context (Fine et al. 2004). This ability of the CNS to change is called plasticity, and means that pathways are not 'hard-wired', so a painful stimulus might not always be detected by the same pathways or in the same way over time (Fine et al. 2004). This is important in the understanding of the generation of central neuropathic pain and central sensitisation, which is discussed later under the heading 'The specific challenge of neuropathic pain'.

It follows from this that different individuals may experience pain from a similar injury in different ways. Some individuals will experience the pain as more severe than others, explained in part by plasticity, the pain pathways or the modulation of the pain experience that can occur in the limbic system and amygdala. It is therefore important for practitioners to avoid being judgemental when someone's experience of cancer-related pain does not correspond to their own view of how the pain is, or, arguably, should be, felt (Arber 2004). An appreciation of some of the complexities of physical pain detection in the nervous system can help us understand that 'pain is whatever the experiencing person says it is, and exists when he says it does' (McCaffery 1968: 8), whilst bearing in mind that exploring and resolving any psychosocial factors in a patient's pain might impact on the level of pain, both experienced and expressed.

Social aspects of pain and pain empathy

It has been shown above how a person in pain can also experience anxiety, fear and alarm, but pain also has a 'social' aspect. People feel alarmed when seeing someone in pain, or about to cause themselves injury or pain, for example, a child reaching a hand out towards a hot kettle, and people instinctively wince at the hard punches whilst watching a boxing match. It is probably natural to feel this 'pain empathy', and natural for the behaviour associated with pain to elicit an empathic response from others (Craig 2004; Sullivan 2008). Using magnetic resonance imaging, Singer et al. (2004) demonstrated that the neural responses of people witnessing others in pain were similar to those of the individuals actually experiencing pain; the responses were not in the pain pathways themselves, but instead in the affective pathways, i.e. those involving mood and feelings associated with pain. It appears that expressing pain and pain empathy is an important part of what makes us human; indeed it has been proposed that both pain behaviours and pain empathy provide important evolutionary survival mechanisms, benefiting the individual in pain, who receives care, support and protection, and 'the group', who are warned of danger in order to avoid harm and protect the vulnerable (Craig 2004; Goubert et al. 2005; Sullivan 2008). Is it any wonder that, when witnessing a loved one in pain, or when hearing about a neighbour with cancer, we feel anxiety, fear and 'pain empathy'?

Some of these concepts are captured in Figure 7.2, which concerns a young woman with cancer pain and the ways in which it impacts on her own and her loved ones' lives as well as on all those who hear about her. The thoughts that she and her family have are repeated time and again by patients with cancer, and will be recognised by people who work with those who experience cancer pain.

Assessment and management of emotional, psychological or spiritual pain

Patients with cancer pain frequently have physical pain, especially in the more advanced stages, but this is almost invariably combined with varying degrees of emotional, psychological or spiritual distress arising from the reality of their condition. A sensitive and detailed assessment of the patient is required to clarify the nature and degree of pain

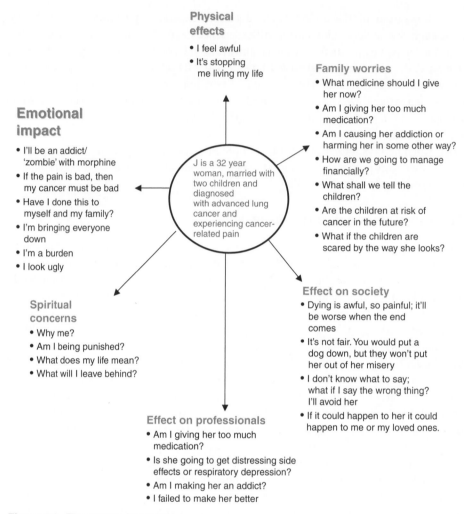

Physical effects
- I feel awful
- It's stopping me living my life

Family worries
- What medicine should I give her now?
- Am I giving her too much medication?
- Am I causing her addiction or harming her in some other way?
- How are we going to manage financially?
- What shall we tell the children?
- Are the children at risk of cancer in the future?
- What if the children are scared by the way she looks?

Emotional impact
- I'll be an addict/ 'zombie' with morphine
- If the pain is bad, then my cancer must be bad
- Have I done this to myself and my family?
- I'm bringing everyone down
- I'm a burden
- I look ugly

J is a 32 year woman, married with two children and diagnosed with advanced lung cancer and experiencing cancer-related pain

Spiritual concerns
- Why me?
- Am I being punished?
- What does my life mean?
- What will I leave behind?

Effect on society
- Dying is awful, so painful; it'll be worse when the end comes
- It's not fair. You would put a dog down, but they won't put her out of her misery
- I don't know what to say; what if I say the wrong thing? I'll avoid her
- If it could happen to her it could happen to me or my loved ones.

Effect on professionals
- Am I giving her too much medication?
- Is she going to get distressing side effects or respiratory depression?
- Am I making her an addict?
- I failed to make her better

Figure 7.2 The reality of total pain.

and emotional suffering experienced. Some patients may deny that they have worries, and express distress using only physical terms, but carers and the healthcare team may notice anxiety or that when distracted the patient moves more freely than would be expected. Occasionally, pain with a large component of emotional distress might fail to improve with analgesics, although the medication regime should be reviewed by a specialist before that conclusion is drawn. In many cases it is clear from a patient's account of their pain that fear is present, and, given the opportunity, patients will often interject descriptions of their physical symptoms with comments such as 'I guess it means I'm dying', 'It's only going to get worse' or 'I don't know why God did this to me'. These issues and the search for meaning need to be recognised and explored, together with relieving the physical pain. Patients' misconceptions can be far more frightening than reality. The experienced nurse can help patients to discuss their concerns and, as part of the caring team, offer advice, support and counselling. Patients need healthcare professionals to treat them as 'whole persons' (Steinhauser et al. 2000). Although clear information and answers are important to them, patients request that communication must be more than this; it involves engaging with them as a person, developing relationships, expressing a sense of caring about what that person is going through (Kimberlin et al. 2004). Allowing time for patients to talk of themselves, their hopes, fears, joys and what makes them unique can help develop the therapeutic relationship and dispel the sense of being just another patient 'lost' among so many.

Spirituality is a notoriously difficult concept to define, but is important to religious and non-religious people alike. Tanyi (2002) described it as an integral part of being human, not a concept interchangeable with religion, but rather a multifaceted dimension linked with a patient's subjective sense of self, and involves searching for meaning in one's life. Importantly, there is evidence that patients would like their healthcare professionals to address their spiritual needs (Wilkinson 2000). With training and a support framework, healthcare professionals may be able to engage with patients' spiritual pain (Mitchell & Gordon 2007; Smith & Gordon 2009). Mitchell and Gordon (2007) describe the importance of 'listening with focus', using a non-judgemental approach to address spiritual distress by recognising and dealing with the 'why' questions with honesty, exploring with the individual why such questions prey on their mind. Patients may initially be reticent about raising some of their emotional, psychological or spiritual concerns with healthcare professionals but as a therapeutic relationship develops this becomes easier. Nurses and other healthcare professionals can sensitively bring about such a conversation by perhaps referring to something a patient said earlier, introducing it with, for example; 'You mentioned you were worried about [. . .]. What worries you about it?' Even when patients do not spontaneously raise issues, it is important to feel able to ask if they have any worries or particular concerns about their pain, with the proviso such that if a healthcare professional feels the discussion has complexities beyond their ability and experience, another member of the team, with greater expertise, will be sought.

Keeping in mind that the experience of physical pain is intimately related to other dimensions as identified in the concept of total pain, as Saunders herself said, 'If physical symptoms are alleviated then mental pain is often lifted also' (Saunders 1963: 746). The chapter will now focus on the assessment and management of physical pain.

Assessment and management of pain

The importance of optimal pain assessment

Assessment is the cornerstone of care and is required to provide a comprehensive understanding of the type and nature of the pain. This is important for two reasons. Firstly, to detect if the cause of the pain is something reversible, even in cancer pain, such as new-onset pleuritic pain with a treatable pulmonary embolus or pneumonia. It is perhaps all too easy to assume that when a patient with cancer complains of pain, the pain will be related to the cancer. However, this is not necessarily always the case. It is therefore important to identify and independently assess each new pain. Second, and equally important, different types of pain can respond to different types of pain relief (Vielhaber &

Portenoy 2002). Analgesics are not necessarily the only solution, and cardinal to optimal pain relief is the recognition that it may be achieved by a wide range of pharmacological and non-pharmacological means. Box 7.1 gives an illustration of how an initial detailed pain assessment is carried out, upon which subsequent assessments can be based and built. Case study 7.1 demonstrates the importance of such a detailed initial pain assessment.

Box 7.1 Pain assessment

Pain assessment is about eliciting from the patient enough about his/her pain to almost feel you know how the pain feels yourself. The favoured medical school mnemonic of SOCRATES, to remind one to ask about all the various aspects of pain, may be a useful aide-memoire, although it must be said that it does not provide a particularly logical sequence for asking questions! The mnemonic is illustrated below, but additional questions are also included for assessing the pain associated with cancer.

How many pains do you have?

Site	Where is your pain?
Onset	When does it come on, what brings it on?
Character	What does the pain feel like when you have it? Then if the patient needs more guidance: Is it a sharp or dull pain? Is it burning or shooting or gnawing? Does it feel like anything you've had before, like a bad toothache?
Radiation	Does the pain go anywhere else?
Associated features	Has anything else unusual happened to your body since you've had this pain?
Timing	How long have you had the pain for? How often do you get the pain? Is it there all the time or does it come and go? How long does it last when it comes? Are there times when it is worse?
Exacerbating/ relieving factors	Is there anything which brings on, worsens or relieves the pain?
Severity	How severe is the pain at its worst (e.g. on a scale of 0–10)? How severe is it most of the time? Are you ever pain-free?
Medication	Do any medications help?
Effect of drugs	Do they help a little, a lot or not at all? Do they take it away completely?
Toxic effects	Are you getting any side effects from your pain killers? Do you get drowsy or muddled with them? Have you any vivid dreams? Are your muscles twitching?
Sleep	Does it affect your sleep?
Worries	Is there anything worrying you about your pain?
Examination	Put the above together with physical examination and diagnosis and site of the tumours.

Notes

- Patients do not always find it easy to describe their pain or to answer questions such as these. The clinician should reassure the patient that they should just do what they can and that there is no 'wrong answer'.
- There are several scales to aid patients with the question of severity. These include simple descriptor scales of 'nil, mild, moderate, severe, very severe' or 'no pain, mild, moderate, horrible, excruciating' or verbal numerical rating scales where patients choose a number on a scale, e.g. 0–10 with 0 being no pain and 10 being the worst pain they could imagine. There are also visual analogue scales, where a patient can circle a number on a scale, or along a line which can then be measured. Each of these have problems, with some patients unable to translate their pain into numerals, disability or visual impairment restricting use of visual analogue scales and descriptors being insensitive to allow assessment of the effect of analgesia as part of ongoing pain assessment (Paice & Cohen 1997). However, a 0–10 numerical rating scale has been shown to be acceptable to most patients and validated in terms of accuracy (De Conno et al. 1994; Paice & Cohen 1997), and is convenient to use in suitable patient. Of course, whichever method is chosen, the same scale should be used for successive assessments in the same patient to allow comparisons over time.
- Multidimensional pain assessment tools which also record site of pain and ask about impact on pain on various social and functional aspects of life have also been developed, though often these are most used in studies. These include the McGill Pain Questionnaire (Melzack 1975), the Brief Pain Inventory (Cleeland 1989) and their shorter forms, amongst others. The Brief Pain Inventory has been translated into many languages. Other scales focus on behaviour to try and assess pain in children (Caraceni et al. 2002) or, in the case of the DOLOPLUS II, those with cognitive impairment (Lefebvre-Chapiro 2001; Hølen et al. 2007).
- However, despite the best efforts it can be difficult to make a pain assessment based on history alone, and in this circumstance the ability to admit the patient to a specialist unit for a team-based pain assessment over several days can be invaluable.

Before progressing to look in detail at the management of pain, there are two other important concepts relating to pain to introduce: 'breakthrough' pain and 'incident' pain.

'Breakthrough' pain

Breakthrough pain is pain which 'breaks through' the effectiveness of the analgesic prescribed. This can occur for several reasons: patients with cancer can have 'good and bad days' and some days the pain is, sadly, worse than normal. Sometimes this is due to a change in activity, position, anxiety, or for no particular reason, or possibly because their cancer has altered in nature. The management of such pain is discussed later under the heading 'The management of breakthrough pain'.

Incident pain

Incident pain is a specific form of breakthrough pain, which occurs only during an aggravating action, such as certain movements (Mercadante et al. 2004), weight bearing, swallowing, coughing (Portenoy & Hagen 1990) and so on. It is therefore relatively predictable in its onset, and often short-lived. Management of incident pain is addressed later under the heading 'The management of incident pain'.

Management of cancer pain

The WHO ladder has proved a critical tool in managing pain associated with cancer. This ladder was first published in 1986 (WHO 1986) and has been widely used since. Simple though it is at first glance, it is not as self-explanatory as it may seem. It is worth taking some time to really understand the WHO ladder and work out what it means in practical terms (see Figure 7.3).

The first thing to note is that the three steps on the ladder correspond to the *severity* of the pain. Of all the questions asked in pain assessment proformas, the WHO ladder only gives guidance about what to do based on the severity of pain. Although this reflects the importance of asking about severity, the other questions are also important, as they help to determine other features of pain, and therefore when to use adjuvant analgesics and non-pharmacological interventions. Adjuvant analgesics are drugs which have a primary indication other than pain, but are analgesic in some painful conditions (Lussier et al. 2004) and can be a valuable addition to opioid medication in cancer pain. These are discussed later under the heading 'The use of adjuvant analgesics'.

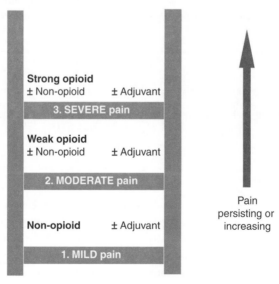

Figure 7.3 A representation of the WHO analgesic ladder for cancer pain.

The WHO ladder is used by starting on the appropriate step according to the severity of the pain. It is important to note that the ladder does not require the clinician to start on the bottom rung and move upwards from there. It is possible, in fact, to start immediately at step three if the pain is severe (Hanks et al 2005). The 'rules' of the ladder state 'by mouth, by the clock and by the ladder', meaning that the medication should be given orally if the patient can swallow and their gastrointestinal tract is intact, it should be given regularly, and one should move up the ladder if pain is still uncontrolled, rather than changing to another medicine on the same level of the ladder.

Step one

Patients with mild cancer-related pain start on step one and would be offered regular paracetamol (1 g four times daily). A non-steroidal anti-inflammatory drug (NSAID) would be considered, such as regular ibuprofen or diclofenac sodium. However, some patients cannot tolerate NSAIDs, developing dyspepsia, peptic ulceration or renal impairment, or there may be an absolute or relative contraindication, such as previous gastric ulceration or renal failure. This unfortunately limits the number of patients who are able to take NSAIDs as part of step one; however, a proton pump inhibitor such as omeprazole can be prescribed to reduce the risk of gastric bleeding (Dickman & Ellershaw 2004). Alternatively, a specialist may suggest using one of the COX-2 antagonist drugs such as celecoxib, which work in a similar way to NSAIDs but with a reduced risk of upper gastrointestinal bleeding (Fitzgerald & Patrono 2001; Dickman & Ellershaw 2004). If the pain persists, or returns despite taking regular paracetamol, and perhaps some NSAID, then it is suggested to move to the second step of the ladder.

Step two

Patients presenting with moderately severe pain will begin at step two and a weak opioid, such as codeine or dihydrocodeine, is administered. An appropriate dose of either codeine or dihydrocodeine is 60 mg four times a day. When moving to this step, patients should still remain on their step one analgesics as paracetamol, NSAIDs and weak opioids all work in different ways, and can help to tackle the pain in different ways. One way is to change a patient's regime from paracetamol to a combination of codeine and paracetamol, such as co-codamol 30 : 500. This strength corresponds to 30 mg codeine and 500 mg paracetamol in each tablet. This means that two tablets four times a day gives a patient the maximum recommended amount of paracetamol and 240 mg codeine daily. Co-codamol 8 : 500 is available but only gives the patient 64 mg codeine daily and is not considered helpful for most cancer patients in pain (clinical guideline 106, SIGN 2008).

Step three

If a patient's pain worsens or persists despite regular weak opioids and non-opioids, then strong opioids should be considered. Any step two analgesics should be discontinued, as weak and strong opioids work through the same mechanism. However, the step one analgesics, paracetamol with or without NSAIDs, should be continued.

The use of strong opioids

General principles

Strong opioids include morphine, oxycodone, diamorphine, fentanyl, alfentanil, hydro-morphone, buprenorphine and methadone. Again, they should be given by mouth if possible, and regularly to ensure adequate analgesic levels. If commenced for a patient who has not previously been prescribed an opioid, a low dose is initially prescribed. The effectiveness is carefully monitored alongside the provision of a 'breakthrough dose' usually calculated as one-sixth of the total daily dose of opioid (Hanks 2001). Strong opioids are adjusted over days and sometimes weeks, until the patient's pain is well controlled without the need for regular breakthrough medication. This process of starting fairly low and building up the dose to match the patient's pain is called titration. Titration relies first, on an effective breakthrough opioid so that the patient does not have to cope with uncontrolled pain if the background opioid dose is too low, and second, on the clinical team performing regular pain assessments and looking for any signs of opioid toxicity (see under heading 'Opioid toxicity').

Prescribing morphine

One of the most commonly used opioids is morphine. In the UK, the oral form is used as two different preparations. The first is a continuous or 'slow release' preparation tablet, usually abbreviated to MST. This form is designed to be given every 12 hours once it is known that the patient requires continuous morphine analgesia. MST actually stands for Morphine Sulphate Tablets, and so more properly a prescriber should stipulate the continuous-release form, perhaps by using a brand name such as MST Continus®. In the remainder of this chapter, MST refers to the continuous oral release form of morphine sulphate.

The liquid oral morphine preparation is the 'normal release' preparation; a commonly used preparation is Oramorph®, which when taken orally achieves a therapeutic effect within about 20 to 30 minutes and should continue to have an effect for several hours. Oramorph can be used either as a breakthrough dose, or, as a safer way of starting opioid therapy, used as a low dose given as needed for pain or on a regular basis, e.g. every 4 hours. It can then be titrated according to the patient's response in terms of pain relief, or omitted or stopped if the patient experiences signs of toxicity.

Most commonly, the two preparations are prescribed together, MST twice daily and Oramorph for breakthrough pain. If several extra doses of Oramorph are being used with good analgesic effect every day and the patient shows no signs of opioid toxicity, the MST can be increased. Often the prescriber will add up the number of extra milligrams of Oramorph which is being taken each day, and simply increase the total MST per day by that same amount, or perhaps a little less. Alternatively, if the patient has not taken break-through doses, despite experiencing continuing pain the MST dose can be increased by a fixed percentage based on the severity of the pain. For example, a patient with moderately severe pain may have the dose increased by 33–50%.

As with other opioids, the breakthrough dose is usually calculated as one-sixth of the total daily dose of opioid (Hanks 2001). For a patient receiving MST 30 mg twice daily, the Oramorph breakthrough dose would be 10 mg to be taken 1–2 hourly if required for pain.

Commencement of morphine

Most patients prescribed an opioid will commence with morphine. Some practitioners will prefer to prescribe initially low-dose regular Oramorph®, such as 5 mg every 4 hours, with a breakthrough dose of 5 mg, though in opioid 'naïve' or sensitive patients they may start with 2.5 mg four times daily. Others will prefer to prescribe MST from the outset. The equivalent of 60 mg codeine given four times daily is approximately 20–30 mg of morphine per day, a figure which surprises many (Persson et al. 1992; Quiding et al. 1993). This means that a patient on regular cocodamol 30 : 500 could be changed to paracetamol plus MST 10–15 mg twice daily with 5 mg Oramorph as required as a breakthrough dose, which may be given as frequently as hourly. Patients and carers are always advised of the signs and symptoms of opioid toxicity, and warned to be alert for its possible occurrence.

Other strong opioids

There are many other strong opioids, all of which have different properties, which can be used to great advantage for individual patients. The process of converting a patient from one opioid to another is called opioid rotation. Table 7.1 summarises some of these opioids and their properties.

Opioid rotation is most often undertaken for two main reasons. First, certain opioids may be tolerated better by some individuals than others (De Stoutz et al. 1995; Mercadante et al. 2009), such that a patient gaining good analgesia from one opioid (e.g. morphine), but with adverse effects, may be converted to another opioid such as oxycodone or fentanyl, with the expectation that the second opioid is better tolerated. This may be due in part to the fact that different opioids are metabolised differently by the body (Lötsch 2005). Second, patients with poor pain control with one opioid may be changed to an alternative opioid in the expectation that they might obtain better analgesia with the second agent (Pasternak 2005).

When moving between different opioids it must be remembered that each form has a different potency on a milligram for milligram basis, and that a conversion factor is required when changing from one form to another. For example, oxycodone given orally is often considered to be 1.5–2 times stronger than oral morphine (Pöyhiä et al. 1993); so MST 30 mg twice daily with 10 mg Oramorph® given 1–2 hourly as required for breakthrough pain is roughly the same as 15–20 mg continuous-release oxycodone (e.g. OxyContin®) given twice daily with 5 mg normal-release oxycodone (e.g. Oxy-Norm®) 1–2 hourly as required for pain. Most people will use the most conservative conversion unless they are very experienced, and the support of an expert should always be sought by less experienced prescribers. However, there is not complete agreement on the relative strengths of different opioids, and different specialists and different regions in the UK may use different conversion factors (Anderson et al. 2001; Pereira et al. 2001). Some suggested conversion factors are given in Table 7.1.

Table 7.1 Opioids and their properties

Name of opioid	Preparations	Some characteristics	References	Potency compared to oral morphine (morphine : opioid equivalence ratio in milligrams)
Oral morphine	Oramorph® ('normal release form', may last approx 4 hours) MST Continus® (12 hourly prep)	Familiar to most prescribers in UK, so more likely to be prescribed in timely fashion Active metabolites are created in the body as the drug is metabolised; these can be both analgesic and cause symptoms of opioid toxicity, such as morphine-6-glucuronide (see text). One metabolite (morphine-3-glucuronide) can inhibit the analgesic action of morphine if present in large amounts. These metabolites will accumulate in patients with renal insufficiency	Anderson et al. 2003; Lötsch 2005	1 : 1*
Parenteral morphine	Morphine sulphate	Can be given as one-off injection, usually subcutaneously Can be used as a continuous infusion in a syringe driver Compatibility data with other drugs in a syringe driver exists Active metabolites as with oral morphine		2 : 1* e.g. 15 mg oral morphine = 7.5 mg parenteral morphine. Some sources use a 3 : 1 conversion ratio
Oral oxycodone	Normal-release form, may last approx 4 hours), e.g. OxyNorm®	Metabolites not thought to be active (though this is controversial) therefore may cause less opioid toxicity than morphine	Hanks et al. 2005; Kalso 2005	2 : 1*

Drug/preparation	Notes	Reference	Equivalence
Continuous-release form, 12-hourly preparation, e.g. OxyContin®	However, clearance is slowed in renal failure so caution should be used. Some patients may prefer it to morphine as they may perceive less stigma associated with the name	Kalso 2005	e.g. 15 mg oral morphine = 7.5 mg oral oxycodone. Some sources say 1.5:1 (e.g. Bruera et al. 1998)
Parenteral oxycodone — e.g. OxyNorm® injection	Can be used as one-off injection or in syringe driver. Increasing compatibility data about mixing with other drugs, but less data available than with morphine	Gagnon et al. 1999	4:1* e.g. 15 mg oral morphine = 3–4 mg SC oxycodone (approx). Some sources say 3:1
Parenteral diamorphine — Diamorphine for injection	High solubility means high doses can be made up into small volumes, so easier for injection and when using high doses in a syringe driver. Traditionally was UK's main parenteral opioid in palliative care, so prescribers may still feel very familiar with this drug. BUT: Only exists in injection form. Similar active metabolites to morphine	Hanks et al. 2005 / Hanks et al. 2005	3:1* e.g. 15 mg oral morphine = 5 mg SC diamorphine
Fentanyl patch — Transdermal patch worn on skin and changed every 3 days	Patch administration aids compliance and is useful in those who cannot swallow. Continuous release means there are no 'wearing off' effects before the next dose is due. Fentanyl not renally excreted so is well tolerated in renal failure	Hair et al. 2008 / Hair et al. 2008	25 µg per hour patch is approx equivalent to 60–90 mg of oral morphine per day*

(continued)

Table 7.1 (*Continued*)

Name of opioid	Preparations	Some characteristics	References	Potency compared to oral morphine (morphine: opioid equivalence ratio in milligrams)
		Fentanyl may be tolerated better in liver failure than other opioids and when other opioids have caused toxicity	Rhee and Broadbent 2007	
		BUT:		
		Takes at least 12–24 hours to provide analgesia when first applied	Lehman & Zech 1992; Kornick et al. 2003; Quigley 2005	
		It should not be used for opioid titration in rapidly changing pain	Lehman & Zech 1992; Hanks et al. 2005	
		Patients may absorb differing amounts from the patch, making exact conversion values difficult to predict (note: a range for morphine conversion is given)		
		It is usually continued when the patient enters the terminal phase and a syringe driver is added as necessary	Ellershaw et al. 2002	
		Another opioid must be used for 'breakthrough' doses – e.g. oral or parenteral morphine or oxycodone	Lehman & Zech 1992	
Subcutaneous or sublingual alfentanil	Injection form can be used sublingually Sublingual spray also available	Specialist drug Fast onset but short acting – may have analgesic effect after 5–15 minutes, but effect wears off after approx 1 hour	NHS Lothian 2009	30 : 1* e.g. 15 mg oral morphine approx = 0.5 mg alfentanil (500 μg alfentanil), given either

Drug		Comments	References	Notes
		One-off doses very useful for 'incident' pain, i.e. short-lived pain which is predictably only present when moving, swallowing, etc. Well tolerated in renal failure and when other opioids have caused toxicity May need to reduce dose in hepatic impairment Can be used as one-off dose or as continuous infusion in syringe driver Useful in syringe driver as high potency enables high-dose opioid to be given in driver BUT: Short-lived effect, so often not useful for 'breakthrough' pain or opioid titration, as very frequent dosing may be required Limited compatibility data with other drugs in syringe driver	NHS Lothian 2009 Dean 2004; Quigley 2005 NHS Lothian 2009	sublingually or subcutaneously
Buccal/sublingual/ nasal fentanyl	Recently licensed for use in UK	Fast acting but short acting – may have analgesic effect after 5–15 minutes, but effect may wear off after approx 1 hour Likely to be useful for 'incident' pain, i.e. short-lived pain which is predictably only present when moving, swallowing, etc. Fentanyl is well tolerated in renal impairment and when other opioids have caused toxicity	Streisand et al. 1998; Blick & Wagstaff 2006 Gardner-Nix 2001; Laverty 2007	No direct conversion data yet published (as of October 2009)
Methadone		Potentially very useful for difficult to control pain; possibly because of its ability to block NMDA receptors (see section on Central neuropathic pain)	Ebert et al. 1995	Can vary widely depending on the individual circumstances

(continued)

Table 7.1 (*Continued*)

Name of opioid	Preparations	Some characteristics	References	Potency compared to oral morphine (morphine:opioid equivalence ratio in milligrams)
		Due to a long half-life and unpredictable inter-individual variability, commencement and titration requires close supervision by a pain specialist experienced in its use	Blackburn et al. 2002	
Oral/SC hydromorphone		High potency useful when high-dose opioid required in syringe driver UK prescribers may be less familiar with this medication	Quigley & Wiffen 2003	Oral hydromorphone 5–7.5 : 1; SC hydromorphone 15 : 1

*NHS Lothian et al. (2009) *Palliative Care Guidelines*.

The management of breakthrough pain

Whenever strong opioids are prescribed, an additional opioid dose to relieve 'breakthrough' pain is also prescribed. This principle of 'anticipatory prescribing' applies not only to pain but also to the management of other symptoms, and is one of the cornerstones of good palliative care. As a general guide, the breakthrough prescription is calculated as *one-sixth* of the total daily dose of opioids prescribed. Some patients may need a little more or a little less and some flexibility is permitted. It is reasonable for patients to take one or two extra breakthrough doses through the day, though if needed more regularly in order to relieve the pain, it would indicate that the background analgesics may need to be increased.

The opioid given for breakthrough pain is usually the same as the one given to achieve background analgesia, but the normal-release form is used. For example, for MST 30 mg twice daily, Oramorph® 10 mg is used; for OxyContin® 15 mg twice daily, OxyNorm® 5 mg is used; for a 24-hour subcutaneous infusion of diamorphine 20 mg in a syringe driver, 3–5 mg of diamorphine subcutaneous injection is used. The breakthrough dose would be prescribed as required every 1–2 hours for pain. It is a common mistake to think that because Oramorph supposedly lasts for 4 hours, it can only be given every 4 hours. As long as the patient has pain *and* the opioid still relieves the patient's pain with no sign of opioid toxicity, more 'breakthrough' Oramorph can be given. However, if the patient is requiring breakthrough analgesia very frequently, such as every hour or two, the analgesic regime should be reviewed.

Transdermal fentanyl (see below) is probably the most obvious exception to the above rules, in that patients will need another opioid to take as breakthrough. Fentanyl patches take approximately 18 hours to achieve 50% of the eventual baseline plasma level (Newshan & Lefkowitz 2001), which raises three considerations: first, full analgesia can take around 24 hours or more to achieve when starting (Kornick et al. 2003; Quigley 2005); second, stopping a fentanyl patch is associated with a delayed end to the analgesic affect (Lehmann & Zech 1992); and third, obviously, patients cannot be prescribed one-sixth of a patch for breakthrough pain. Oramorph® or normal-release oxycodone is usually prescribed for breakthrough pain if tolerated, and occasionally sublingual or buccal fentanyl if advised by a pain specialist. The correct breakthrough dose for a 25 µg/hour fentanyl patch is approximately 15 mg of Oramorph, though this will depend on the individual response of each patient (see Table 7.1).

The management of incident pain

Normal-release morphine or oxycodone is commonly used prior to movement for incident pain. However, they can take some time to come into effect, for the patient to move with ease, and for some patients the persisting effects of the opioid can cause side effects and drowsiness once the movement is over (Hanks 1991; Mercadante 1997). Sublingual or buccal fentanyl and alfentanil can be tried as alternatives under specialist guidance, as they are rapid and short-acting opioids (Blick & Wagstaff 2006). Sometimes specialists may try adjuvant analgesics such as gabapentin or ketamine for preventing pain on movement, particularly pain due to bone metastases (Jackson et al. 2001; Caraceni et al. 2008; Mercadante et al. 2009).

Side effects of opioid analgesics

Side effects of opioids include constipation, nausea and itching, which can be widespread or sometimes may just be an irritatingly itchy nose! Opioid-induced constipation is very common, and patients should have access to regular aperients (SIGN 106 guideline) as opioids cause slow bowel transit, increase tone in the lower bowel sphincter and, because the stool is in the colon for a longer period, more water is absorbed and it becomes hardened (Liu & Wittbrodt 2002; Kurz & Sessler 2003). This two-fold problem requires aperients which act as a softener such as sodium docusate and a stimulant such as bisacodyl (SIGN, 2008), taking care that the stimulant does not cause colic pains. A good choice for patients with end-stage cancer is co-danthramer, as it contains both a softener and a stimulant. However, attentive nursing care is important as codanthramer can cause rashes if the stool is left in contact with the skin (Lennard-Jones 1994), and is best avoided in those patients with no sensation of passing stool, such as those with spinal cord compression.

Opioid-induced nausea is generated in the brain at the chemoreceptor trigger zone via the neurotransmitter, dopamine; the best antiemetics to use are therefore those that act at that site such as metoclopramide, domperidone, haloperidol or levomepromazine (Twycross & Wilcox 2001). The choice will depend on a careful assessment of the patient, bearing in mind the presence of other conditions and any contraindications.

Opioid-induced itching is a difficult symptom to treat, and if changing the opioid is not effective then various interventions can be tried. These range from soothing baths and lotions such as simple calamine, oatmeal or menthol, and antihistamines, to the more effective 5-hydroxytryptophan-3 (5HT3) antagonist and antiemetic, ondansetron (Fransway & Winkelmann 1998; Twycross et al 2003). Unfortunately the latter may also cause constipation (Aapro 2005; Sykes 2006).

Nurses have an important role in detecting and assessing the severity and distress caused by side effects. Communicating with patients with empathy and understanding and assisting patients with procedures in an attempt to minimise their discomfort is fundamental. Sometimes cooling the air, changing the position of the patient and spending time interacting with the patient may help distract the patient and thereby alleviate some of their distress.

Opioid toxicity

The aim in controlling pain using opioids is always to achieve optimal analgesia with a minimum of side effect and without causing toxicity. Unfounded worries about opioid toxicity may needlessly hinder timely and effective pain control by practitioners and patients alike. However, the reality of toxicity can be distressing and, at worst, dangerous for patients, so it should never be ignored. This makes understanding opioid toxicity extremely important, particularly for nurses and junior doctors who may be the first to observe and detect the signs of toxicity.

Opioid toxicity should not be confused with the *side effects* of opioids. The cause of opioid toxicity depends on the patient. The patient may simply have been prescribed too much opioid or, if the pain is only partially responsive to opioid, as analgesia is not achieved, opioids just accumulate. There may also be an accumulation of opioid metabolites. Some opioids are metabolised by the body into a series of compounds which are then excreted by the kidneys. Some of these metabolites are active, particularly those of morphine and diamorphine (Lötsch 2005). If these metabolites build up they produce the same effect as too much opioid. Many opioids are cleared by the kidneys, so the opioid and its metabolites will also accumulate if a patient becomes dehydrated or has or develops renal impairment. In such situations, opioids are prescribed which are not excreted via the kidneys. As a general rule, morphine should be avoided in renal failure, with fentanyl or alfentanil being appropriate alternatives. It should also be remembered that serious opioid toxicity can occur if the pain is suddenly controlled by a different means, for example after radiotherapy, nerve block or addition of an adjuvant (Mercadante & Portenoy 2001a).

The spectrum of signs and symptoms of opioid toxicity include seeing 'shadows' at the peripheries of the visual fields, varying degrees of drowsiness, vivid 'real' dreams at night, myoclonic muscle twitching, feeling vague, disorientated, muddled or confused (Quigley 2005), and eventually reduced consciousness and even respiratory depression if left untreated. Toxicity usually develops gradually, although occasionally a patient can be extremely sensitive to opioids, reinforcing the wisdom of beginning opioids at a low dose, particularly in opioid-naïve patients (Mercadante et al. 2006). Fears of giving Oramorph® to patients on opioids and in pain, and causing immediate respiratory depression, are unfounded as long as the opioids are initiated and titrated properly (Ravenscroft & Schneider 2000; Hanks et al. 2005). Notwithstanding this, staff, patients and their families should all be alert for the early signs of opioid toxicity whilst titrating a patient's opioid, as, when mild, patients often ignore these signs. It is good practice to ask about such possible symptoms at regular intervals as they can develop unexpectedly if the patient suddenly becomes physiologically less able to clear the opioids from their system (Kinghorn & Gaines 2007).

The management of opioid toxicity

There is a balance to be achieved between the analgesic effects and the unwanted 'toxic' effects when using opioids; too little opioid leaves the patient with untreated pain, too much can cause sedation and confusion (Fallon and O'Neill 1998). As indicated above, it is always important that the patient's hydration is optimal and maintained. When opioid toxicity occurs this may require support with parenteral fluids (Bruera et al. 1995).

- If the patient is pain-free, the probability is that too much opioid has been prescribed and should be reduced by one-third (Indelicato & Portenoy 2002; NHS Lothian et al. 2009).
- If a patient requires opioid to relieve pain and the additional opioid doses completely relieve their pain, despite signs and symptoms of opioid toxicity, it is likely that the patient has opioid-responsive pain but has metabolite accumulation. In this case, changing to another opioid should be considered (Indelicato & Portenoy 2002; Mercadante et al. 2009).
- If the pain is uncontrolled and the breakthrough opioid doses are only partially effective or ineffective, an adjuvant analgesic should be considered, although a trial of a different opioid may sometimes be considered.

All such decisions will, as indicated above, depend on ongoing careful pain assessment. Rarely, a patient may unexpectedly become so opioid toxic that the respiratory rate reduces to less than 8 breaths per minute and the level of consciousness falls concomitantly. Specialist help should be sought and a dilute solution of low doses of the opioid antagonist naloxone may be cautiously administered intravenously, with increments of 40–80 μg until the patient's respiratory rate improves, regardless of whether or not the patient awakens or becomes alert. Alternatively an intramuscular dose of 100 μg may be given if intravenous access is not easily obtainable. It must be remembered that too great a dose may improve the consciousness level but will also reverse the analgesic effect, and while the naloxone is still active, the returning pain will be resistant to subsequent opioids. This emphasises the need for specialist advice and written protocols in this situation (NHS Lothian et al. 2009).

Changing the route of opioid administration

Patients with cancer pain may reach a stage where the oral route of opioid administration is no longer appropriate, for example, if a patient can no longer swallow due to tumour obstruction, or the patient is vomiting, or because he or she is in the last stages of their illness and is no longer sufficiently alert to take tablets consistently. The choice is commonly that of a 24-hour subcutaneous infusion in a syringe driver. It is important to recognise that opioids may be more potent when the route is changed. For instance, morphine given as an injection, whether intravenously, intramuscularly or subcutaneously, is approximately twice as potent as when given orally (see Table 7.1). As an example, a regimen of 30 mg of MST twice daily (60 mg per day) would be changed to 30 mg of subcutaneous morphine as a 24-hour infusion in a syringe driver. The breakthrough dose would be 5 mg morphine given as a subcutaneous injection 1–2 hourly as required for pain.

Misconceptions about strong opioids

It is always important to address any misconceptions about opioids on the part of patient and family. For trust to be established in the use of these potent medications, the time spent ensuring full understanding of any potent medication is invaluable. As indicted at the outset of this chapter, the lay person, and even many healthcare professionals, may have worrying misconceptions about the use of opioids, fearing oversedation or the individual being no longer 'themselves', and may even fear that opioids cause death (Jacobsen et al. 2007; Vallerand et al. 2007; Al-Atiyyat 2008). What is often not fully realised is that when someone with cancer approaches the end of their life, the natural process is often to become increasingly tired, to do less and sleep more as their consciousness gradually decreases. Symptoms such as pain, agitation and nausea can disturb this and prevent a peaceful sleep, and although the medications given for these can contribute to the reduced level of consciousness, it is usually not the medications that are primarily causing this as the end of life approaches. Understanding this as a healthcare professional and explaining the situation to patients and their relatives can help them to appreciate the value of opioids. Of course, many individuals at an earlier stage in their cancer journey, although they might know their lives are limited, might not be ready to discuss end-of-life issues, even as part of an explanation about opioids, and such readiness must be sensitively assessed.

Another commonly cited concern associated with the use of morphine is addiction. There are several important distinctions between opioid use for pain and the addiction of opioid abuse. The first is the psychological addiction. Portenoy (1990) described addiction to opioids as being characterised by behaviour indicative of psychological dependence and a compulsive use of the drug, with associated drug-related activity. In contrast, cancer patients prefer to continue to take opioid to prevent recurrence of the pain, but if the pain can be controlled by other means, opioids may be reduced and even sometimes discontinued (Portenoy 1990; O'Neill & Fallon 1997). The caveat is that patients' bodies do become 'used to' the opioid, developing 'physical tolerance', and if the opioids are discontinued too suddenly, a physical withdrawal reaction may be experienced. Care is therefore taken to only gradually reduce the prescribed opioids when a patient's pain experience improves through other means, such as nerve blocks, surgery or radiotherapy (Portenoy 1990; O'Neill & Fallon 1997). However, this physiological tolerance is very different from the psychological addiction of opioid misuse when reducing and stopping opioids is notoriously difficult.

Additionally, when patients are prescribed morphine for pain, they are taking this purely for pain, and not for some other psychological secondary gain, and so their bodies will respond differently to those of substance misusers. In substance misuse, the individual takes the opioid to experience a 'high' or euphoric effect, and increasing amounts will be required to continue to get the euphoric effect as tolerance increases (Cornwell 1993). By contrast, euphoria is rarely reported in patients receiving opioids for the relief of pain (Portenoy 1996). Patients with cancer-related pain do not seem to become tolerant to the analgesic effects of opioids, and so do not usually require higher doses unless their pain actually worsens (Portenoy 1996; O'Neill & Fallon 1997).

The use of adjuvant analgesics

This is the part of the WHO ladder which might almost look like an afterthought in its simplicity. However, it is in fact where the complexity of achieving optimal analgesia may be seen. Although many different types of pain can be completely controlled with opioids without unwanted 'toxic' effects or the use of adjuvants, some cannot (Vielhaber & Portenoy 2002; Lussier et al. 2004); in these cases, if the opioids continue to be increased, patients will show all the hallmarks of unacceptable opioid toxicity before pain relief is achieved (Portenoy et al. 1990). In such cases adjuvant analgesics are invaluable.

An adjuvant is a medication primarily indicated for other reasons but which also has an analgesic effect (Lussier et al. 2004). Adjuvants are usually used in conjunction with opioids, and are nowadays often considered as 'co-analgesics', sometimes used as first-line therapy, particularly in neuropathic pain (Dworkin et al. 2003; McGeeney 2008). They can be used at all stages of the WHO ladder. Choosing and using adjuvant analgesics depends on a skilled pain assessment.

Some examples of adjuvant medication include:

- Corticosteroids have been shown to reduce spontaneous discharge in injured nerves (Mercadante & Portenoy 2001c) and are effective at reducing inflammation and tumour-related oedema. This makes them useful in the treatment of neuropathic pain, headache due to brain metastases, and liver capsule pain due to liver metastases (Watanabe & Bruera 1994). High-dose dexamethasone (8–16 mg) is widely used in palliative care thanks to its long duration of action, making it suitable for morning administration, particularly as corticosteroids can interfere with sleep. For most patients, the aim is to reduce the dose over time, aiming for the lowest dose which still controls symptoms, in order to minimise the side effects, which can include proximal myopathy, psychosis and weight gain (Fine et al. 2004).

- For neuropathic pain the anticonvulsant medications gabapentin and pregabalin are often employed. Originally designed to act via the inhibitory neurotransmitter, gamma-aminobutyric acid (GABA), it appears they are actually more likely to act through other mechanisms, probably by binding to specific calcium channels and thus interfering with nerve conduction (Maneuf et al. 2001; Stahl 2004; Taylor 2009). Gabapentin is started at 100–300 mg at night and titrated gradually to optimal effect over days and weeks, to a dose of between 300 mg and 1800 mg daily in three or four divided doses, or even higher under specialist supervision. Its main side effects are drowsiness and dizziness, but if titrated slowly and carefully, it is usually well tolerated (Fine et al. 2004; Lussier et al. 2004).

- Amitryptiline is a tricyclic antidepressant, with properties effective in relieving neuroptathic pain, used at much lower doses than those used to treat depression. It antagonises many neurotransmitters, which are thought to interfere with the process of nerve conduction but which also account for its many side effects such as dry mouth and sedation, which can limit its acceptability and use (Stahl 2000; McGeeney 2004).

- Ketamine is an *N*-methyl-ᴅ-aspartate (NMDA) antagonist, particularly useful in centrally mediated neuropathic pain (see below under the heading 'Central neuropathic pain'). It is a specialist drug, which can be given as constant or 'burst' therapy, orally or parenterally, and can help to abolish central sensitisation (see below under the heading 'Central neuropathic pain') and improve the responsiveness of the pain to opioid (Jackson et al. 2001; Bell et al. 2003; Good et al. 2005). Its side effects include severe hypertension and mood and psychotomimetic effects, and patients need to be carefully monitored during titration (Campbell-Fleming & Williams 2008).

- Parenteral lidocaine (intravenous bolus, or subcutaneous infusion) is sometimes used by specialists in a controlled environment for severe, intractable and neuropathic pain. It blocks sodium channels and therefore interferes with the action potential and signal along pain nerves (Ferrini 2000; Ferrini & Paice 2004; Fine et al. 2004).

- Of course there are other medications which can help different pains such as hyoscine (hydrobromide or butylbromide), which is an anticholinergic smooth muscle relaxant, and will help the pain of gastrointestinal colic, by diminishing spasm (Ripamonti 1994). If tolerated, NSAIDs can have a particular role in metastatic bone pain (Mercadante et al. 1999), as can intermittent intravenous bisphosphonate, for metastatic bone pain in certain types of cancer (Mannix et al. 2000). Although not commonly considered an adjuvant, there is even an argument for calling complementary therapies such as acupuncture an adjuvant therapy.

- Oncological treatment such as radiotherapy and certain chemotherapy can be useful in palliation of pain and potentially thought of as adjuvant therapy (Fine et al. 2004) (see below, under 'Cancer therapies and the management of pain').

The specific challenge of neuropathic pain

Neuropathic pain is present in up to 40% of cancer pain syndromes (Caraceni & Portenoy 1999), and, as it is managed in a different way from other pain, it is important that it is understood and recognised. Nociceptive pain, described earlier under the heading 'Pain pathways', is detected within a normal nervous system, as most types of pain are detected. However, sometimes the nerves which make up the pain system become damaged or distorted, causing an abnormal signal to reach the brain. This may result in pain being perceived in the absence of a stimulus, or in response to a normally non-painful stimulus (McGeeney 2008). It may even be that although there was originally a nociceptive pain, the experience of pain persists long after the 'cause' has gone. This is neuropathic pain, the name meaning that it is pain originating from or within an abnormal nervous system.

There are two main types of neuropathic pain: peripheral neuropathic pain, where the nerve which carries the impulses to the spinal cord is damaged and central neuropathic pain, where the spinal cord and/or brain is damaged or distorted in some way. Neuropathic pain poses a challenge as it is often only partially responsive to opioids (Portenoy et al. 2005). It is here that certain adjuvant medications can be particularly beneficial.

Peripheral neuropathic pain

A peripheral nerve can easily be damaged by tumour in a patient with cancer, and damaged nerves can spontaneously discharge, or discharge with very little stimulation (Paice 2003). There are several indications in a pain assessment which suggest neuropathic pain (Fine et al. 2004):

- It often 'shoots', 'like an electric shock', along the course of a nerve (rather like the pain of sciatica).
- Because the fibres that sense temperature often run alongside the pain fibres, patients may describe neuropathic pain as being burning, cold or tingling.
- It may be in an area of obvious nerve dysfunction if the tumour has damaged motor and sensory nerves, or even just felt in an area where the skin is more numb, has 'pins and needles' sensations, is very painful to the lightest of touches, or the patient cannot detect changes in temperature in that area, all of which are clues that the pain may be neuropathic.
- Because most patients have not previously experienced neuropathic pain, they often do not have anything with which to compare the pain and find it difficult to describe.
- Because the pain starts by direct irritation of the pain nerve, it 'bypasses' the pain receptors, and can send a maximal signal to the spinal cord. This means that the pain severity can seem out of proportion compared to what might be expected.
- Finally, as indicated, neuropathic pains are often not well controlled by opioids alone. When any pain is unresponsive to opioids or a patient becomes easily toxic despite trying a variety of opioids, the possibility of neuropathic pain should be considered.

Peripheral neuropathic pain can be treated with tricyclic antidepressants, such as low-dose amitryptiline, or an anticonvulsant such as carbamazepine or gabapentin, the latter of which has been licensed for neuropathic pain, making it a popular prescribing choice, and patients seem to tolerate these well if started at a low dose and titrated slowly (Lussier et al. 2004). Patients may find it helpful to think of neuropathic pain as that due to overactive nerves and the adjuvant drugs used to treat the pain as active in 'calming down' the nerve activity, although such drugs are normally for conditions such as depression or epilepsy. Although this is a simplistic explanation, many of these drugs indeed act to interrupt the signal along the pain nerves: lidocaine and phenytoin are sodium channel antagonists and thus inhibit the action potential along the nerve (Moshe 2000; Devor 2006); gabapentin and pregabalin are thought now to act through other mechanisms (Maneuf et al. 2001, Stahl 2004); probably by binding to specific calcium channels (Taylor 2009); amitryptiline antagonises many neurotransmitters, which are thought to interfere with the process of nerve conduction but which also account for its many side effects (Stahl 2000).

Central neuropathic pain

Due to the ability of the CNS to change over time, termed 'plasticity', the CNS can become more sensitive to the input it receives from the peripheral nervous system (Mercadante & Portenoy 2001b). It is thought that when pain is unremitting and uncontrolled for any length of time and pain fibres are persistently stimulated, receptors for NMDA can be activated (Herrero et al. 2000), making the central neurons hyperexcitable, altering the function of the dorsal horn cells (Attal & Bouhassira 1999) such that a much stronger signal is transmitted to the brain. In addition, there are likely to be many other chemical changes involving excitatory neurotransmitters. This abnormal state is called central sensitisation (Dworkin et al. 2003). Some pain fibres which normally only respond to non-painful stimuli (Aβ fibres) may 'rewire' to another part of the spinal cord which normally detects painful stimuli via pain fibres (Aδ and C fibres) (Fine et al. 2004).

For the individual, distressing features become evident. Previously innocuous stimuli are now perceived as painful (allodynia), weakly painful stimuli may be detected as very painful (hyperalgesia), a painful stimulus may be felt very deeply, persisting over time (hyper-pathia), or the site of the pain may widen so that it is felt over a larger area. Worse still, because the CNS detects more pain, the NMDA receptors are further activated and an ever-increasing spiral of distress is created (Herrero et al. 2000). Rapid and effective control of pain is therefore the most effective way to prevent the development of central sensitisation. In addition, it should be noted that opioids are generally less able to control pain mediated by activated NMDA receptors, and central sensitisation often results in opioid-resistant pain.

It is possible to interrupt central sensitisation by 'aggressive' pain control measures or by using drugs such as ketamine, which blocks the action of NMDA (Lussier et al. 2004), or methadone, a potent, long-acting opioid with some NMDA-blocking activity (Gorman et al. 1997). The use of these medications requires specialist expertise. (See Case study 7.1, which illustrates the assessment and management of a patient with neuropathic pain.)

Other pain-relieving measures

Cancer therapies and the management of pain

Radiotherapy can be a very useful treatment for pain, particularly when patients have discrete sites of tumour-associated pain, such as isolated bony metastases (Price et al. 1986; McQuay et al. 2000). However, there is a limit to the number of times an area can be treated with radiotherapy, and some tumours are more radiosensitive than others. This means that the analgesic benefit of radiotherapy can differ from one tumour type to another. The oncologist will be able to discuss the relative merits of utilising radiotherapy for pain, particularly in a patient who may be struggling with adverse effects from analgesics. Chemotherapy can occasionally be considered for some suitable patients with cancer pain although the patient's ability to tolerate this must be carefully considered on each occasion.

Complementary and alternative therapy

Informally, individuals have always used non-pharmacological methods such as rubbing or massaging painful areas, or using warmth or cold to relieve pain. Indeed, there is some evidence for the benefits of massage, heat and acupuncture in the relief of cancer pain (Weiger et al. 2002; Fellowes, 2004; Liu & Fawcett 2008). Of course there are other complementary therapies which anecdotally some patients report as helpful, for which high-quality evidence of their efficacy has not been found, such as reiki, reflexology and hot stone therapy. Unfortunately the evidence base for complementary therapy in terms of large-scale double-blind randomised controlled trials is poor, due mainly to methodological problems such as finding an adequate placebo, the individualised nature of each therapy and funding issues (Nahin & Strauss 2001).

There are guidelines for the use of complementary therapies in cancer patients, including comprehensive guidelines from the Prince's Foundation for Integrated Health, which covers topics such as ensuring massage is not performed on patients with low platelets, directly over an area of cancer or bony metastases, or over a suspected deep venous thrombosis (Prince's Foundation for Integrated Health and National Council for Hospice and Specialist Services 2003). As long as safety guidelines are adhered to and the patient gains benefit, there is no reason for patients not to try certain complementary therapies, although these are often not provided within the National Health Service.

Acupuncture in particular is gaining more favour within the medical population when practised as the so-called 'western approach acupuncture', where an orthodox clinical diagnosis is made, and acupuncture provided (Filshie 2004; White et al. 2008). Acupuncture is thought to work by causing the endogenous release of a variety of substances, including 'natural' opioids (Filshie 2004). Some studies have found that when the opioid antagonist, naloxone, is given to patients with electro-acupuncture-induced analgesia, the pain returns (Han & Sun 1990). Leng (1999) audited the use of acupuncture in a palliative care service and found it to be clinically useful in patients with cancer pain: 62% of patients with pain had a good or excellent response to acupuncture, although the greatest benefits were with pain of musculoskeletal origin. However, in common with other complementary therapies, large randomised controlled trials have not been conducted.

Although many patients feel that herbal medication is 'natural' and therefore harmless, some remedies contain potent chemicals. It must be noted that many of our traditional medicines, including digoxin, quinine and atropine, originated from plants (Rates 2001). In addition, herbal medication can potentiate or reduce the effect of other prescribed medication, to potentially dangerous effect (Ernst 2001). It is therefore necessary for patients to discuss the possibility of their use with their medical team as well as a fully trained herbal practitioner before commencement of herbal therapies. Homeopathic intervention, whereby a prepared tincture is said to act by an increase in potency with serial dilution, may also be considered. However, Ernst (2001) argues that such remedies are so dilute that there is probably no pharmacologically active substance left in the solution to interfere with the prescribed medication, and may therefore be used alongside conventional medicine if the patient feels homeopathy is of benefit.

Other means of relieving pain focus on essential communication and interpersonal skills and in harnessing the individual's own psychological resources to ease pain. Such interventions include relaxation techniques, guided imagery and simple distraction techniques. Ensuring that patients feel secure and have trust in those working with them to relieve pain is essential to optimal pain relief. Also not to be forgotten are the simple caring, comfort measures integral to the nurse's role.

Relieving pain at the end of life

Pain in patients whose life is nearing its end requires a different form of intervention from that described above. The most important aim at this stage is to maximise the comfort of the patient and for them to be entirely pain-free. Some of the adverse effects of medications described above may be of secondary importance when the state of consciousness of the patient is already lowered. Most patients' pain relief can be maintained with an opioid, either alone or in combination with a benzodiazepine, even if they are no longer able to take other medications. It is of importance to recognise that many patients who are at the end of life may experience 'terminal agitation', a severe restlessness that can coexist alongside pain or opioid toxicity, or may be worsened by pain or opioid toxicity (De Stoutz et al. 1995). Such agitation should be carefully assessed alongside any pain and, if no easily reversible cause is found, it is best treated with a subcutaneous infusion of a benzodiazepine such as midazolam. If the patient remains agitated, levomepromazine, a useful agent in agitated, terminally ill patients, may be administered in larger doses than those used for nausea (O'Neill and Fountain 1999; 12.5–50 mg is commonly used in such circumstance, rather than the much smaller doses of 2.5–5 mg used for nausea (Kennett et al. 2005; NHS Lothian 2009). The reader is referred to Chapter 12 for a detailed exploration of end-of-life cancer care.

Conclusion

The management of a patient with cancer-related pain can be complex. Identification of the different types of physical pain a patient is experiencing is key to successful management, but equally crucial is the recognition that both physiological and psychosocial factors are involved in the experience of pain. Healthcare professionals have a myriad of pharmacological and non-pharmacological resources at their disposal, though none may be individually perfect. However, with careful and compassionate assessment and team-working between the patient, family, generalist doctors and nurses, specialist doctors and nurses, social workers, chaplain and the wider multidisciplinary team, it should be possible to achieve the alleviation of pain for patients with cancer and enable them, even in advanced disease, to maintain a desired quality of life.

Case study 7.1   Mrs D: assessing and managing her cancer pain

Mrs D was a 74-year-old woman who attended her general practitioner, complaining of pain. She had been diagnosed with colon cancer two years previously, and now had been diagnosed with bone and lung metastases from which she was currently asymptomatic. She had had vague intermittent abdominal pain, thought to be tumour-related with a neuropathic component, for which she was taking gabapentin 600 mg at night, MST 30 mg twice daily, and Oramorph® 10 mg when she needed it for pain. This regime had so far kept her comfortable. As she also lived with type 2 diabetes, she was being visited twice a week by her district nurse to check her blood sugar whilst taking the corticosteroid dexamethasone (4 mg) to improve her appetite and sense of wellbeing. After initial social pleasantries, the following is her initial pain assessment.

Initial pain assessment

GP	Mrs D
Where is the pain?	(pointing to circular area lateral mid thigh) 'Right here in the middle of my right thigh.'
Does it go anywhere else?	'No, not really. It just seems to be here, really deep inside.'
Is it there all the time or does it come and go?	'No, it's sore all the time, but it's worse when I stand on the leg.'
Does anything make the pain worse or better?	'Well, it gets really bad when I stand on the leg. It eases when I sit down. Sometimes I forget about it when my family visit, but not always.'
And what does the pain feel like?	'Oh, it is very sore.'
Is it a dull sore, like an ache, or is it sharp?	'Well most of the time it is a deep achy soreness, but it's sharp like a knife when I stand on it.'
You said it's very sore. How severe is the pain – out of ten, if 1 is like a scratch and 10 is the worst pain you could imagine?	'It's about 4 or 5 when I'm sitting here in the chair, and when my district nurse makes me comfortable with cushions, but it's 9 out of 10 when I stand up to move about and try to do things.'
Does your Oramorph help the pain?	'It does help but not completely. I'm taking it about three, maybe four, times a day, but it makes me feel sleepy when I take it that much. It doesn't help much with the standing up pain.'

On examination, the lateral right mid-femur area was tender to firm palpation but there was no altered sensation in that area. The pain corresponded to the areas of known metastatic bone disease on her last bone scan.

Likely pain diagnosis: Bone pain secondary to bone metastases.

Management decisions, rationales and effectiveness

Mrs D's GP discussed her case with the community palliative care specialist nurse associated with the local hospice as to how to optimise her quality of life. Mrs D refused the suggested radiotherapy, despite reassurances that this would likely be a gentle treatment and unlikely to cause ill effects; she was influenced by the memories of her late husband, who had 'suffered with chemotherapy and radiotherapy when he had cancer' although she could not remember any details of his cancer or why radiotherapy was given. The NSAID, diclofenac sodium, was prescribed for the bone pain, which helped to alleviate her background pain. The morphine was changed to oxycodone as it was felt the former would cause toxic effects if the dose were increased. OxyContin® 15 mg twice daily and 5 mg OxyNorm® as needed were commenced. In the first instance, Mrs D was advised to use OxyNorm® prior to planned movement for her incident pain. Mrs D quickly became more comfortable. Although sublingual alfentanil was considered for this incident pain for its faster onset and shorter duration of action, it was not tried, as taking OxyNorm prior to movement worked well for Mrs D without causing excessive sedative effects. She remained comfortable and independent at home for two further months before needing further medical input.

Two months later Mrs D was visited at home by her district nurse, who found her not only in severe pain but also sleepy and muddled. The district nurse suspected opioid toxicity due to the presence of new pain, unrelieved by OxyNorm. It was arranged for Mrs D to be seen at home by her GP and specialist community palliative care nurse.

Pain assessment

Doctor and nurse	Mrs D
Exactly where is the pain?	'It's my left leg, all over, even down to my toes.'
Does it go anywhere else?	'No, not really. Just the leg.'
Does it start all over your leg, or does it start in one place and spread out?	'It starts all over the back of my thigh, then it spreads all over my thigh, then spreads all down my leg and all round it.'
Is it there all the time or does it come and go?	'It's not always there, but it suddenly comes and is really sore for ages.'
Does anything set off the pain?	'No, it just seems to come.'

And what does the pain feel like; is it a sharp pain or a dull pain?

'Well, I don't know. It's really hard. It feels . . . weird. . . burning, but not on my skin, deep inside. It feels like. . . sunburn but on the inside. And it's a really sore burning.'

How often are you getting the pain, and how long does it last?

'It's coming three or four times a day and can last for an hour. Nothing can distract me from this pain.'

You said it's very sore. How severe is the pain – out of ten, if 1 is like a scratch and 10 is the worst pain you could imagine?

'I'd say 12 out of 10! It feels like I'm on fire. But there's nothing there you know; it's not even hot when you touch it.'

Does your Oramorph® help the pain?

'No, not at all. Nothing helps. I just think it's going to get worse and worse, and nothing will take it away, and I'm going to die like this.'

Does your leg feel weak?

'My leg is a bit weaker I think, though it might just be the pain. I certainly don't want to go walking on it, put it that way.'

Have you any back pain? How are your bowels and bladder?

'My bowel and bladder are fine. I've always got a bit of back pain, it's called old age. Can't you sort out my pain now?'

Pain diagnosis: Neuropathic leg pain, possibly due to spinal cord compression, possibly due to pelvic lymph node compression of leg nerves.

Management decisions, rationales and effectiveness

Importantly, Mrs D's district nurse had suspected that this was a new pain and alerted her doctor and specialist nurse, which was crucial in this case. As Mrs D was known to have bone metastases and as she now had new neuropathic pain and possibly leg weakness, there was a possibility that she had spinal metastases and the potentially serious complication of spinal cord compression (SCC); an emergency, as SCC can lead to irreversible loss of leg movement and loss of bowel and bladder function if not relieved quickly. Mrs D was immediately given high-dose corticosteroids, 16 mg dexamethasone, to reduce any tumour-associated oedema which would exacerbate any compression. It was suggested she was immediately admitted to the local acute hospital for a magnetic resonance imaging (MRI) scan of her spine with a view to offering radiotherapy. Although she still had reservations about accepting radiotherapy, after careful explanation and discussion of her current condition and because of the trust established with her care team she could now accept its real benefits. Fortunately, no SCC was found and the cause of her neuropathic pain was therefore thought to be secondary to local lymph node compression. After a few days, the decision was made to transfer her to the hospice for their specialised expertise in pain control and end-of-life care. Mrs D herself felt she had become frail over the previous few weeks and that her time was 'short'; she was now clear that what mattered most to her was to be free from pain.

She continued to receive the high-dose steroid initially, in case inflammation was worsening her neuropathic pain. As she was already taking gabapentin this was increased towards a maximum dose. This provided some analgesia, but the titration process was taking too long without affording her good analgesia. The opioid breakthrough she was using was only partially helpful and caused sedation. She was therefore started on a subcutaneous infusion of ketamine, which helped her pain greatly, and made her OxyNorm 'work again'. Mrs D also found comfort and relaxation from her daughter giving her gentle massage, employing soothing aroma-therapy oils.

In the following weeks, Mrs D became weaker and her previously well-controlled pain became severe, with little relief gained from increasing ketamine. She was agitated, wishing only to be pain-free. 'I don't care if I am sleepy.' She was given increased doses of diamorphine and midazolam, and she slept more peacefully and without pain. She died peacefully ten days later, with her family present.

References

Aapro M (2005) 5-HT-3 receptor antagonists in the management of nausea and vomiting in cancer and cancer treatment. *Oncology* **69**: 97–109.

Al-Atiyyat NMH (2008) Patient-related barriers to effective cancer pain management. *Journal of Hospice & Palliative Nursing* **10**(4): 198–204.

Amunts K, Kedo O, Kindler M, et al. (2005) Cytoarchitectonic mapping of the human amygdala, hippocampal region and entorhinal cortex: intersubject variability and probability maps. *Anatomy and Embryology (Berl)* **210**(5–6): 343–52.

Andersen G, Christrup L, Sjogren P (2003) Relationships among morphine metabolism, pain and side effects during long-term treatment: An update. *Journal of Pain and Symptom Management* **25**(1): 74–91.

Anderson R, Saiers JH, Abram S, Schlicht C (2001) Accuracy in equianalgesic dosing: Conversion dilemmas. *Journal of Pain and Symptom Management* **21**(5): 397–406.

Attal N, Bouhassira D (1999) Mechanisms of pain in peripheral neuropathy. *Acta Neurologica Scandinavica Suppl* **173**: 12–24.

Arber A (2004) Is pain what the patient says it is? Interpreting an account of pain. *International Journal of Palliative Nursing* **10**(10): 491–6.

Bell RF, Eccleston C, Kalso E (2003) Ketamine as adjuvant to opioids for cancer pain: A qualitative systematic review. *Journal of Pain and Symptom Management* **26**(3): 867–75.

Blackburn D, Somerville E, Squire J (2002) Methadone: an alternative conversion regime. *European Journal of Palliative Care* **9**: 93–6.

Blick SKA, Wagstaff AJ (2006) Fentanyl Buccal Tablet in breakthrough pain in opioid-tolerant patients with cancer. *Drugs* **66**(18): 2387–93.

Bruera E, Franco JJ, Maltoni M, Watanabe S, Suarez-Almazor M (1995) Changing pattern of agitated impaired mental status in patients with advanced cancer: Association with cognitive monitoring, hydration, and opioid rotation. *Journal of Pain and Symptom Management* **10**(4), 287–91.

Bruera E, Belzile M, Pituskin E, et al. (1998) Randomized, double-blind, cross-over trial comparing safety and efficacy of oral controlled-release oxycodone with controlled-release morphine in patients with cancer pain. *Journal of Clinical Oncology* **16**: 3222–9.

Campbell-Fleming JM, Williams A (2008) The use of ketamine as adjuvant therapy to control severe pain. *Clinical Journal of Oncology Nursing* **12**(1): 102–7.

Caraceni A, Portenoy RK (1999) An international survey of cancer pain characteristics and syndromes. IASP Task Force on Cancer Pain. International Association for the Study of Pain. *Pain* **82**(3): 263–74.

Caraceni A, Cherny N, Fainsinger R, et al. and the Steering Committee of the EAPC Research Network (2002) Pain measurement tools and methods in clinical research in palliative care: Recommendations of an Expert Working Group of the European Association of Palliative Care. *Journal of Pain and Symptom Management* **23**(3): 239–55.

Caraceni A, Zecca E, Martini C, Pigni A, Bracchi P (2008) Gabapentin for breakthrough pain due to bone metastases. *Palliative Medicine* **22**(4): 392–3.

Carrasquillo Y, Gereau RW (2007) Activation of the extracellular signal-regulated kinase in the amygdala modulates pain perception. *Journal of Neuroscience* **27**(7): 1543–51.

Clark D (1999) 'Total pain', disciplinary power and the body in the work of Cicely Saunders, 1958–1967. *Social Science & Medicine* **49**(6): 727–36.

Cleeland CS (1989) Measurement of pain by subjective report. In: Chapman CR, Loeser JD (eds) *Advances in Pain Research and Therapy*, Volume **12**: Issues in Pain Measurement. New York: Raven Press, pp. 391–403.

Cleeland CS (1984) The impact of pain on the patient with cancer. *Cancer* **54**: 2635–41.

Colvin LA, Lambert DG (2008) Editorial I. Pain medicine: advances in basic sciences and clinical practice. *British Journal of Anaesthesia* **101**(1): 1–4.

Cornwell V (1993) Illegal narcotic use. In: Cornwell A, Cornwell V (eds) *Drugs, Alcohol and Mental Health*, 2nd edn. Cambridge: Cambridge University Press, p. 42.

Craig KD (2004) Social communication of pain enhances protective functions: A comment on Deyo, Prkachin and Mercer (2004). *Pain* **107**: 5–6.

Dean M (2004) Opioids in renal failure and dialysis patients. *Journal of Pain and Symptom Management* **28**(5): 497–504.

De Conno F, Caraceni A, Gamba A, et al. (1994) Pain measurement in cancer patients: a comparison of six methods. *Pain* **57**: 161–6.

De Stoutz ND, Bruera E, Suarez-Almazor M (1995) Opioid rotation for toxicity reduction in terminal cancer patients. *Journal of Pain and Symptom Management* **10**(5): 378–84.

Devor M (2006) Sodium channels and mechanisms of neuropathic pain. *Journal of Pain* **7**: S3–12.

Dickman A, Ellershaw J (2004) NSAIDS: gastroprotection or selective COX-2 inhibitor? *Palliative Medicine* **18**: 275–86.

Dworkin RH, Backonja M, Rowbotham MC, et al. (2003) Advances in neuropathic pain: diagnosis, mechanisms, and treatment recommendations. *Archives of Neurology* **60**: 1524–34.

Ebert B, Andersen S, Krogsgaard-Larsen P (1995) Ketobemidone, methadone and pethidine are non-competitive N-methyl-D-aspartate (NMDA) antagonists in the rat cortex and spinal cord (Letter). *Neuroscience* **187**: 165–8.

Ellershaw JE, Kinder C, Aldridge J, Allison M, Smith JC (2002) Care of the dying: Is pain control compromised or enhanced by continuation of the fentanyl transdermal patch in the dying phase? *Journal of Pain and Symptom Management* **24**(4): 398–403.

Ernst E (2001) Herbal and non-herbal medicine. In: Ernst E, Pittler MH, Stevinson C, White A, Eisenberg D (eds) *The Desktop Guide to Complementary and Alternative Medicine: An Evidence-Based Approach*. London: Mosby.

Fallon MT, O'Neill B (1998) Opioid toxicity should be managed initially by decreasing the opioid dose (letter). *BMJ* **317**: 81.

Fellowes D (2004) Aromatherapy and massage for symptom relief in patients with cancer. *Cochrane Database of Sytematic Reviews* **2**: CD002287.

Ferrini R (2000) Parenteral lidocaine for severe intractable pain in six hospice patients continued at home. *Journal of Palliative Medicine* **3**(2): 193–200.

Ferrini R, Paice JA (2004) How to initiate and monitor infusional lidocaine for severe and/or neuropathic pain. *Journal of Supportive Oncology* **2**(1): 90–4.

Filshie J, Thompson JW (2004) Acupuncture. In: Doyle D, Hanks G, Cherny N, Calman K (eds) *Oxford Textbook of Palliative Medicine*, 3rd edn. Oxford: Oxford University Press.

Fine PG, Miaskowski C, Paice JA (2004) Meeting the challenges in cancer pain management. *Journal of Supportive Oncology* **2** (suppl 4): 5–22.

Fitzgerald GA, Patrono C (2001) The coxibs, selective inhibitors of cyclooxygenase-2. *New England Journal of Medicine* **345**(6): 433–42.

Fransway AF, Winkelmann RK (1998) Treatment of pruritus. *Seminars in Dermatology* **7**: 310–25.

Gagnon B, Bielech M, Watanabe S, Walker P, Hanson J, Bruera E (1999) The use of intermittent subcutaneous injections of oxycodone for opioid rotation in patients with cancer pain. *Supportive Care in Cancer* **7**(4): 265–70.

Gardner-Nix J (2001) Oral transmucosal fentanyl and sufentanil for incident pain (letter). *Journal of Pain and Symptom Management* **22**(2): 627–30.

Good P, Tullio F, Jackson K, Goodchild C, Ashby M (2005) Prospective audit of short-term concurrent ketamine, opioid and anti-inflammatory ('triple-agent') therapy for episodes of acute on chronic pain. *Internal Medicine Journal* **35**: 39–44.

Gorman AL, Elliott KJ, Inturrisi CE (1997) The *d*- and *l*- isomers of methadone bind to the non-competitive site on the *N*-methyl-aspartate (NMDA) receptor in rat forebrain and spinal cord. *Neuroscience Letters* **223**(1): 5–8.

Goubert L, Craig KD, Vervoort T, et al. (2005) Facing others in pain: the effects of empathy. *Pain* **118**: 285–8.

Hair PL, Gillian M, Keating GM, McKeage K (2008) Transdermal matrix fentanyl membrane patch (Matrifen®) in severe cancer-related chronic pain. *Drugs* **68**(14): 2001–9.

Han JS, Sun S (1990) Differential release of enkephalin and dynorphin by low and high frequencies electroacupuncture in the central nervous system. *Acupuncture: The Scientific International Journal (New York)* **1**(1): 19–27.

Hanks GW (1991) Opioid-responsive and opioid-non-responsive pain in cancer. *British Medical Bulletin* **47**: 718–31.

Hanks GW (2001) Morphine and alternative opioids in cancer pain: The EAPC recommendations. *British Journal of Cancer* **84**: 587–93.

Hanks G, Cherny NI, Fallon M (2005) Opioid analgesic therapy. In: Doyle D, Hanks G, Cherny N, Calman K (eds) *Oxford Textbook of Palliative Medicine*, 3rd edn. Oxford: Oxford University Press.

Herrero JF, Laird JMA, Lopez-Garcia JA (2000) Wind-up of spinal neurones and pain sensation: much ado about something? *Progress in Neurobiology* **61**: 169–203.

Hølen JC, Saltved I, Fayers PM, Hjermstad MJ, Loge JH, Kaasa S (2007) Doloplus-2, a valid tool for behavioural pain assessment? *BMC Geriatrics* **7**: 29.

Indelicato RA, Portenoy RK (2002) Opioid rotation in the management of refractory cancer pain. *Journal of Clinical Oncology* **20**(1): 348–52.

Jacobsen R, Sjøgren P, Møldrup C, Christrup L (2007) Physician-related barriers to cancer pain management with opioid analgesics: a systematic review. *Journal of Opioid Management* **3**(4): 207–14.

Jackson K, Ashby M, Martin P, Pisasale M, Brumley D, Hayes B (2001) 'Burst' ketamine for refractory cancer pain: an open-label audit of 39 patients. *Journal of Pain and Symptom Management* **22**: 834–42.

Kalso E (2005) Oxycodone. *Journal of Pain and Symptom Management* **29**(5 Suppl): S47–56.

Kennett A, Hardy J, Shah S, A'Hern R (2005) An open study of methotrimeprazine in the management of nausea and vomiting in patients with advanced cancer. *Supportive Care in Cancer* **13**: 715–21.

Kimberlin C, David Brushwood D, Allen W, Radson E, Wilson D (2004) Cancer patient and caregiver experiences: communication and pain management issues. *Journal of Pain and Symptom Management* **28**(6): 566–78.

Kinghorn S, Gaines S (2007) Pain control. In: Kinghorn S, Gaines S (eds) *Palliative Nursing: Improving End Of Life Care*, 2nd edn. London: Churchill Livingstone, p. 36.

Kornick CA, Santiago-Palma J, Moryl N, Payne R, Obbens EAMT (2003) Benefit-risk assessment of transdermal fentanyl for the treatment of chronic pain. *Drug Safety* **26**(13): 951–73.

Kline RH, Wiley RG (2008). Spinal μ-opioid receptor-expressing dorsal horn neurons: role in nociception and morphine antinociception. *Journal of Neuroscience* **28**(4): 904–13.

Kurz A, Sessler DI (2003) Opioid-induced bowel dysfunction: pathophysiology and potential new therapies. *Drugs* **63**: 649–71.

Laverty D (2007) Actiq: an effective oral treatment for cancer-related breakthrough pain. *British Journal of Community Nursing* **12**(7): 311–16.

Lefebvre-Chapiro S (2001) The DOLOPLUS 2 scale – evaluating pain in the elderly. *European Journal of Palliative Care* **8**: 191–4.

Lehmann KA, Zech D (1992) Transdermal fentanyl: clinical pharmacology. *Journal of Pain and Symptom Management* **7**(3 suppl): S8–16.

Lennard-Jones J (1994) Clinical aspects of laxatives, enemas and suppositories. In: Kamm M, Lennard-Jones J (eds) *Constipation*. Petersfield, UK: Wrightson Biomedical Publishing, pp. 327–41.

Leng G (1999) A year of acupuncture in palliative care. *Palliative Medicine* **13**: 163–4.

Levin DN, Cleeland CS (1985) Public attitudes toward cancer pain. *Cancer* **56**: 2337–9.

Liu M, Wittbrodt E (2002) Low-dose oral naloxone reverses opioid induced constipation and analgesia. *Journal of Pain and Symptom Management* **23**(1): 48–53.

Liu Y, Fawcett TN (2008) The role of massage therapy in cancer pain: a review of the evidence. *Nursing Standard* **22**(21): 35–40.

Lötsch J (2005) Opioid metabolites. *Journal of Pain and Symptom Management* **29**(5 suppl): S10–24.

Lussier D, Huskey AG, Portenoy RK (2004) Adjuvant analgesics in cancer pain management. *Oncologist* **9**: 571–91.

Maneuf YP, Hughes J, McKnight AT (2001) Gabapentin inhibits the substance P-facilitated K-(+)-evoked release of [(3)H]glutamate from rat caudial trigeminal nucleus slices. *Pain* **93**: 191–6.

Mannix K, Ahmedzai SH, Anderson H, Bennett M, Lloyd-Williams M, Wilcock A (2000) Using bisphosphonates to control the pain of bone metastases: evidence-based guidelines for palliative care. *Palliative Medicine* **14**(6): 455–61.

McCaffery M (1968) *Nursing Practice Theories Related to Cognition, Bodily Pain and Man–Environment Interactions*. Los Angeles: University of California.

McGeeney BE (2008) Adjuvant agents in cancer pain. *Clinical Journal of Pain* **24**(4 Suppl): S14–20.

McQuay HJ, Collins SL, Carroll D, Moore RA (2000) Radiotherapy for the palliation of painful bone metastases. *Cochrane Database of Systematic Reviews* **2**: CD001793.

Melzack R, Wall PD (1965) Pain mechanisms: a new theory. *Science* **150**(3699): 971–9.

Mercadante S (1997) Malignant bone pain: pathophysiology and treatment. *Pain.* **69**(1–2): 1–18.

Mercadante S, Casuccio A, Agnello A, Pumo S, Kargar J, Garofalo S (1999) Analgesic effects of nonsteroidal anti-inflammatory drugs in cancer pain due to somatic or visceral mechanisms. *Journal of Pain and Symptom Management* **17**(5): 351–6.

Mercadante S, Portenoy RK (2001a) Opioid poorly-responsive cancer pain. Part I: Clinical considerations. *Journal of Pain and Symptom Management* **21**(2): 144–50.

Mercadante S, Portenoy RK (2001b) Opioid poorly-responsive cancer pain. Part 2: Basic mechanisms that could shift dose response for analgesia. *Journal of Pain and Symptom Management* **21** (3): 255–64.

Mercadante S, Portenoy RK (2001c) Opioid poorly-responsive cancer pain. Part 3: Clinical strategies to improve opioid responsiveness. *Journal of Pain and Symptom Management* **21** (4): 338–54.

Mercadante S, Villari P, Ferrera P, Casuccio ABS (2004) Optimization of opioid therapy for preventing incident pain associated with bone metastases. *Journal of Pain and Symptom Management* **28**(5): 505–10.

Mercadante S, Villari P, Ferrera P, Arcuri E, David F (2009) Case Report. Opioid switching and burst ketamine to improve the opioid response in patients with movement-related pain due to bone metastases. *Clinical Journal of Pain* **25**(7): 648–9.

Melzack R (1975) The McGill Pain Questionnaire: major properties and scoring methods. *Pain* **1**(3): 277–99.

Millan M (1999) The induction of pain: an integrative review. *Progress in Neurobiology* **57**: 1–164.

Mitchell D, Gordon T (2007) Making sense of spiritual care. In: Kinghorn S, Gaines S (eds) *Palliative Nursing: Improving End of Life Care*, 2nd edn. London: Churchill Livingstone Elsevier.

Moshe SL (2000) Mechanisms of action of anticonvulsant agents. *Neurology* **55**(suppl 1): S32–40.

Nahin RL, Strauss SE (2001) Research into complementary and alternative medicine: problems and potential. *BMJ* **322**(7279): 161.

Newshan G, Lefkowitz M (2001) Transdermal fentanyl for chronic pain in AIDS: a pilot study. *Journal of Pain and Symptom Management* **21**(1): 69–77.

NHS Lothian in partnership with NHS borders and NHS Lanarkshire (2009) *Palliative Care Guidelines*, 3rd edn. http://www.palliativecareguidelines.scot.nhs.uk/.

O'Neill B, Fallon M (1997) ABC of palliative care: Principles of palliative care and pain control. *BMJ* **315**: 801–4.

O'Neill J, Fountain A (1999) Levomepromazine (methotrimeprazine) and the last 48 hours. *Hospital Medicine* **60**: 564–7.

Paice JA, Toy C, Shott S (1998) Barriers to cancer pain relief: fear of tolerance and addiction. *Journal of Pain and Symptom Management* **16**(1): 1–9.

Paice JA, Cohen FL (1997) Validity of a verbally administered numeric rating scale to measure cancer pain intensity. *Cancer Nursing* **20**(2): 88–93.

Paice JA (2003) Mechanisms and management of neuropathic pain in cancer. *Journal of Supportive Oncology* **1**(2): 107–19.

Pasternak GW (2005) Molecular biology of opioid analgesia. *Journal of Pain and Symptom Management* **29**(5 Suppl): 2–9.

Pereira J, Lawlor P, Vigano A, Dorgan M, Bruera E (2001) Equianalgesic dose ratios for opioids: A critical review and proposals for long-term dosing. *Journal of Pain and Symptom Management* **22**(2): 672–87.

Persson K, Hammarlund-Udenaes M, Mortimer Ö, Rane A (1992) The postoperative pharmacokinetics of codeine. *European Journal of Clinical Pharmacology* **42**: 663–6.

Portenoy RK (1989) Cancer pain epidemiology and symptoms. *Cancer* **63**(11 suppl): 2298–307.

Portenoy RK (1990) Chronic opioid therapy in nonmalignant pain. *Journal of Pain and Symptom Management* **5**(1 suppl): S46–62.

Portenoy RK, Hagen NA (1990) Breakthrough pain: definition, prevalence and characteristics. *Pain* **41**: 273–81.

Portenoy RK, Foley KM, Inturrisi CE (1990) The nature of opioid responsiveness and its implications for neuropathic pain; new hypotheses derived from studies of opioid infusions. *Pain* **43**(3): 273–86.

Portenoy RK (1996) Opioid therapy for chronic non-malignant pain: a review of the critical issues. *Journal of Pain and Symptom Management* **11**(4): 203–17.

Portenoy RK, Forbes K, Lussier D, Hanks G (2005) Difficult pain problems: an integrated approach. In: Doyle D, Hanks G, Cherny N, Calman K (eds) *Oxford Textbook of Palliative Medicine*, 3rd edn. Oxford: Oxford University Press.

Pöyhiä R Vainio A, Kalso E (1993) Oxycodone: an alternative to morphine for cancer pain. A review. *Journal of Pain and Symptom Management* **8**: 63–7.

Price P, Hoskin PJ, Easton D, Austin D, Palmer S, Yarnold JR (1986) Prospective randomised trial of single and multifraction radiotherapy schedules in the treatment of painful bone metastases. *Radiotherapy and Oncology* **6**: 247–55.

Prince's Foundation for integrated Health and National Council for Hospice and Specialist services (2003) *National Guidelines for the Use of Complementary Therapies in Supportive and Palliative Care.* Available at http://www.fih.org.uk/information_library/publications/health_-guidelines/complementary.html (accessed October 2009).

Quiding H, Lundqvist G, Boréus LO, Bondesson U, Ohrvik J (1993) Analgesic effect and plasma concentrations of codeine and morphine after two dose levels of codeine following oral surgery. *European Journal of Clinical Pharmacology* **44**: 319–23.

Quigley C, Wiffen P (2003) A systematic review of hydromorphone in acute and chronic pain. *Journal of Pain and Symptom Management* **25**(2): 169–78.

Quigley C (2005) The role of opioids in cancer pain. *BMJ* **331**(8): 825–9.

Ravenscroft P, Schneider J (2000) Bedside perspectives on the use of opioids: transferring results of clinical research into practice. *Clinical and Experimental Pharmacology and Physiology* **27**: 529–32.

Rates SMK. (2001) Plants as source of drugs. *Toxicon* **39**(5): 603–13.

Rhee C, Broadbent AM (2007) Palliation and liver failure: Palliative Medications Dosage Guidelines. *Journal of Palliative Medicine* **10**(3): 677–85.

Ripamonti C (1994) Management of bowel obstruction in advanced cancer patients. *Journal of Pain and Symptom Management* **9**(3): 193–200.

Saunders C (1963) Distress in dying. (Letter) *BMJ* **2**: 746.

Saunders C (1964) The symptomatic treatment of incurable malignant disease. *Prescribers' Journal* **4**(4): 68–73.

Saunders C (1966) The care of the dying. *Guy's Hospital Gazette* **80**: 136–42.

Saunders C (1996) Into the valley of the shadow of death: a personal therapeutic journey. *BMJ* **313**: 1599–601.

Scottish Intercollegiate Guideline Network (2008) *Clinical Guideline 106. Control of pain in patients with cancer.* Edinburgh: SIGN Secretariat. Available at http://www.sign.ac.uk/guidelines/fulltext/106/index.html.

Singer T, Seymour B, O'Doherty J, Kaube H, Dolan RJ, Frith CD (2004) Empathy for pain involves the affective but not sensory components of pain. *Science* **303**: 1157–62.

Smith T, Gordon T (2009) Developing spiritual and religious competencies in practice: pilot of a Marie Curie blended learning event. *International Journal of Palliative Nursing* **15**(2): 86–93.

Stahl SM (2000) *Essential Psychopharmacology: Neuroscientific Basis and Practical Applications*, 2nd edn. Cambridge: Cambridge University Press, pp. 218–22.

Stahl SM (2004) Anticonvulsants and the relief of chronic pain: pregabalin and gabapentin as alpha (2)delta ligands at voltage-gated calcium channels. *Journal of Clinical Psychiatry* **65**: 596–7.

Steinhauser KE, Christakis NA, Clipp EC, McNeilly M, McIntyre L, Tulsky JA (2000) Factors considered important at the end of life by patients, family, physicians, and other care providers. *Journal of the American Medical Association* **284**: 2476–82.

Streisand JB, Busch MA, Egan TD, Gaylord Smith B, Gay M, Pace NL (1998) Dose proportionality and pharmacokinetics of oral transmucosal fentanyl citrate. *Anesthesiology* **88**: 305–9.

Sullivan MJL (2008) Toward a biopsychomotor conceptualization of pain: implications for research and intervention. *Clinical Journal of Pain* **24**(4): 281–90.

Sykes NP (2006) The pathogenesis of constipation. *Journal of Supportive Oncology* **4**: 213–18.

Tanyi RA (2002) Towards clarification of the meaning of spirituality. *Journal of Advanced Nursing* **39**(5): 500–9.

Taylor CP (2009) Mechanisms of analgesia by gabapentin and pregabalin: calcium channel α_2-δ [$Ca_v\alpha_2$-δ] ligands. *Pain* **142**(1–2): 13–16.

Thomason TE, McCune JS, Bernard SA, Winer EP, Tremont S, Lindlay CM (1998) Cancer Pain Survey: Patient-centred isssues in control. *Journal of Pain and Symptom Management* **15**(5): 275–84.

Twycross R, Greaves MW, Handwerker H, Jones EA, LIbretto SE, Szepietozski JC, Zylicz Z (2003) Itch: scratching more than the surface. *QJM: An International Journal of Medicine* **96**(1): 7–26.

Twycross R, Wilcox A (2001) Alimentary symptoms. In: Twycross R, Wilcox A (eds) *Symptom Management in Advanced Cancer*, 3rd edn. Oxford: Radcliffe Medical Press.

Vallerand AH, Collins-Bohler D, Templin T, Hasenau SM (2007) Knowledge of and barriers to pain management in caregivers of cancer patients receiving homecare. *Cancer Nursing* **30**(1): 31–7.

Ventafridda V, Tamburini M, Caraceni A, DeConno F, Naldi F (1987) A validation study of the WHO method for cancer pain relief. *Cancer* **59**(4): 850–6.

Vielhaber A, Portenoy RK (2002) Advances in cancer pain management. *Haematologic and Oncologic Clinics of North America* **16**: 527–41.

Watanabe S, Bruera E (1994) Corticosteroids as adjuvant analgesics. *Journal of Pain and Symptom Management* **9**(7): 442–5.

Weiger WA, Smith M, Boon H, Richardson MA, Kaptchuk TJ, Eisenberg DM (2002) Advising patients who seek complementary and alternative medical therapies for cancer. *Annals of Internal Medicine* **137**(11): 889–903.

White A, Cummings M, Filshie J (2008) *An Introduction to Western Medical Acupuncture*. Churchill Livingstone Elsevier.

Wilkinson S (2000) Spiritual recognition within palliative care. *International Journal of Palliative Nursing* **6**(1): 4.

Woolf C, Mannion RJ (1999) Neuropathic pain: aetiology, symptoms, mechanisms and management. *Lancet* **353**: 1959–64.

World Health Organization (1986) *Cancer Pain Relief*. Geneva: WHO.

Zaza C, Baine N (2002) Cancer pain and psychosocial factors: a critical review of the literature. *Journal of Pain and Symptom Management* **24**(5): 526–42.

Zech DF, Grond S, Lynch J, Hertel D, Lehmann KA (1995) Validation of World Health Organization Guidelines for cancer pain relief, a 10 year prospective study. *Pain* **63**, 65–76.

Chapter 8

Cancer-related fatigue

Antonia Dean

We all feel fatigue, usually on a daily basis, and numerous research studies suggest that it is one of the most common symptoms that the population as a whole will experience (Hotopf 2004). Some of us feel constantly fatigued and, in the days before acronyms were strongly discouraged, TATT (tired all the time) was a regular feature in the general practitioner's (GP) notes.

Fatigue is also one of the symptoms most commonly reported by patients with cancer, although prevalence rates vary widely (Stone 2002). Cancer-related fatigue has been defined as more severe, more unrelenting and more distressing than the fatigue experienced by healthy people (Holley 2000). In the past few years there has been a swell of research interest in the condition. The number of people diagnosed with cancer is increasing, but as treatments become more effective, people are often living for longer but sometimes with debilitating symptoms. Research is increasingly focusing, not only on living longer with cancer, but on living better and on the reduction of symptoms such as cancer-related fatigue (Fawcett & Dean 2004).

Whether research into cancer-related fatigue has benefited the patient is debatable. Certainly people are often warned that their treatment may cause fatigue. However, my current experience of work on a breast cancer telephone helpline, speaking to patients across the United Kingdom, is that there is very little in place to help people who are living with fatigue. Many interventions for cancer-related fatigue are non-pharmacological, and embracing such therapies may require a change in thinking from the belief that relief from such symptoms can be found only in some form of medication – 'a pill for every ill'.

This chapter will look to address the potential causes and management of cancer-related fatigue and discuss how the National Health Service (NHS) might offer a service that incorporates a wider range of therapeutic interventions that acknowledge the 'survivorship' agenda for those living with cancer. It will also be argued that there is therefore a necessity for national guidelines synthesising all the available evidence to ensure best practice and help healthcare professionals manage cancer-related fatigue in their patients.

Perspectives on Cancer Care. Edited by Josephine (Tonks) N. Fawcett and Anne McQueen
© 2011 Blackwell Publishing Ltd

Definitions of cancer-related fatigue

Fatigue is inherently a subjective experience, which makes both definition and measurement difficult, something which has been identified many times over. The American National Comprehensive Cancer Network (NCCN) describes fatigue as:

> a distressing, persistent, subjective sense of tiredness or exhaustion related to cancer or cancer treatment that is not proportional to recent activity and interferes with usual function.
>
> NCCN (2008: MS-2)

It is questionable whether tiredness needs to interfere with function to be classed as legitimate fatigue, although certainly most studies of the patient experience suggest normal function is usually impaired (Ream & Richardson 1997; Rosman 2009).

Holley (2000) offers a more emotive description:

> More energy draining, more intense, longer lasting, more severe and more unrelenting when compared with 'typical' fatigue.
>
> Holley (2000: 87)

As with pain, fatigue occurs when the patient says it does; the patient is the expert in defining the nature and intensity of their own fatigue and the effect it has on their life. Perhaps one of the difficulties in fully recognising and treating cancer-related fatigue is that we, as healthcare professionals, all have our own experiences and understanding of fatigue. We know what it feels like to be tired and this may lead some practitioners to underestimate the effect of cancer-related fatigue which, according to participants in Wu and McSweeny's study, is 'so much more than being tired' (2007: 117).

The experience of cancer-related fatigue

The literature identifies that almost all areas of a person's life can be affected by cancer-related fatigue. These include (Holley 2000; Barsevick et al. 2001; Armes 2004):

- physical domain;
- psychological domain;
- social domain;
- spiritual domain;
- cognitive domain;
- sense of self.

In addition, although it could easily be incorporated within the categories above, the effect of fatigue on a person's sexual function should also be specifically considered (Dean 2008). This is only very rarely mentioned within the literature but, given the propensity of many cancers, such as breast, prostate or the gynaecological cancers, to have a negative impact on sexuality, it is important to acknowledge the probable effects of this very common symptom on the intimate relationships of cancer patients.

Being fatigued often means that people cannot live their lives in the way they would like to. It may be that they struggle to do their job, look after their children, socialise or exercise. After recently facilitating a workshop about fatigue for a group of women with breast cancer, one woman told me she struggled to find the energy to sit up straight, let alone manage anything other than the most basic of activities. This can lead to a feeling that the essence of self has been eroded, as demonstrated by Ream and Richardson (1997: 49): 'Why can't I be me again? That's all I want, to be me again.'

It has been reported that patients with cancer-related fatigue will often receive very little support in managing their symptoms (Stone et al. 2000). In some cases it seems that even a basic acknowledgement of the condition is lacking, leading patients to wonder if the symptoms they experience are caused by some personal weakness on their part:

> What a difference it would have made if my fatigue had been acknowledged! What validation I would have had . . . I am totally convinced that an acknowledgment of my fatigue would have alleviated many of its excesses. I was doing my utmost – a healthy diet, meditation, counselling, as much exercise as I could manage, and lots more besides – to cope with my fatigue. I needed to know that my exhaustion wasn't the result of a want of imagination or some other lack in me or my attitude.
>
> Gilbert (2003: 4)

A qualitative study of disease-free cancer patients in the Netherlands, who experienced persistent fatigue 7–10 years after their treatment, found that participants struggled to gain a medical diagnosis of fatigue which they perceived would legitimise their symptoms in the eyes of friends, family and colleagues. For several participants a medical diagnosis was also desired to support claims for disability allowances (Rosman 2009).

Curt and Johnston (2003) report that surveys of American and Irish patients have demonstrated that a significant minority of cancer patients have such severe fatigue that it leaves them wanting to die. Clearly the impact of fatigue cannot be underestimated.

Assessing and measuring cancer-related fatigue

Fatigue is a complex, subjective symptom, making measurement very difficult. However, as Stone (2002) noted, pain, breathlessness and nausea are all subjective symptoms so this is not an isolated problem. Indeed there is no lack of scales with which to measure fatigue, rather an inelegant over-sufficiency. Thus cross-comparison between research studies is almost impossible due to the myriad of methods used in assessment. These include the Revised Piper Fatigue Scale (Piper et al. 1998), the Fatigue Symptom Inventory (Hann et al. 1998) and the Multi-dimensional Fatigue Inventory (Smets et al. 1995). Most scales will ask a variety of questions about the physical, cognitive and emotional domains of fatigue, to which the patient responds using a numerical or linear scale to rate severity.

Many of these scales are extremely long and designed for research purposes only. However, while research would benefit enormously from having a single scale with which to measure fatigue, it is equally important that a recognised method of assessing fatigue is developed for use in clinical practice. Nurses have become accustomed to asking their patients to score their pain out of 10, re-evaluating after provision of analgesics. While a more comprehensive assessment is often needed to determine the cause and most appropriate treatment for fatigue, one feels that a simple way of assessing fatigue may have the best chance of being used in busy, resource-stretched hospitals and clinics.

Studies looking at treatment-related fatigue often fail to include a baseline measure of fatigue prior to treatment starting, or an age-matched healthy control group. Consequently, the validity of results could be questioned (Richardson 2004). Prospective research prior to diagnosis would be very difficult to perform. Long-term follow-up is usually absent and many studies are retrospective, relying on participants' ability to recall their symptoms. Measuring and assessing fatigue accurately may be further compromised by the phenomenon of 'response shift'. If patients have experienced severe fatigue during treatment, this may affect the way they perceive subsequent levels of fatigue, or the way they recall previous levels (Visser et al. 2000).

Causes and mediators of cancer-related fatigue

Treatment-related fatigue

Many of the most common treatments for cancer are known to cause fatigue. Patients will usually be offered a variety of treatment modalities, making it difficult to assess the contribution of each in causing fatigue, particularly in patients experiencing fatigue that persists long after treatment has ceased.

Radiotherapy and chemotherapy have been the most well researched, although the mechanisms by which they cause fatigue are still not fully understood. A number of theories have been proposed. These include the suggestions that cancer treatments, and the cancer itself can increase brain serotonin (5-HT) levels leading to a functional disruption of the hypothalamic–pituitary–adrenal (HPA) axis. This is thought to affect many areas including sleep, the maintenance of circadian rhythms, memory, muscle function, mood and hormonal regulation (Ryan et al. 2007). More specifically the HPA axis is also involved in the regulation of the stress hormone, cortisol, output of which has been observed to be lower in a group of fatigue sufferers who had previously been treated for breast cancer (Bower et al. 2005). Cancer treatment is also associated with higher levels of inflammatory mediators called cytokines which may affect fatigue, and this is discussed in more depth below.

There has been less focus on treatment modalities such as hormone therapy, biological therapies and surgery, but evidence suggests these may also contribute towards a patient's fatigue (Payne et al. 2008; Lin et al. 2008). It is possible that the mechanism by which this occurs is indirect. For example, hormone therapy may cause side effects such as hot flushes and night sweats which can interfere with a patient's ability to get a restful night's sleep.

Pain, both acute and chronic, can cause patients to experience sleep disturbance, which leads to fatigue (see Chapter 7). It is therefore important that pain is assessed and properly treated if fatigue is to be effectively managed (NCCN 2008). Pain can result from the cancer itself or from the short and long term effects of surgery. Other treatments such as radiotherapy can also cause pain due to tissue damage. Pain can result from inflammation in the immediate period during and after treatment, but some patients will also experience long-term pain due to nerve damage caused by radiotherapy. Some chemotherapy agents can also cause peripheral nerve damage.

Chemotherapy regimes can vary considerably depending on the site of disease, and studies report slightly different patterns of fatigue. It is also difficult to compare across studies as a variety of measures of fatigue have been used. However, several studies report that fatigue is worse at the beginning of the chemotherapy cycle but may decline towards the end (Pickard-Holley 1991; Richardson et al. 1998). Some patients will continue to experience significant fatigue for many months, or even years, after treatment although there are few research studies providing the results of long-term follow-up of fatigue following chemotherapy. There is also very little information as to which chemotherapy regimes are particularly prone to cause fatigue in the patient, and this is an area which warrants further study. Given the wide range of chemotherapeutic agents and combinations available, it seems unlikely that that this need will be addressed comprehensively in the near future. Much of the research on cancer fatigue has used participants with breast cancer, so it is also important that future research also focuses on other types of cancer.

While the treatments themselves appear to have a significant long-term effect on feelings of fatigue, other side effects of treatment may also be contributory factors. Particularly for patients having chemotherapy or for those with gastrointestinal cancers, nausea and vomiting can be very distressing side effects. Nausea and vomiting are also very common in patients with advanced cancer (Millership 2003). The physical effort of frequent vomiting is tiring, and if the patient is unable to maintain a sufficient nutritional intake over time, fatigue can develop. There is now a huge choice of antiemetics, so patients should be encouraged to report uncontrolled nausea or vomiting swiftly since, once the cause of nausea has been established, an alternative drug will often ensure that symptoms are controlled if initial antiemetic therapy fails to help.

Anaemia, resulting from a reduced amount of circulating red blood cells or concentration of haemoglobin, may also cause feelings of fatigue. Chemotherapy patients will usually have blood tests, including haemoglobin estimation, prior to each cycle so anaemia may be discovered and treated at this point. Patients who are experiencing fatigue, but have not recently had a full blood count taken, may benefit from a full blood count to rule out anaemia as a possible contributing factor.

There is little agreement on the magnitude of fatigue typically experienced by patients receiving radiotherapy. Again, it is difficult from the research available to extrapolate if the site or dose of radiotherapy is significant. Smet et al. (1998a) measured levels of fatigue in 250 cancer patients, with a variety of diagnoses, receiving adjuvant radiotherapy, and found that 46% of patients reported fatigue to be among the top three symptoms causing them the most distress. Patients undergoing radiotherapy will often find that fatigue will commence from their first treatment and continue to intensify as treatment progresses, until it reaches a plateau between the second and fourth week (Richardson 2004). A study measuring fatigue levels in cancer patients nine months after completing radiotherapy found that fatigue levels in participants did not appear to be greater than for the general population, although 34% of participants reported that fatigue post-treatment was worse than they had anticipated (Smets et al. 1998b).

The role of cytokines

Cytokines are proteins that are thought to contribute to the development of cancer by mediating communication between cells. They exist normally in the body as part of the body's inflammatory immune response, but levels are increased in people with cancer. Their mechanism in contributing to cancer-related fatigue is not fully determined but it has been proposed that they may have an impact on neurotransmitters and endocrine pathways (Anisman et al. 1996). Cytokines are thought to build up as a result of their release in response to cell damage, suggesting a potential role in fatigue caused both by treatment and by advanced cancer. However, studies examining the role of cytokines in fatigue have not been consistent in their results, leaving much still to be understood (Ahlberg et al. 2003).

Cytokines may also influence the development of cancer cachexia (Ahlberg et al. 2003). Cachexia is the tem used to describe the extreme loss of weight, weakness and muscle wastage often found in people with advanced cancer. Such cachexia may be linked to the fatigue experienced by people in the later stages of their illness. The malnutrition and raised metabolic level associated with cachexia may also affect fatigue. Cachexia is difficult to treat, as the ideal would be to treat the causative factor: the cancer itself. However, given that cachexia will usually occur in the late stages of advanced cancer, when active treatment is often not an option, other strategies have been tried with only with limited success. These have included nutritional management, progestational steroids (discussed below) and fish oils containing eicosapentaenoic acid (EPA) (Miller et al. 2009).

Fatigue caused by the cancer itself

As discussed above, there are biological reasons why cancer may inherently cause fatigue. However, as with the treatment-related factors, there are also metastatic disease-related causes which may affect perception of fatigue.

Many patients, particularly those with either primary or metastatic disease in the lungs, experience breathlessness. Breathlessness can also be caused by symptoms of advanced disease such as ascites, superior vena cava obstruction or tumour embolism. In addition, treatment-related factors such as radiation-induced lung fibrosis can also contribute to breathlessness (Bredlin 2003). Breathlessness can be difficult to treat, but depending on the cause, symptoms can often be managed with procedures such as pleurodesis, which seals the space between the pleural layers where pleural effusion is present, opioids to reduce respiratory effort, or oxygen therapy or breathing exercises to make respiratory effort more efficient.

Pain, nausea and vomiting are also frequently experienced by patients with advanced cancer, and these symptoms can contribute to fatigue by interrupting restful sleep in the case of pain, and by malnutrition, dehydration and exhaustion in the case of nausea and vomiting. Effective palliative care is crucial in managing these distressing symptoms.

Where the cancer is advanced, decisions must be made with the patient about what attempts are made to treat certain symptoms. For example, a patient may be fatigued and malnourished due to bowel obstruction caused by primary or secondary disease. It may not be possible, or appropriate, to attempt to resolve the obstruction surgically or medically, and some symptoms such as fatigue may be accepted as inevitable by both healthcare professionals and patients in the very late stages of disease.

Depression and fatigue

There appears to be a complex relationship between depression and fatigue. Evidence suggests that the two conditions frequently coexist, and a number of researchers have called for depression, fatigue and insomnia to be considered as a 'symptom cluster' when they exist together rather than as separate entities (Donovan and Jacobsen 2007).

It is difficult to separate cause and effect. Depression could cause fatigue or fatigue could be a symptom of depression. Diagnostic criteria for depression include a lack of energy (World Health Organization 2007). It would also be plausible, given the patient's experience of fatigue, if this were to lead to feelings of depression. Equally there might be an unknown independent factor causing both. For example, cytokines have been associated with both fatigue and depression (Seruga et al. 2008). However, there has been little support for the theory that fatigue could be treated with antidepressants. Results have been better when psychological support is offered (see below).

Management of cancer-related fatigue

A variety of approaches can be tried to alleviate cancer-related fatigue, and these will be more or less appropriate depending on the cause of the fatigue (if this can be ascertained), the stage of the cancer and the preferences of the patients themselves. For example, a patient with very advanced cancer may be unable to consider methods such as exercise or keeping a fatigue diary, but may be willing to try a pharmacological approach. Conversely, for a patient who has been successfully treated for primary cancer and could reasonably be expected to live for many years, it may be more prudent to concentrate, at least initially, on non-pharmacological methods which would not carry with them the potential for side effects, particularly with long-term use. In the sections below, both pharmacological and non-pharmacological methods of management will be discussed, with a summary of the evidence for each approach.

Pharmacological methods

A number of pharmacological methods have been employed to combat cancer-related fatigue.

Psychostimulant medication

Psychostimulants are drugs that are prescribed to produce wakefulness and arousal and to stimulate behaviour. Most research studies involve a very small numbers of participants, thereby limiting the confidence with which we can interpret the data; however, methylphenidate, Ritalin®, is probably the best-studied in relation to cancer-related fatigue. A small-scale study by Roth et al. (2006) in men with prostate cancer compared fatigue scores in 14 participants who had been given methylphenidate and 15 who had been given a placebo. It is of note that six patients in the methylphenidate arm and one patient in the control arm withdrew from the study. For those who completed the study, 73% of those who received methylphenidate had a significant reduction in fatigue levels compared with a 23% improvement in the control group. Other trials have also suggested there may be a benefit to using methylphenidate for fatigue (Bruera et al. 2006; Hanna et al. 2006) in patients with both primary and advanced cancer. A recent Cochrane review concluded that, while the research was encouraging, more was needed to clarify the role of methylphenidate in this area (Minton et al. 2008). In contrast, the American NCCN guidelines suggest that methylphenidate should be considered for treating cancer-related fatigue in adults after other causes of fatigue have been ruled out (NCCN 2008). However, side effects from psychostimulant drugs are not insubstantial and can include agitation, anorexia, headache, hypertension, arrhythmias and palpitations. In the case of advanced cancer, symptom control and quality of life are paramount, so any significant side-effect burden would need to be very carefully considered before prescribing methylphenidate. This is also equally true for patients with primary cancer, particularly given the potential need for long-term treatment of fatigue.

Antidepressant medication

As discussed previously, the relationship between fatigue and depression has been considered and has led researchers to question whether antidepressants, particularly selective serotonin reuptake inhibitors (SSRIs) may help treat cancer-related fatigue. However, results have not been encouraging, with studies failing to show a difference in fatigue scores when an antidepressant was compared with placebo (Morrow et al. 2003; Roscoe et al. 2005; Stockler et al. 2007).

However, if a patient has been assessed as clinically depressed, fatigue may be a symptom of their depression and an antidepressant medication may be helpful in these circumstances (Brietbart & Alici 2008).

Corticosteroid medication

Due to the long-term side effects of corticosteroids such as muscle wastage, it would not be appropriate to prescribe these on a long-term basis for patients with a primary cancer. There is very little data looking at the effects of such steroids on fatigue for patients with advanced cancer, although many patients take them for other reasons such as to relieve the symptoms of cerebral oedema or spinal cord compression. Bruera et al. (1985) demonstrated a short-term increase in activity levels in patients with advanced cancer receiving methylprednisolone, and there is belief amongst many clinicians that corticosteroids can be helpful in enhancing feelings of wellbeing at the end of life (Lundström & Fürst 2006). In some situations, even a few days of enhanced energy levels can make a great difference, as is illustrated in Case study 8.1.

Case study 8.1 Mrs B

Mrs B, aged 65, had metastatic ovarian cancer with spread to her bowel, peritoneal cavity and liver. She had ascites, meaning her abdomen was distended with fluid despite an ascitic drain which had remained in place for several days. As a result she was breathless and had a poor appetite. She felt constantly fatigued and lacked the energy to do anything other than move from bed to commode when necessary. Mrs B's daughter was due to be married and her mother was keen to attend the church service but was uncertain if she could manage this. After a long discussion with her palliative care consultant, Mrs B was started on a short course of dexamethasone to see if this would give her a boost and allow her to attend the wedding. Although she reported the steroids made her feel slightly agitated, she was able to go to the wedding which was a great source of comfort to both Mrs B and her daughter.

Progestational steroids

While there is some evidence to suggest that progestational steroids such as megestrol acetate may have an effect on stimulating appetite and feelings of wellbeing in advanced cancer, there is not currently sufficient evidence to support giving this class of drugs in the hope of relieving cancer-related fatigue (Minton et al. 2008).

Haemopoietic growth factors

As the name suggests, these agents stimulate the production of red blood cells. A Cochrane review examined the evidence for two haemopoietic growth factor drugs: erthyropoietin and darbopoietin. Most studies looked at anaemic patients receiving chemotherapy, and both drugs demonstrated small but significant beneficial effects on fatigue in this setting (Minton et al. 2008).

Non-pharmacological methods

Exercise

Though it may seem somewhat counter-intuitive, a strong evidence base is developing for the use of exercise in the management of cancer-related fatigue. It is not clear how exercise benefits people with fatigue. Various theories have been suggested. One posits that patients become 'deconditioned' by long periods of inactivity during and after cancer treatment. This leads to muscle wastage which then causes the patient to require more energy to perform physical tasks. This, in turn, leads to a cycle of worsening fatigue, and it is proposed that exercise could break this cycle (Dimeo et al. 1997). Other theories emphasise the effect of blood oxygenation from increased ventilation and cardiac output, or the increased production of exercise-induced endorphins which may affect perception of fatigue (Porock & Fu 2004).

Most research in this area has looked at breast cancer patients at various points during and after treatment. However, there have been promising studies with patients with other malignancies. A small randomised controlled study of men with prostate cancer receiving radiotherapy found that both aerobic and resistance exercise improved fatigue levels in the short term, and that resistance exercise improved both strength and quality of life in the longer term (Segal et al. 2009).

A Cochrane review of exercise for the management of cancer-related fatigue in adults found that exercise appeared to have a beneficial effect in most studies included in the review. However, it recommended that more research was needed on the type, intensity and timing of the exercise required. The review also called for more research on the effects of exercise on different cancer subtypes (due to the emphasis to date on breast cancer) and on different stages of cancer (Cramp & Daniel 2008).

Many studies involve participants exercising in a group, and it is possible that part of the therapeutic effect derives from being in a group with peers. However, there have been studies where participants were given a home exercise programme to follow, and reported a positive effect on fatigue (e.g. Pinto et al. 2005). The participants in the exercise arm of this study were also given telephone-based motivational counselling to support the exercise intervention, so it remains difficult to be sure of the actual cause of the improvement.

Certain factors need to be considered when advising those with cancer fatigue about exercise. Those with advanced cancer, depending on the stage of their illness and how symptomatic they are may be unable to take part. Patients who are immunocompromised, such as those receiving chemotherapy, need to be advised to be careful when blood counts are low. For example, swimming pools may be best avoided in this group of patients due to the risk of infection. Patients at risk of or suffering from lymphoedema require education on avoiding over-exertion of the affected limb. Patients with weakened skeletons due to primary or secondary cancer in the bones should be cautioned to avoid high-impact activity. Those with primary or secondary lung disease may benefit from being taught breathing techniques to help with breathlessness. In short, the patient's pathology and range of symptoms must be taken into account when recommending an exercise programme, and referral to a physiotherapist for specialist advice may be appropriate. Once certain safety considerations have been accounted for, exercise is generally free of serious side effects, is low-cost and has other health benefits, making it an ideal primary strategy for many people suffering from cancer-related fatigue (see Case study 8.2).

Case study 8.2   Mr H

Mr H was a 31-year-old man who had received chemotherapy and radiotherapy for stage 2 Hodgkin lymphoma. Six months following the end of his treatment he reported to his GP that he still felt very tired and this was affecting both his performance at work and his social life. After the results of initial blood tests were revealed to be normal, Mr H's GP recommended a programme of exercise. Mr H mentioned that he used to enjoy golf, so his GP suggested that he take this up again, perhaps asking some of his friends if they would like to join him. Mr H had to build up gradually and, although at first he was unable to complete a full round of golf, this improved over a few months. Mr H reported that his energy levels were still not what they had been prior to treatment, but he felt so much better for the exercise and planned to continue.

Fatigue diaries

Fatigue diaries encourage patients to keep a record of their levels of fatigue over a period of time. Such a record allows them to note if there is a pattern to their fatigue. It may be worse in the morning but better in the afternoon, for example. Some activities may tire individuals more than others, and keeping a diary can help patients gain a greater understanding of their fatigue, around which they are then more easily able to plan what is important to them. An illustration might be that they may wish to organise their social activities for when they expect to have the most energy. Macmillan Cancer Support provides a fatigue diary that can be downloaded from their website for patients to use for this purpose (Macmillan Cancer Support 2008) although patients can of course compile a diary in any format they prefer. Fatigue diaries may also help patients discuss their symptoms with their healthcare professionals, which in turn may help the latter with assessment.

The notion of energy conservation

A study by Barsevick et al. (2004) found that patients undergoing chemotherapy, radiotherapy or both derived a small but significant benefit from receiving three telephone calls, on the subject of energy conservation, from an oncology nurse during their first five weeks of treatment. The aim of energy conservation is for the patient to use their energy judiciously, avoiding unnecessary activities and finding ways to reduce their energy output, such as by prioritisation or delegation, allowing them to feel less fatigued for the activities they value. A number of practical tips can be suggested, as listed in Box 8.1 and illustrated in Case study 8.3.

Box 8.1   Practical tips for energy conservation in cancer-related fatigue

- For those that are employed, consider requesting to work from home a few days per week to avoid travelling, allowing them to work and rest when they feel appropriate.
- Discussion with friends and family about which tasks might be delegated.
- Internet shopping.
- Making double portions of meals to allow half to be frozen for another occasion.
- Using a bathrobe rather than a towel to help drying after showers or baths.
- Sitting down for tasks such as ironing.

Case study 8.3   Miss C

Miss C was a 37-year-old with primary breast cancer. She received surgery, chemotherapy and trastuzumab. She was an active user of Internet discussion forums and posted to others about her experiences. She had remained fatigued after treatment, and found her fatigue was worse in the evenings. She had tried moving her schedule around to accommodate her symptoms but this had not been successful, as her main aim was to spend more time with her two young children who were not back from school until the late afternoon. She wrote in the Internet forum that she had been 'saved' by employing a cleaner who was able to do the majority of the housework, leaving her with slightly more energy to enjoy her children in the evening.

The use of distraction techniques

There is some evidence to suggest that distraction, for example, music, games or other activities that focus the attention away from the symptoms being experienced, can help people manage their fatigue (Richardson & Ream 1997). This could be suggested to patients, alongside other strategies to reduce fatigue. However, given the concerns of patients such as Gilbert (2003) that their fatigue was not adequately acknowledged by healthcare professionals, it is important to ensure that mentioning distraction techniques is not perceived as belittling or failing to acknowledge and address the patient's symptoms.

Sleep 'hygiene'

Cancer patients often struggle to sleep well. Particularly during active treatment, sleep may be difficult to achieve due to a variety of factors such as postoperative discomfort, anxiety, hospitalisation and medication side effects such as the wakefulness that can be caused by corticosteroids. However, in the longer term, fatigue may cause patients to nap during the day. This may affect night-time sleep quality; patients should be advised to avoid long naps and be encouraged to experiment to see if staying awake during the day helps with sleep at night. Patients can also be provided with more general information about aiding restful sleep such as keeping bedrooms dark, cool, quiet and free from stimulating distractions such as television or computers (Macmillan Cancer Support 2008).

Supportive interventions and fatigue

Support alone seems to have a beneficial effect on patients who are living with fatigue. Badger et al. (2005) found that patients with breast cancer who received telephone counselling reported lower levels of fatigue than those who did not.

In a study of patients receiving chemotherapy, participants were randomly allocated to either 'usual care' or to an intervention group which, over three months, provided them with a fatigue diary, an information pack and monthly visits from a support nurse (Ream et al. 2006). The information pack contained educational advice on exercise, distraction, energy conservation, relaxation and sleep hygiene techniques. The nurse assessed levels of fatigue and provided support and coaching in order to help patients cope more effectively. The intervention group reported lower levels of fatigue with a reduction of impact on activities they classed as important. They were also found to be less depressed, anxious and distressed than the control group. There are difficulties in evaluating this kind of intervention: it was not possible to blind the participants and researchers as to who was in the experimental group. It is also impossible to decide the precise cause of any effect. Whether it was the education, the support element or the diaries, or indeed the sum total of these which provided the benefit to the participants cannot be determined. However, given our knowledge of the various techniques that can be employed to manage fatigue, it seems perhaps foolish not to evaluate them together. Fatigue is multifactorial in its aetiology, and patients require both information and support to guide them through the strategies available to them (see Case study 8.4).

Case study 8.4   Mrs D

Mrs D had received surgery and chemotherapy for invasive bladder cancer. She spoke to her nurse specialist about her symptoms of fatigue. She was frequently tearful throughout the conversation, describing how she 'hated living like this'. Her nurse suggested various interventions but Mrs D became frustrated, saying she had tried everything and nothing made any difference. Her nurse referred her to the hospital's counsellor, suspecting Mrs D was displaying signs of depression. After six sessions of counselling, Mrs D told her nurse that she still felt the same symptoms of fatigue but recognised how helpful the counsellor had been in assisting her to explore her feelings about her cancer and treatment. Mrs D requested details of her local cancer support group, which her nurse provided.

Discussion

Cancer-related fatigue management: challenges and possible solutions

Most of the evidence on cancer-related fatigue indicates that we are not dealing with it very well. A survey to investigate cancer patients' perceptions of fatigue and its management found that 58% of the 576 patients who responded to the survey reported that fatigue affected them 'somewhat or very much'. Fatigue had not been reported to the hospital doctor in 52% of cases and only 14% had received support, treatment or advice about how to manage their fatigue (Stone et al. 2000). More must be done to encourage reporting of symptoms of fatigue by patients with cancer, many of whom, it seems, perceive fatigue as inevitable. Moreover, it is imperative that patients who report fatigue receive help to reduce their symptoms.

While some of the pharmacological approaches to managing fatigue seem encouraging and require more research, it appears that strategies based on support, education and exercise carry the most promise at present. This poses some difficulty. Particularly after initial cancer treatment has finished, patients may be called to follow-up appointments periodically, but otherwise they are commonly instructed to get in touch with their team if any problems occur, and are not necessarily in regular contact with their hospital. Managing fatigue seems to require the practitioner to be something of a coach: encouraging, educating and motivating. Compared to their oncology nurse colleagues, nurses working in primary care, cardiology and other fields where lifestyle change is important to recovery are perhaps more accustomed to working with patients in this way.

It certainly seems reasonable that, as people live for longer with cancer, rehabilitation should become an increasing part of the role of people who care for those with cancer. However, in practice this may prove challenging. Many nurse specialists report that they feel overstretched as it is, struggling to find time to care for their existing caseload. A 2004 survey conducted among breast care nurses by the charity, Breast Cancer Care, found that 40% of those surveyed did not feel there was a sufficient number of nurses in their area to cope with demand; 20% reported they did not have time to talk through the written information they provide; and another 20% did not have the time to sit with patients to provide basic psychological support (Royal College of Nursing and Breast Cancer Care 2004). Other cancer types have even less specialist nurse provision than breast cancer, suggesting that, with current numbers, specialist nurses may struggle to take on the additional workload. A study by Leary et al. (2008) estimated that a lung cancer nurse specialist in England currently works around 317 hours unpaid overtime per year.

If fatigue were truly recognised as the burden on patients that it appears to be, and if we were committed to improving the quality of life of cancer patients, then there might be opportunities to deliver services differently, perhaps more creatively. With an increasing emphasis on providing care local to the patient, it seems possible that rehabilitation programmes could be run in the community. In the same way that interventions for smoking cessation can be run by experienced practice nurses, groups could be set up for patients with cancer to help manage their fatigue.

- Patients could be individually assessed to establish a baseline for their fatigue and to identify any potentially correctable causes such as pain or anaemia.
- Education could be provided in groups on ways of managing fatigue including practical tips on energy conservation and the promotion of fatigue diaries.
- Exercise classes could be offered to teach safe techniques to gradually increase levels of activity.
- Exercise prescriptions could be written for those who wish to exercise at home or for those who live in a remote location where frequent travel to a central location is difficult.
- Telephone follow-up could be offered.

The *Cancer Reform Strategy* (Department of Health 2007) suggests that there is a will at government level to consider a different way of working with cancer patients, and more creative strategies are being suggested for meeting the long-term needs of cancer survivors, such as the examples given below. Information prescriptions should set a standard for the level of information to be provided during and after a cancer diagnosis, which may benefit patients struggling with fatigue. The National Cancer Survivorship Initiative, a recommendation of the Cancer Reform Strategy, is to consider a wide range of approaches working across primary, secondary, tertiary and voluntary sectors including:

> best practice regarding care planning for survivorship. This is likely to include formal assessments of a patient's needs and preferences for care at the completion of treatment and what role the patient wishes to take in managing their own care.
>
> DH (2007: 81.

These approaches include rehabilitation programmes, psychological support and expert patient programmes (DH 2007). A number of pilot projects are to be carried out, the results of which could be used to influence those commissioning health and social care.

An initiative at a London hospital has seen breast and prostate cancer patients enrolled in a project called 'Surviving Cancer, Living Life' aimed at improving the quality of life for cancer survivors (Richardson et al. 2008). Nurses are trained in telephone motivational interviewing techniques and use these skills to work with patients to help them in a number of areas. These include managing symptoms, making healthy lifestyle choices, maintaining treatment compliance and understanding their own health concerns. The patient is typically called weekly for a month, then fortnightly, then monthly.

Depending on the results of projects such as the one mentioned above, there may be a brighter future for the management for fatigue. If there were a structure in place that assessed cancer patients for fatigue, informed them as to evidence-based methods to help combat fatigue, and supported and empowered them over time to make healthy choices, then there is hope that fatigue will start to become adequately managed.

Fatigue, then, can be seen as part of the wider survivorship agenda, and perhaps its management can be seen within this broader context. Patients with cancer can suffer a range of side effects which can persist long after treatment has finished, including cognitive dysfunction, sexual dysfunction, pain, poor body image and psychological distress. There is increasingly more interest in developing care plans for cancer survivors to help them manage symptoms themselves and identify when to seek help (DH 2008). Care plans can also help deliver some much-needed standardisation in the follow-up care of patients after cancer treatment.

The Edmonton Fatigue Framework (Olson et al. 2008), although focusing on patients with advanced cancer, aims to propose a model which the authors hope will promote further research linking fatigue to other processes such as sleep, nutrition, cognitive function and muscle strength. As research advances and we understand more about the complex relationships between symptoms and their causes, it may help us design a more integrated approach to managing fatigue.

Healthcare commissioning may also be aided if fatigue is seen, not in isolation, but as one of the many symptoms that patients may need help and support to live with. 'Follow-up' care needs to be designed with this in mind. There may be opportunities for creative partnership working between the NHS and the voluntary sector. For some time charities have been designing and running programmes to help people with a diagnosis of cancer to live well after treatment, and often have considerable expertise in this area (Breast Cancer Care 2009). Patient-led courses such as those designed by the Expert Patient Programme could also assist with the design of future interventions (Expert Patient Programme 2009). While the Expert Patient Programme does not provide the medical information that would be necessary to help patients understand more about the long-term side effects of treatment, it aims to facilitate confidence in self-management of health in its participants which would be vitally important when helping patients with cancer-related fatigue. Those who have attended an Expert Patient course report attending the emergency department, outpatient department or GP less often (Expert Patient Programme 2009) and it would be interesting, when piloting interventions to manage fatigue and other long-term symptoms, to monitor the effect of intervention on attendance at other services.

For patients with advanced disease, careful assessment is important to help ensure the most appropriate recommendations. Many patients can live with metastatic cancer for some time, and if symptoms are controlled, can hope to remain active for as long as possible in this period. Interventions such as those suggested above could be tailored for this population, just as for patients with primary disease. However, once disease has progressed to the stage where the patient is approaching the end of life, then the decision must be made in consultation with the patient and his or her family, to cease trying to manage the fatigue with active strategies and allow 'the natural decline towards death' (Porock 2003). Initiatives such as the Liverpool Care Pathway (LCP) can help nurses ensure that symptoms that indicate a patient is near death are recognised and treated where necessary (Marie Curie Palliative Care Institute Liverpool 2009). The ambitious aims of the LCP to provide a framework which delivers improvements in end-of-life care at a national level are inspirational when considering a national response to managing fatigue. While the LCP deals with a discrete time period (the last days and hours of life), the principles involved would help create a template by means of which healthcare professionals could be guided through evidence-based recommendations for fatigue (see Chapter 12).

Prior to developing care plans or a framework for managing fatigue, it would be helpful to synthesise available evidence into a set of national guidelines to assist healthcare professionals in assessing the current evidence when treating patients with cancer-related fatigue, and to ensure greater consistency in care. As previously referred to, guidelines exist in other countries such as the NCCN clinical practice guidelines in America. Separate provisions are given for children, adults receiving treatment, adults post-treatment and those with advanced cancer, to ensure that recommendations are appropriate for the patient's clinical situation. While fatigue is mentioned in several of the guidance documents issued by the National Institute of Clinical Excellence (NICE) there is no overall appraisal looking at the optimal management of cancer-related fatigue. A document such as this, setting out best practice, might also assist in service development if it were demonstrated that the treatment of fatigue is falling far short of what would be classed as ideal.

It is a potentially exciting time to be involved in caring for patients with cancer. It feels as if there is change in the air (see Chapter 1). We can no longer provide treatment with the intent to cure cancer without considering the symptoms that patients will be left with after treatment stops. Equally, for those with advanced disease, palliative care cannot only encompass those symptoms which can be easily dealt with pharmacologically.

Our responsibility does not stop when the consent form for treatment is signed. Survival rates remain crucially important, but the way people live with, and after, cancer requires our attention and, equally important, our resources. We must ensure that life after a diagnosis of cancer is a life worth living.

Conclusion

It has been identified that fatigue is a very common problem for people with cancer. Incidence is expected to grow as cancer rates increase and mortality rates decrease. Fatigue can be caused by factors related to the cancer itself, but treatment has also been shown to have a significant impact on fatigue, with chemotherapy and radiotherapy having a demonstrably negative effect on energy levels for a considerable length of time after treatment. The relationship between depression and fatigue is less clear; the two frequently coexist but medical treatment of depression appears to have very little effect on fatigue.

Indeed, with the exception of treating anaemia, pharmacological management of fatigue has yet to deliver any long-term solutions, though patients with advanced disease may obtain a short-term increase in wellbeing from corticosteroids. Research is ongoing into a number of agents, including stimulants such as methylphenidate. A more promising strategy appears to be the non-pharmacological approaches to helping patients live with fatigue. These include exercise, psychological support and energy conservation.

The current interest in 'survivorship' may pave the way towards better care for patients with primary cancer-related fatigue. There are government-led initiatives to improve the experience of patients living with cancer, and a real acknowledgement exists that the current structure of patient follow-up may not be enough to meet their needs. Nurses may find there are opportunities to deliver patient care in new ways, perhaps with the NHS and voluntary sector working in closer partnership. Survivor care plans may provide a framework to guide the development of new services to provide patients with the education and support they require to manage their fatigue. It is also important that those with advanced cancer are not forgotten, as striving towards a good quality of life in this patient population is paramount. Initiatives such as the Liverpool Care Pathway suggest that nationalised standards of care are achievable, and may pave the way towards better symptom control for all patients with cancer.

References

Ahlberg K, Ekman T, Gaston-Johansson F, Mock V (2003) Assessment and management of cancer-related fatigue in adults. *Lancet* **362**: 640–50.

Anisman H, Baines MG, Berczi I, et al. (1996) Neuroimmune mechanisms in health and disease, 2: disease. *Canadian Medical Association Journal* **155**: 1075–82.

Armes J (2004) The nature of fatigue. In: Armes J, Krishnasamy M, Higginson I (eds) *Fatigue in Cancer*. Oxford: Oxford University Press.

Badger T, Segrin C, Meek P, Bonham E (2005) Profiles of women with breast cancer: Who respond to a telephone interpersonal counseling intervention? *Journal of Psychosocial Oncology* **23**(2–3): 79–99.

Barsevick A, Whitmer K, Walker L (2001) In their own words: using the common-sense model to analyze patient descriptions of cancer-related fatigue. *Oncology Nursing Forum* **28**(9): 1368–9.

Barsevick A, Dudley W, Beck S, et al. (2004) A randomised clinical trial of energy conservation for cancer-related fatigue. *Cancer* **100**: 1302–10.

Bower JE, Ganz PA, Dickerson SS, Petersen L, Aziz N, Fahey JL (2005) Diurnal cortisol rhythm and fatigue in breast cancer survivors. *Psychoneuroendocrinology* **30**(1): 92–100.

Breast Cancer Care (2009) Support days and activities. http://www.breastcancercare.org.uk/.

Bredlin M (2003) Breathlessness. In: O'Connor M, Aranda S (eds) *Palliative Care Nursing: A Guide to Practice*, 2nd edn. Oxford: Radcliffe Medical Press.

Brietbart W, Alici Y (2008) Pharmacologic treatment options for cancer-related fatigue. *Clinical Journal of Oncology Nursing* **12**(5): 27–36.

Bruera E, Roca E, Cedaro I, Carraro S, Cacon R (1985) Action of oral methylprednisolone in terminal cancer patients: a prospective randomised double-blind study. *Cancer Treatment Reports* **69**(7–8): 751–4.

Bruera E, Valero V, Driver L, et al. (2006) Patient-controlled methylphenidate for cancer fatigue: a double blind, randomised, placebo-controlled trial. *Journal of Clinical Oncology* **24**(13): 2073–78.

Cramp F, Daniel J (2008) Exercise for the management of cancer-related fatigue in adults (review). *Cochrane Database of Systematic Reviews* **2**: CD006145.

Curt G, Johnston P (2003) Cancer fatigue: the way forward. *Oncologist* **8**(suppl 1): 27–30.

Dean A (2008) Supporting women experiencing sexual problems after treatment for breast cancer. *Cancer Nursing Practice* **7**(8): 29–33.

Department of Health (2007) Cancer Reform Strategy. London: DH.

Department of Health (2008) National Cancer Survivorship Initiative Newsletter – Autumn 2008, Issue 1. http://www.dh.gov.uk/en/Publicationsandstatistics/Publications/PublicationsPolicyAnd Guidance/DH_088879.

Dimeo F, Fetscher S, Lange W, et al. (1997) Effects of aerobic exercise on the physical performance and incidence of treatment-related complications after high-dose chemotherapy. *Blood* **90**: 3390–4.

Donovan KA, Jacobsen PB (2007) Fatigue, depression, and insomnia: evidence for a symptom cluster in cancer. *Seminars in Oncology Nursing* **23**(2): 127–35.

Expert Patient Programme (2009) *About expert patients.* http://www.expertpatients.co.uk/public/ default.aspx?load=ArticleViewer&ArticleId=500.

Fawcett TN, Dean A (2004) The causes of cancer-related fatigue and approaches to its treatment. *Professional Nurse* **19**(9): 503–7.

Gilbert M (2003) A survivor's journey: one woman's experience with cancer-related fatigue. *Oncologist* **8** (Suppl 1): 3–4.

Hann DM, Jacobsen PB, Martin SC, Kronish LE, et al. (1998) Measurement of fatigue in cancer patients: development and validation of the Fatigue Symptom Inventory. *Quality of Life Research* **7**(4): 301–10.

Hanna A, Sledge G, Mayer MI, et al. (2006) A phase 11 study of methylphenidate for the treatment of fatigue. *Supportive Care in Cancer* **14**(3): 210–15.

Holley S (2000) Cancer-related fatigue: suffering a different fatigue. *Cancer Practitioner* **8**(2): 87–95.

Hotopf M (2004) Definitions, epidemiology, and models of fatigue in the general population and in cancer. In: Armes J, Krishnasamy M, Higginson I (eds) Fatigue in Cancer. Oxford: Oxford University Press.

Leary A, Bell N, Darlison L, Guerin M (2008) An analysis of lung cancer clinical nurse specialist workload and value. *Cancer Nursing Practice* **7**(10): 29–33.

Lin NU, Carey LA, Liu MC, Younger J, et al. (2008) Phase 11 trial of lapatinib for brain metastases in patients with human epidermal growth factor receptor 2-positive breast cancer. *Journal of Clinical Oncology* **26**(12): 1993–9.

Lundström SH, Fürst CJ (2006) The use of corticosteroids in Swedish palliative care. *Acta Oncologica* **45**(4): 430–7.

Macmillan Cancer Support (2008) *Fatigue Diary.* http://www.cancerbackup.org.uk/Resourcessup-port/Symptomssideeffects/Fatigue/Copingathome/FatigueDiary.pdf.

Marie Curie Palliative Care Institute (2009) *Liverpool Care Pathway for the Dying Patient.* http:// www.mcpcil.org.uk/liverpool_care_pathway.

Miller C, Reid J, Porter S (2009) The challenges of managing cachexia in advanced cancer. *Cancer Nursing Practice* **8**(4): 24–7.

Millership R (2003) Nausea and vomiting. In: O'Connor M, Aranda S (eds) *Palliative Care Nursing: A Guide to Practice*, 2nd edn. Oxford: Radcliffe Medical Press.

Minton O. Stone P, Richardson A, Sharpe M, Hotopf M (2008) Drug therapy for the management of cancer-related fatigue (review). *Cochrane Database of Systematic Reviews* 1: CD006704.

Morrow GR, Hickok JT, Roscoe JA, et al. (2003) Differential effects of paroxetine on fatigue and depression: a randomised, double-blind trial from the University of Rochester Cancer Center Community Clinical Oncology Program. *Journal of Clinical Oncology* 21(24): 4635–41.

National Comprehensive Cancer Network (2008) *Cancer-related fatigue: clinical practice guidelines in oncology.* www.nccn.org.

Olson K, Turner AR, Courneya KS, et al. (2008) Possible links between behavioral and physiological indices of tiredness, fatigue, and exhaustion in advanced cancer. *Supportive Care in Cancer* 16(3): 215–16.

Payne JK, Held J, Thorpe J, Shaw H (2008) Effect of exercise on biomarkers, fatigue, sleep disturbances, and depressive symptoms in older women with breast cancer receiving hormone therapy. *Oncology Nursing Forum* 35(4): 635–42.

Pickard-Holley S (1991) Fatigue in cancer patients- a descriptive study. *Cancer Nursing* 14(1): 13–19.

Pinto BM, Frierson GM, Rabin C, Trunzo JJ, Marcus BH (2005) Home-based physical activity intervention for breast cancer patients. *Journal of Clinical Oncology* 23(15): 577–87.

Piper BF, Dibble SL, Dodd MJ, et al. (1998) The revised Piper Fatigue Scale: psychometric evaluation in women with breast cancer. *Oncology Nursing Forum* 25(4): 677–84.

Porock D (2003) Fatigue. In: O'Connor M, Aranda S (eds) *Palliative Care Nursing: A Guide to Practice*, 2nd edn. Oxford: Radcliffe Medical Press.

Porock D, Fu M (2004) The therapeutic effects of exercise on fatigue. In: Armes J, Krishnasamy M, Higginson I (eds) *Fatigue in Cancer*. Oxford: Oxford University Press.

Ream EK, Richardson A (1997) Fatigue in patients with cancer and chronic obstructive airways disease: a phenomenological enquiry. *International Journal of Nursing Studies* 34(1): 44–53.

Ream EK, Richardson A, Alexander-Dann C (2006) Supportive intervention for fatigue in patients undergoing chemotherapy: a randomised controlled trial. *Journal of Pain and Symptom Management* 31(2): 148–61.

Richardson A (2004) A critical appraisal of the factors associated with fatigue. In: Armes J, Krishnasamy M, Higginson I (eds) *Fatigue in Cancer*. Oxford: Oxford University Press.

Richardson A, Ream EK (1997) Self-care behaviours initiated by chemotherapy patients in response to fatigue. *International Journal of Nursing Studies* 34: 35–43.

Richardson A, Ream EK, Wilson-Barnett J (1998) Fatigue in patients receiving chemotherapy: patterns of change. *Cancer Nursing* 21(1): 17–30.

Richardson A, Griffin M, Miller C, McNeil I (2008) Living life after cancer treatment: a nurse-led support service. *Cancer Nursing Practice* 7(10): 36–8.

Roscoe JA, Morrow GR, Hickok JT, et al. (2005) Effect of paroxetine hydrochloride (Paxil) on fatigue and depression in breast cancer patients receiving chemotherapy. *Breast Cancer Research and Treatment* 89(3): 243–9.

Rosman S (2009) 'Recovered from cancer but still ill': strategies used to legitimise extreme persistent fatigue in disease-free cancer patients. *European Journal of Cancer Care* 18: 28–36.

Roth AJ, Nelson CJ, Rosenfeld B, et al. (2006) Randomised controlled trial testing methylphenidate as treatment for fatigue in men with prostate cancer (Abstract 275). *Journal of Clinical Oncology*. ASCO Prostate Cancer Symposia, 231.

Royal College of Nursing and Breast Cancer Care (2004) *Time to Care: Maintaining Access to Breast Care Nurses. Policy Briefing.* http://www.rcn.org.uk/__data/assets/pdf_file/0008/78641/002494.pdf.

Ryan JL, Carroll JK, Ryan EP, Mustian KM, Fiscella K, Morrow GR (2007) Mechanisms of cancer-related fatigue. *Oncologist* 12 (Suppl 1): 22–34. Review.

Segal RJ, Reid RD, Courneya KS, et al. (2009) Randomised controlled trial of resistance or aerobic exercise in men receiving radiation therapy for prostate cancer. *Journal of Clinical Oncology* **27**(3): 344–51.

Seruga B, Zhang H, Bernstein LJ, Tannock IF (2008) Cytokines and their relationship to the symptoms and outcome of cancer. *National Review of Cancer* **8**(11): 887–99.

Smets EM, Garssen B, Bonke B, De Haes J (1995) The Multidimensional Fatigue Inventory (MFI) psychometric qualities of an instrument to assess fatigue. *Journal of Psychosomatic Research* **39**(3): 315–25.

Smets EM, Visser MR, Willems-Groot AF, et al. (1998a) Fatigue and radiotherapy: (A) experience in patients undergoing treatment. *British Journal of Cancer* **78**(7): 899–906.

Smets EM, Visser MR, Willems-Groot AF, et al. (1998b) Fatigue and radiotherapy: (B) experience in patients 9 months following treatment. *British Journal of Cancer* **78**(7): 907–12.

Stockler MR, O'Connell R, Nowak AK, et al. (2007) Effect of sertraline on symptoms and survival in patients with advanced cancer, but without major depression: a placebo-controlled double-blind randomised trial. *Lancet Oncology* **8**(7): 603–12.

Stone P (2002) The measurement, causes and effective management of cancer-related fatigue. *International Journal of Palliative Nursing* **8**(3): 120–8.

Stone P, Richardson A, Ream A, et al. (2000) Cancer-related fatigue: inevitable, unimportant and untreatable? Results of a multi-centre patient survey. *Cancer Fatigue Forum Annals of Oncology* **11**(8): 971–5.

Visser MR, Smets EM, Spranhers MA, de Haes J (2000) How response shift may affect the measurement of change in fatigue. *Journal of Pain and Symptom Management* **20**(1): 12–18.

World Health Organization (2007) Mental and behavioural disorders: mood (affective) disorders. *ICD-10*. F32, Chapter V. http://www.who.int/classifications/apps/icd/icd10online/.

Wu HS, McSweeney M (2007) Cancer-related fatigue: 'It's so much more than being tired.' *European Journal of Oncology Nursing* **11**(2): 117–25.

Chapter 9

The clinical research nurse in cancer clinical trials

Patricia B. Campbell

From its inception, nursing has been a practice discipline with a focus on holistic care of the sick and infirm. It has drawn on the relevant knowledge and skills of other disciplines to inform and improve the quality of care and the nursing profession itself. Over the years nursing has responded to social and scientific developments and to advances in technology. The work of nurses extends across the healthcare spectrum, from prevention through acute and long-term care to rehabilitation and to care at the end of life. Social and technological change has opened up many new opportunities for nurses to extend their roles and to develop new roles, applying their special nursing knowledge and skills in the wide remit of healthcare.

This chapter explores the nature of clinical trials in cancer research and the roles of the clinical research nurse within clinical trials. It discusses the role of the nurse in providing and communicating complex trial and treatment information for patients and families, broken down and paced to meet individual needs. The chapter explores the role of the nurse as pathfinder: helping patients negotiate the web of information and services available to them, and examines the relationships developed between patients and research nurses in the clinical trial setting. In addition the chapter also discusses the direct caregiver role and the provision of expert care.

Clinical research nurses are registered nurses employed at research sites to facilitate and conduct any phase of a clinical trial. The input of the research nurse in clinical trials is associated with improved clinical trial quality, because of their skill in communication, education, recruitment and ensuring patient compliance (Spilsbury et al. 2007). Even though the role of the research nurse in cancer care has been known for over 40 years, in the grand scheme of things research nursing is still in its formulative stage. A look at the time line in Boxes 9.1a–c shows that the role of the research nurse in clinical trials is still evolving, and has a way to go to maturity.

The role of the clinical trial research nurse has been one of evolution, from its earliest incarnation in the United States in the 1960s as part of the early clinical trials of chemotherapy (Deinenger 2008), to present day, where it is still constantly evolving (Molin & Arrigo 1995). The primary role in the early days was that of direct caregiver, with

Perspectives on Cancer Care. Edited by Josephine (Tonks) N. Fawcett and Anne McQueen
© 2011 Blackwell Publishing Ltd

Box 9.1a The history of clinical trials: key dates

- **1747** James Lind first documented comparative study using citrus in the treatment of scurvy.
- **19th** century utilised basic trial concepts in the development of drugs and vaccines (smallpox, diphtheria and cholera).
- Early **20th century** studies focused on the prophylaxis and treatment of infectious diseases.
- **1948** First placebo-controlled randomised trial using streptomycin for the treatment of tuberculosis.
- **1954** First randomised trial in cancer treatment comparing two chemotherapy regimens in the treatment of acute leukaemia.

Source: Breslin (2008)

Box 9.1b The history of clinical trials: key developments in ethical issues

- **1947** Establishment of ethical principles to guide the use of human subjects in experimentation (Nuremburg Code).
- **1964** Specific guidelines for physicians conducting human research (Declaration of Helsinki).
- **1996** International Conference on Harmonisation (ICH) established good clinical practice (GCP) guidelines for research in human subjects.
- **2004** Medicines for Human Use (Clinical Trials) Regulations 2004 (SI 2004/1031) that implement the European Clinical Trials Directive (2001) came into force in the UK and provides the legal framework to ensure:
  1. standardisation of procedures for ethics and competent authorities;
  2. GCP standards for conducting clinical trials;
  3. Good Manufacturing Practice (GMP) standards for medicines used in clinical trials;
  4. inspections against internationally accepted standards of GCP and GMP, supported by enforcement powers.

Source: Breslin (2008), MHRA (2009)

few other elements included. Now, as clinical trials have become more complex, roles have expanded beyond essential nursing care skills. The research nurse's role is now multi-faceted, and comprises several sub-roles that may be present individually or combined to meet the complex needs of the patient and family involved in a clinical trial. Several sources cite these sub-roles: educator, patient advocate, protocol manager (Ocker & Plank 2000), direct care giver, coordinator of care and research, administrator of research resources and participation in the conduct of the study (Di Giulio et al. 1996). This chapter focuses on the roles of direct care provider, advocate (pathfinder) and educator.

Box 9.1c The history of clinical trials: the research nurse

- **1960s** First roles for research nurses developed in the United States, during early clinical trials in chemotherapy, and arose from a need to develop new knowledge, skills and collaborative practices with oncologists caring for patients in clinical trials (Deininger, 2008).
- **1980s** Central role of the research nurse in clinical trials was fully described and responsibilities were made explicit.
- **1990s** European Organisation for Research and Treatment of Cancer (EORTC) oncology nurse study group survey discussed the involvement of nurses in clinical trials.
- **2000** With the implementation of the National Cancer Plan in the UK (2000) and increased funding for clinical trials in cancer care, demand for clinical research nursing posts within the National Health Service greatly increased.

Preparation of research nurses

Raybuck (1997) discussed the qualities integral to the role of research coordinator as that of excellent clinical judgement related to the specialty area, knowledge of sound ethical principles upon which to practise, as well as excellent communication and organisation skills. These qualities can be applied across all the sub-roles, and are, of course, necessary qualities for nurses practising in any area, at any level.

Educational preparation is essential for further development of the role. Some authors suggest that research nurses are not well prepared for the role. Raja-Jones (2002) suggests that better preparation in research methodology would give research nurses a fuller understanding of protocols and an ability to manage more effectively the problems that can arise from clinical trials. While Groer and Krebs (1998) stated that any specific training and educational needs can be met on the job, Raybuck (1997) asserted that a Masters degree gives the research nurse the necessary clinical, leadership and research skills to collaborate with other healthcare professionals in the area of clinical drug trials. There are postgraduate programmes in clinical research nursing in both the United States and the United Kingdom. Cancer research nurse positions have traditionally been held by nurses with specialty backgrounds such as in oncology that have incorporated the research component (Wheeler 1991; Ocker & Plank 2000). Having a theoretical knowledge of the disease process and the ability to manage the disease process and complications allows the research nurse to understand objectives and endpoints of studies, as well as to evaluate the tasks required to answer the research question(s) (Kenkre & Chatfield 2004).

The position of research nurse may be appropriate for a first-level registered nurse with relevant experience, demonstrating the appropriate competencies and skills for the job and clinical setting. The candidate should be educated to degree level (or working towards) and will be required to demonstrate excellent teamworking skills and the ability to work using their own initiative. In addition to being experienced in caring for patients with cancer, many job descriptions require candidates to have completed an appropriate adult cytotoxic chemotherapy administration programme. In addition, education, training and mentorship will be provided from within the experienced team once an appointment has been made (NHS Lothian 2008).

'A sound knowledge of Good Clinical Practice (GCP), Research Governance, Data Protection and the regulatory frameworks that guide clinical trials is essential and will be provided as mandatory training within 3 months of employment' (University of Edinburgh 2009). There are opportunities in the current environment for nurses prepared at either a first degree, baccalaureate or masters degree level within the field of research nursing (Molin & Arrigo 1995). The Royal College of Nursing (RCN) competency documents state that competencies as well as educational level should determine the role of the research nurse (see Box 9.2).

Box 9.2 Competencies for the clinical trials research nurse

Competency 1: To demonstrate knowledge and understanding of the evolution of clinical research.
Competency 2: To apply knowledge and skills in the clinical research environment.
Competency 3: To work within, and adhere to, the requirements of research ethics, research governance and legislation.
Competency 4: To understand the principles and practice of obtaining valid informed consent.

Source: Royal College of Nursing (2008)

The purpose of a competency is to enable an individual to understand expectations for the position, identify personal development and educational needs, and provide evidence of achievements to support career development and progression. Competencies are necessary to shape nursing work in all clinical and practice settings. As practitioners acquire new skills, knowledge, understanding and confidence in their field of practice, they are able to demonstrate how they meet increasingly challenging levels of competence (RCN 2008). There are skills and personal attributes necessary to fill the role of the clinical research nurse and these are considered to be effective listening and interpersonal skills, time management skills, ability to prioritise workload, information technology (IT) skills, willingness to take responsibility and work collaboratively to deliver solutions to difficult problems. In addition the person must be highly organised, methodical and precise. Perhaps most importantly, the research nurse must exhibit flexibility and the ability to adapt to change (University of Edinburgh 2009). Kenkre and Foxcroft (2001) cite skills and expertise required for research nursing as reliability, organisation, communication, motivation, self-discipline and critical thought. The clinical research nurse therefore is required to be well-educated and up-to-date in professional issues; she or he would benefit from having an inquiring mind and being well motivated to work independently but in collaboration with professional colleagues as part of the multidisciplinary team. Indeed, Chatfield (2008) proposes that the research nurse should consider postgraduate education in clinical research at the Master's level, progressing to doctoral research, in order to gain and develop the skills for career progression for a research, developmental and educational role within the research project team.

Phases of clinical trials in cancer care

Cancer research nurses work with patients participating in clinical trials in most phases of drug development, generally divided into four phases (see Box 9.3). Phase I trials are most intensive with phase III and phase IV being the least intensive, in terms of one-to-one interaction between the patient and nurse. As the phases of drug development are discussed further, the reasons for this will become clear.

Box 9.3   Framework for drug development trials

Phase I: Clinical pharmacology and toxicity, dose finding (maximum tolerated dose).
Phase II: initial investigation of treatment activity, continuing collection of safety
    information.
Phase III: comparison of novel therapy to current standard treatment.
Phase IV: post marketing surveillance.

Source: Girling et al. (2003)

Phase I trials

Classic phase I clinical drug trials utilise the new agent for the first time in humans. In patients with cancer, this is usually when they are no longer responding to standard therapeutic options. These studies are often of high risk and, in reality, generally are of little direct benefit to the patient. In fact, the key issue that patients must understand when deciding to enter a phase I trial is that there is little chance that the investigative agent will actually help them. While there is always hope that it will provide some benefit, the purpose of a phase I drug trial is to determine the maximum tolerated dose of the agent and to develop a safety profile for the drug. There is a higher potential for risk since all that is known about the new drug comes from animal or laboratory studies (Kerr et al. 2006). 'Dose finding' in phase I studies is usually carried out by means of a dose escalation scheme, the first dose, based on preclinical data, is usually one-tenth of the maximum tolerated dose in mice and so is a minute fraction of what is thought to be the active dose in humans (Jenkins & Hubbard 1991).

While the drug being investigated may provide minimal therapeutic benefit to the patients, it does offer them several other benefits and reasons for participating. One of the primary reasons that patients participate in early-phase drug trials is an altruistic one. Many patients speak of the desire to give something back to the health service, to help other patients in the future and to advance medical science. Other reasons include those of needing to take a chance, to continue to do something positive for themselves. Although the chances of benefit from phase I investigative agents cited in the literature range between 3% and 5%, Kerr et al. quote a statement from the husband of a cancer patient:

> Even if the doctors had told us she had only a 1% chance of benefit, we would have done the trial. She was young, we had children, and she wanted to take any chance at all.
>
> Kerr et al. (2006: 12)

There are intangible, unmeasurable benefits of participating in a phase I trial. Because protocols for phase I trials usually include at least a weekly clinical review (sometimes more frequent) the patient is monitored quite closely. For most patients this gives them an added sense of security in that they are able to contact the research nurse and access the research team if at any time they feel that they are unable to manage their symptoms at home. Because little will be known about the trial drug, there is the potential for quite toxic side effects that must be anticipated and then managed by the research team. The patient may have multiple medical comorbidities that also must be managed.

There are other types of trials that do not fit into the classic drug development schema described above. One of these is the 'phase I absorption, distribution, metabolism and excretion (ADME)/extension' trial. These are studies where more is known about the agent because it has already gone through the classic phase I dose escalation part of the process. This type of study gives patients the opportunity to participate and receive new drugs in the very early phase of their development, when the patient may derive some benefit as more information is available about the agent, including therapeutic doses, side-effect profiles and the tumour types in which they exhibit activity. ADME studies use a radio-labelled formulation of the drug in development to track its metabolism and excretion through the body. This type of study requires a real commitment from the patient to participate, as the study usually includes an inpatient stay of about a week and collection of all bodily fluids to measure the excreted radiation and determine the metabolism and excretion of the drug. After the inpatient part of the study has taken place the patient is usually eligible to receive the non-radioactive formulation of the phase I agent in the extension part of the study. This type of study also requires coordination skill on the part of the research nurse.

The education, direct care provision and coordination aspects of the research nurse's role are the components most frequently called into play in a phase I trial. As direct caregivers, nurses may help to plan the investigational study and are often seen as consultants to the principal investigator in planning treatment. Clinical research nurses may also administer the phase I agent and are the most likely to observe and detect expected and unexpected side effects, either at the acute or chronic stage. Research nurses also play an integral part in the management of complications and are instrumental in the development of symptom management guidelines (Payne & Bruso 2001). Coordination of care and services between different groups involved in the patient's care is also critical.

The patient's general practitioner needs to be kept apprised of developments in the patient's care and their status while participating in a trial. Nurses may be asked to monitor other medical conditions that may or may not be related to the patient's trial treatment. While the patient's consultant may be responsible for providing the actual written communication to the general practitioner, it is the responsibility of the research nurse to ensure that events such as clinic appointments and scans trigger the letters (SE-Scotland Cancer Research Network Standard Operating Procedure 212, 2008). The research trial nurses may also be the point of contact for general practitioners and other healthcare providers in the community, for questions regarding an individual patient's progress on the phase I trial. Cancer trials nurses also ensure that information is collected regarding events that may occur in the patient's home community, often many miles from the trial's centre. For example, if the patient is hospitalised in a local general hospital the research nurse would liaise with the medical team in the local community to obtain the information about the patient's hospitalisation and subsequent aftercare. While the nurse fulfils this function for any phase of clinical trial, it is especially important when dealing with novel agents which may be of unknown toxicity.

The role of educator is also a vitally important aspect of the work of nurses who participate in phase I trials. A cancer research trial nurse is the ideal person to reinforce information about the protocol and the science behind it and to answer questions as treatment progresses. This is part of their role in the informed consent, which is an ongoing process from study start until the results are published. Research nurses must be able to write and produce educational materials for patient and family education, and also educational tools for teaching other healthcare professionals involved in the patient's care (Payne & Bruso 2001).

Phase II trials

Once phase I trials have determined the maximum tolerated dose and therefore its therapeutic dose, the first real evaluation of the drug's anti-tumour activity comes with phase II trials (Girling et al. 2003). A phase II trial may be the first time a patient encounters the concept of randomisation, and the research nurse needs to have a clear understanding of randomisation and the appropriate way to explain this concept to the patient and their family. Randomisation is done to avoid bias, and the aim is to make sure that patients assigned to treatment groups are balanced for both known and unknown factors that could affect their response to treatment (Girling et al. 2003). Lesley Fallowfield and her colleagues have done considerable work on the subject of clinical trials, randomisation and how to effectively communicate this to patients (Jenkins et al. 2005). They state that giving complex information, and explaining the concept of randomisation in simple terms, is not an easy task for healthcare professionals. If communication is ineffective the patient will not understand the experimental nature of the trial, will not understand that there are other available treatment options outside the trial, and will be unable to give true informed consent. It is important to remember that an essential part of information giving is pacing it at the right level for the patient and their family (Jenkins et al. 2005). The nurse must ensure that the patient and their family understand the information provided, including randomisation, and so Fallowfield and Jenkins recommend these key points to remember when explaining trials to patients (Fallowfield 1993; Fallowfield & Jenkins 2006):

- Establish patient's own knowledge base
- Signpost where the interview is going
- Summarise and check understanding regularly

- Outline conventional – 'gold standard' – treatment
- Describe 'uncertainty' and scope for improvement in currently available treatment
- Describe the structure of the trial options, which includes non-participation
- Don't hard-sell trial participation
- Explain risks, benefits and side effects
- Explain randomisation explicitly
- Stress that participation is voluntary
- Provide opportunities for further discussion with the research nurse
- Give the patient written information
- Make sure the patient understands that they have time to consider options
- Validate patient understanding
- Support their decision and thank them for considering the trial.

The components of the role of research nurses in the phase II stage of trials are similar to those in phase I. However, the research nurse does not necessarily deliver the drug treatment or provide the direct, hands-on care. It may be delegated to a group of competent nursing colleagues who are experienced in chemotherapy administration and who provide this service on a daily basis. The research nurse is responsible for working to a set of tight eligibility criteria for study entry, ensuring that patients have the same medical characteristics and the same medical condition. This may involve knowledge and deep understanding of pathological grading and staging as well as tumour histology and surgical procedures, to ensure that the selected patients meet the study entry criteria. The knowledge required by the cancer research nurse becomes sub-specialised, dependent on the type of studies the nurse is working with or the disease subtype that is being worked with.

Phase II trials may take several months or several years to complete, depending on what is being studied (Kerr et al. 2006). This may leave the research nurse with a large caseload of patients, ranging from those in treatment to those in long-term follow-up. In this circumstance the research nurse is dealing with patient issues related to the acute side effects of treatment, long-term effects of treatment, and patients who are progressing on treatment or are in the follow-up period, and must therefore have a wide range of knowledge and resources in order to manage patients over such a time span. In this way, the research nurse's role parallels that of the clinical nurse specialist. In fact, the cancer research nurse is a specialist nurse in his or her own right. The title of specialist nurse implies expertise in not only the clinical setting but in three or four sub-roles as well. The sub-roles of educator, consultant and manager, similar to the research nurse's sub-roles already discussed, are part of many graduate programmes that prepare clinical nurse specialists (Arena & Page 1992). In other nursing specialties outside of cancer care, research nurses are developing their roles in much the same manner. For example, in diabetes care in the United Kingdom the role of the research nurse is often embedded in the role of the diabetes specialist nurse (Chester et al. 2007).

Phase III trials

The main purpose of a phase III trial is to test a new treatment against a standard intervention for a specific disease. Phase III trials identify the effectiveness, dosing regimens and routes of administration of the new treatment. One hopes, when carring out a phase III trial, that the trial treatment can offer more than the standard treatment, or that it is less toxic than the standard treatment (Kerr et al. 2006). Because the treatments in phase III are well understood by this point in the drug development process, the risk to the patient is considered to be much lower. Phase III trials have large numbers of patients enrolled into them and are usually run in a large number of centres over a long period of time (usually years). Often, because these studies recruit such large numbers, patient contact with the research nurse is limited both in duration and in scope. The research nurse may have either limited or no direct care provision for this group of patients, but is still responsible for patient recruitment and education regarding the trial requirements, coordination of scans and other investigations, and shared management of the patient with the centre administering the treatment. The research nurse may provide a consultation link to the patient's own general practitioner, who may play a greater role in the care of the patient at this stage. Phase III trials are often randomised. As already mentioned, randomisation is an important concept, but may be difficult for some patients to accept. Patients may have already decided that the 'new' treatment is their preferred treatment and may not be willing to be randomised or to accept the results of the randomisation. It is the research nurse who must unpick this tangle, and sort out all the misconceptions so that the patient is truly informed and committed to participation in the clinical trial (McEvoy et al. 1991).

Phase IV trials

Phase IV trials are usually conducted after the investigative agent has been licensed and marketed. They may be conducted either in hospitals or GP practices. These trials may be done as a condition of licensing the new treatment, for example, to obtain more information about side effects and their frequency now that the drug is being used in a larger patient population. They may also be carried out to see if there are other applications for the agent, or to compare it with a competitor's product to see if there are advantages of one preparation over another. Pharmaco-economic assessment may also be included as part of a phase IV trial (Kerr et al. 2006). The cancer research nurse does not usually provide care for patients participating in these trials.

The nurse–patient relationship in cancer clinical trials

The importance of communication with the patient, to ensure their understanding and their commitment in clinical trials, has been explained above. However, holistic care of patients with cancer also involves interaction with and support of the patient's family or carers. The relationship formed and developed among these individuals can be thought of as a partnership; it is dynamic and is largely dependant on the nurse's interpersonal skills (McQueen 2000).

Thorne and Robinson (1988) have written about the evolving relationships between healthcare providers and patient's carers in the setting of chronic illness. Their analysis described an evolving process comprising three stages that they have labelled naïve trusting, disenchantment and guarded alliance. Naïve trusting is described as the feeling of the patient's family that the healthcare provider has the patient's best interests at heart. Disenchantment occurs when the family realises that there is a difference in the perception of the healthcare provider and the carers of just what the best interests of the patient are. Guarded alliance is the culmination of the process whereby trust is regained on an informed level and allows cooperative care of the patient that embraces both the medical perspective and the family's perspective. The hallmarks of this behaviour are active information seeking, stating perspectives and expectations more clearly, and promotion of mutually satisfying care through negotiation (Thorne & Robinson 1988). In thinking about the interactions between research nurses and their cancer patients this model has some validity. There are phases of relationship development and there is always a tentative period where the patient and the nurse learn about each other and learn to trust each other. This, however, is not naïve trust. It is trust of a different nature, and patients say things like:

> You make me feel so safe. I wish I could take you home with me.
> You were all so kind and caring; you calmed our fears and made [. . .] feel safe.
> Thanks and love. . .
>
> (personal, unpublished correspondence)

This is trust that can both honour and burden the research nurse. Especially when breaking bad news, such as that of disease progression or the patient having to stop trial treatment, this trust is put to the test. Nurses have an important role in the process of disclosure of bad news, and providing support and information following such a disclosure (Thorne & Robinson 1988). The research nurse may feel that the 'side' has let the patient down, and may feel a sense of failure. Fallowfield et al. (2001) surveyed a large number of senior cancer nurses, who indicated that managing personalities and reactions was one of the most challenging communication problems they faced. Breaking bad news was also a problem identified by this group of nurses.

Not only does the clinical research nurse care for the patient, but she or he may find themselves engaged in a caring relationship for the patient's significant others. Nurses have described how important it is for them to gain family trust in order for them to carry out their caring role. They also acknowledged the emotional demands placed on them in caring for families (Stayt 2009).

Emotional labour in clinical trials nursing

Emotional labour pervades the work of clinical trials nursing; for example, in working with patients where the intervention may be of little benefit to their medical condition, where options for treatment are running out and when confronted with ethical dilemmas relevant to their care. In practical terms, emotional labour has been identified as an important component of the process of breaking bad news (Arber & Gallagher 2003). Emotional labour is a concept first described by Hochschild and it has continued to be developed by other theorists such as James (1992), McQueen (1997; 2000; 2004) and Stayt (2009). This concept has also been explored by Aranda as the presentation of the appropriate face that becomes a commodity that can be considered labour or work. This face denies what the nurse may be thinking or feeling (Aranda 2001).

Historically, emotions have been professionalised to present an impersonalised approach of medicine to staff and patients (Gray 2009). McQueen discusses how the breaking down of these professional barriers has potentially led to better patient care and job satisfaction, but has left nurses more exposed to emotional stress and emotional exhaustion (McQueen 1997). There is a price that is exacted by the clinical research nurse for the nature of the relationships that are developed with patients who participate in cancer clinical trials. The ethical and emotional dilemmas that nurses face every day in their work influence the quality of nurse–patient relationships and can take their toll on the nurse, through stress-related illness and burnout (Gray 2009). Work-related stress developing from close interpersonal contact with patients with cancer and their families may result in physical, emotional, social and spiritual problems for the nurses caring for them. The result of this cumulative distress on the nurse and the effect on her care has historically been referred to as burnout. However, the result of the workplace ramifications of sadness and despair on nursing staff are not really revealed in this term. Compassion fatigue appears to be a more descriptive term (Aycock & Boyle 2009). The physical and psychological manifestations of burnout and compassion fatigue have been described by nurses and run the gamut from headaches and muscular pain to irritability, worry, insomnia and overwhelming fatigue. These descriptions reveal the ound suffering of nurses caring for patients (Ekstedt & Fagerberg 2003).

The word 'care' is derived from an Old English word which means sorrow and anxiety. Caring for cancer patients at any stage in their journey implies that there will be moments of worry and anxiety about treatment outcomes on the part of the nurse providing the care for the patient. It is the nature of the emotional rapport developed between trials patients and their nurses that can make small worries develop into profound suffering and lead to the illness, depression and despair exhibited by a trials nurse with compassion fatigue.

Aranda (2001) describes the development of cancer nurses' close relationships with patients as a hidden practice, one that should be talked about and described. She describes how nurses learn from these interactions, making it easier to understand the patient's feelings and to be responsive to the patient's needs. Her paper discusses both the positive and negative aspects of the relationship between patient and cancer nurse: the positive and negative benefits of emotional labour (Aranda 2001). Emotional labour is generally thought of as hard work that takes time and requires considerable knowledge and expertise in the practitioner, but because it seems invisible, there is a risk that it will be underestimated and discounted (Skilbeck & Payne 2003). Despite all the negatives implied in the issues of emotional labour, burnout and compassion fatigue, one author titled a paper 'Only one who burns can burn out' (Weber-Pillar 2009). This is true of the cancer trials nurse; he or she has that burning scientific interest, the desire to be on the cutting edge of treatment, the need to care for a complex and interesting group of patients and take the clinical trial journey with them.

Emotional intelligence

The term 'emotional intelligence' was developed by Mayer and Salovey in 1997. They described it as perceiving emotions, integrating them into thought processes, understanding emotions and managing emotions to stimulate both emotional and intellectual growth (Morrison 2008). Gooch (2006) discusses that in Goleman's theory (Emmerling & Goleman 1993) emotional intelligence involves self-awareness, mood management, self-motivation, empathy and managing relationships. (See also Chapter 10.) Emotional intelligence and the qualities associated with it can be advantageous to nurses as they cope with the emotional 'ups and downs' inherent in their work.

Kenny et al. (2007) suggest that reflective practice and clinical supervision provide effective mechanisms for the exploration of emotions and a means for developing emotional intelligence. Emotional intelligence is also supported by informal peer support and feedback (McQueen 2000) and, according to Kenny et al. (2007), support by management is necessary for nurses providing psychosocial care for patients with cancer. While it is recognised that those within the management structure should support the emotional work of nurses and foster emotional intelligence, it has been found that most support for emotional work has come from colleagues or friends (McQueen 1997).

Hill and MacArthur (2006) discuss that many clinical trials nurses work in isolation and are line managed by a non-nursing manager. Therefore, clinical trials nurses do not typically have access to supervision, informal peer support, expert modelling, coaching or mentoring to help them manage the emotional stressors and situational issues and encourage the development of emotional intelligence. Hill and MacArthur, (2006) argue that research nurses should have access to clinical supervision, and it should be integrated into a job plan for continual professional development and support. A Research Nurse Forum was organised in NHS Lothian (Scotland) in order to take forward some of the recommendations of Hill and MacArthur's work. The forum membership comprised research nurses from within all the organisations aligned to NHS Lothian that employ research nurses (NHS, universities and charities). This was an attempt to bring together research nurses in all specialties, working within teams or in isolation, to discuss common issues, to provide educational and networking opportunities and to provide informal peer support. The group meets quarterly. Hill has gone on to develop a Scotland-wide clinical trials group, the Scottish Research Nurse and Coordinators Network (SRNCN), for the same purposes as the local forum. The organisation has a website that includes a message board and job postings. The need for access of clinical research nurses to colleagues for discussion and support is therefore recognised, and moves are afoot to address this for the benefit of the nurses and the care they provide.

The clinical trials nurse as cancer nursing researcher

Nursing research in the clinical area is designed to improve the quality of care delivered to patients (Polit et al. 2001). Parahoo (2006) describes the need for nurses to participate and lead on research in order to contribute to practice by providing an insight and understanding of their practice and to test the effectiveness of the care they provide. At the outset of this chapter, the role of the nurse as researcher was identified as undergoing evolution. Previously the nurses were seen simply as data collectors for physicians doing research, but now oncology nursing practice has benefited from the contributions of trials nurses, developing symptom management interventions that have been validated and are effective (McEvoy et al. 1991). The increasing recognition of the importance of research in undergraduate and postgraduate nursing education has enabled nurses to take a more informed, active role in medical research and to demonstrate their initiative in developing research studies with a particular focus on nursing.

It is becoming more common that clinical trials also contain a nursing element or companion study. The companion study is usually derived from the primary trial but asks a particular nursing question. These studies may explore a number of methods from qualitative research, such as ethnographic and phenomenological approaches (Ferrell & Cohen 1991). Clinical trials nurses are perfectly poised to lead on companion studies, and this may lead to future funding opportunities for independent cancer nursing research as the nurse establishes a track record of publications and presentations.

Conclusion

Clinical research in cancer care is a long and complex process that takes place in a variety of clinical settings along the continuum of care. Nurses play a key role in the successful design, implementation and evaluation of clinical research. The nurse in the research setting has the opportunity to develop and utilise advanced skills and knowledge that are not always necessary in other healthcare settings. Not only does the nurse have the chance to participate in the development of new drugs and treatments for cancer, but also has the opportunity to provide expert care, emotional support and perhaps even hope, to patients and their families. It is both an awesome responsibility and a great honour to be able to travel this part of the cancer journey with patients and it is the journey, not necessarily the outcome, that matters.

Clearly this work requires special knowledge and skills for competence in the technical care of the patients. In addition there is a need to be able to engage in emotional work in the care and support of patients and in communication with patients and their relatives. To this end it would seem advantageous for research nurses in cancer care to operate with a high level of emotional intelligence if this can offer some protection for their personal, emotional wellbeing.

Emotional intelligence can be acquired and developed with support from managers and through activities such as reflection and clinical supervision. Supporting the cancer research nurse to support the patient can lead to enhanced patient care and improved job satisfaction. This is an exciting time to participate in clinical trials nursing in cancer care. Clinical research nurses have the ability through the work that they do to play a key role in transforming future healthcare and cancer treatment for more patients than they might imagine, as well as for the single patient in their care.

References

Aranda S (2001) Silent voices, hidden practices: exploring undiscovered aspects of cancer nursing. *International Journal of Palliative Nursing* 7(4): 178–85.
Arber A, Gallagher A (2003) Breaking bad news revisited: the push for negotiated disclosure and changing practice implications. *International Journal of Palliative Nursing* 9(4): 166–72.

Arena D, Page N (1992) The impostor phenomenon in the clinical nurse specialist role. *Image: Journal of Nursing Scholarship* **24**(2): 121–5.

Aycock N, Boyle D (2009) Interventions to manage compassion fatigue in oncology nursing. *Clinical Journal of Oncology Nursing* **13**(2): 183–91.

Breslin S (2008) History and background of clinical trials. In: Klimazewski AD, Bacon M, Deininger HE, Ford BA, Westendorp JG (eds) *Manual of Clinical Trials Nursing*, 2nd edn. Pittsburgh, PA: Oncology Nursing Society, pp. 3–9.

Chatfield D (2008) Role of the specialized neuro-intensive care nurse in neuroscience research. *European Journal of Anaesthesiology* **25** (Suppl 42): 160–3.

Chester P, Kennedy ED, Hynd S, Matthews DR (2007) Clinical research networks in diabetes: the evolving role of the research nurse. *European Diabetes Nursing* **4**(1): 10–13.

Deininger HE (2008) Specialization in clinical trials nursing. In: Klimazewski AD, Bacon M, Deininger HE, Ford BA, Westendorp JG (eds) *Manual of Clinical Trials Nursing*, 2nd edn. Pittsburgh, PA: Oncology Nursing Society, pp. 353–6.

Di Giulio P, Arrigo C, Gall H, Molin C, Nieweg R, Strohbucker B (1996) Expanding the role of the nurse in clinical trials: The nursing summaries. *Cancer Nursing* **19**(5): 343–7.

Emmerling R, Goleman D (2003) Emotional Intelligence: Issues and common misunderstandings. *Issues and Recent Developments in Emotional Intelligence* **1**(1), available at http://www.eiconsortium.org (accessed 27 August 2009).

Ekstedt M, Fagerberg I (2003) Lived experiences of the time preceding burnout. *Journal of Advanced Nursing* **49**(1): 59–67.

Fallowfield L (1993) Giving sad and bad news. *Lancet* **341**(8843): 476–8.

Fallowfield L, Jenkins V (2006) Key points when discussing RCTs. *Talking About Randomised Clinical Trials: PowerPoint Presentation for Facilitators*. Course materials, Facilitator Training Course, 2006 (http://www.lifesci.sussex.ac.uk).

Fallowfield L, Saul J, Gilligan B (2001) Teaching senior nurses how to teach communication skills in oncology. *Cancer Nursing* **24**(3): 185–91.

Ferrell B, Cohen M (1991) Companion studies. *Seminars in Oncology Nursing* **7**(4): 252–9.

Girling D, Parmar M, Stenning S, Stephens R, Stewart L (2003) *Clinical Trials in Cancer*. Oxford: Oxford University Press.

Gooch S (2006) Emotionally smart. *Nursing Standard* **20**(51): 20–2.

Gray B (2009) The emotional labour of nursing. 1: exploring the concept. *Nursing Times* **105**(8): 26–9.

Groer M, Krebs D, Elson G (1998). A new path: Looking ahead. *American Journal of Nursing* **98**: 16B–16D.

Hill G, MacArthur J (2006) Professional issues associated with the role of the research nurse. *Nursing Standard* **20**(39): 41–7.

James N (1992) Care = organisation + physical labour + emotional labour. *Sociology of Health and Illness* **14**(4): 488–509.

Jenkins J, Hubbard S (1991) History of clinical trials. *Seminars in Oncology Nursing* **7**(4): 228–34.

Jenkins V, Fallowfield L, Solis-Trapala I, Langridge C, Farewell V (2005) Discussing randomised clinical trials in cancer therapy: evaluation of a Cancer Research UK training programme. *BMJ* **330**(7488): 400.

Jenkinson C, Burton J, Cartwright J, et al. (2005) Patient attitudes to clinical trials: development of a questionnaire and results from asthma and cancer patients. *Health Expectations* **8**: 244–52.

Kenkre J, Chatfield D (2004) Study site co-ordinator/clinical research nurse: a career for nurses in the pharmaceutical industry? *Clinical Research Focus* **15**(8): 5–9.

Kenkre J, Foxcroft D (2001) Career pathways in research: clinical research. *Nursing Standard* **16**(5): 41–4.

Kenny A, Endacott R, Botti M, Watts R (2007) Emotional toil: psychosocial care in rural settings for patients with cancer. *Journal of Advanced Nursing* **60**(6): 663–72.

Kerr DJ, Knox K, Robertson DC, Stewart D, Watson R (2006) *Clinical Trials Explained: A Guide to Clinical Trials in the NHS for Healthcare Professionals.* Malden, MA: Blackwell Publishing.

Mayer J, Salovey P (1997) What is emotional intelligence? In: Salovey P, Sluyter D (eds) *Emotional Development and Emotional Intelligence: Educational Implications.* New York: Basic Books.

McEvoy M, Cannon L, McDermott M (1991) The professional role for nurses in clinical trials. *Seminars in Oncology Nursing* **7**(4): 268–74.

McQueen A (1997) The emotional work of caring, with a focus on gynaecological nursing, *Journal of Clinical Nursing* **6**(3): 233–40.

McQueen A (2000) Nurse–patient relationships and partnership in hospital care. *Journal of Clinical Nursing* **9**(5): 723–31.

McQueen A (2004) Emotional intelligence in nursing work. *Journal of Advanced Nursing* **47**(1): 101–8.

Medicines and Heathcare Products Regulatory Agency (2009) www.mhra.gov.uk (accessed August 2009).

Meredith C, Symonds P, Webster L, et al. (1996) Information needs of cancer patients in west Scotland: cross sectional survey of patients' views. *BMJ* **313**(7059): 724–6.

Molin C, Arrigo C (1995) Clinical trials and quality of life assessment. *European Journal of Cancer* **31**(suppl 6): S8–10.

Morrison J (2008) The relationship between emotional intelligence competencies and preferred conflict-handling styles. *Journal of Nursing Management* **16**: 974–83.

NHS, Lothian (2008) Oncology research nurse, job description. Unpublished material.

Ocker B, Plank D (2000) The research nurse role in a clinic-based oncology research setting. *Cancer Nursing* **23**(4): 286–92.

Parahoo K (1997) *Nursing Research: Principles, Process and Issues.* London: Macmillan.

Payne Y, Bruso P (2001) Gene therapy. In: Rieger P (ed.) *Biotherapy: A Comprehensive Overview,* 2nd edn. Philadelphia: Jones & Bartlett, pp. 353–6.

Polit D, Beck C, Hungler B (2001) *Essentials of Nursing Research.* Philadelphia: Lippincott.

Raja-Jones H (2002) Role boundaries – research nurse or clinical nurse specialist? A literature review. Journal of Clinical Nursing **11**: 415–20.

Raybuck JA (1997) The clinical nurse specialist as research coordinator in clinical drug trials. *Clinical Nurse Specialist* **11**(1): 14.

Royal College of Nursing (2008) *Competency Framework for Clinical Research Nurses version 1.* London: RCN.

Scottish Research Nurse and Coordinators Network (SRNCN) www.srncn.scot.nhs.uk.

Skilbeck J, Payne S (2003) Emotional support and the role of the clinical nurse specialists in palliative care. *Journal of Advanced Nursing* **43**(5): 521–30.

Spilsbury K, Petherick E, Cullum N, Nelson A, Nixon J, Mason S (2007) The role and potential contribution of clinical research nurses to clinical trials. *Journal of Clinical Nursing* **17**(4): 549–57.

Stayt L (2009) Death, empathy and self preservation: the emotional labour of caring for families of the critically ill in adult intensive care. *Journal of Clinical Nursing* **18**: 1267–75.

Thorne SE, Robinson CA (1988) Health care relationships: the chronic illness perspective. *Research in Nursing and Health* **11**: 293–300.

University of Edinburgh (2009) Senior research nurse job description. *Oncology.*

Weber-Pillar M (2009) 'Only one who burns can burn out': caregivers and burnout syndrome in health care careers. [German] *Kinderkrankenschwester* **28**(6): 234–9.

Wheeler V (1991) Preparing nurses for clinical trials: the cancer center approach. *Seminars in Oncology Nursing* **7**(4): 275–9.

Further reading

Association of the British Pharmaceutical Industry (2007) Guidelines for Phase I Clinical Trials. Available at http://www.abpi.co.uk.

Butler L, Degner L, Baile W, SCRN Communication Team, Landry, M. (2005) Developing communication competency in the context of cancer: a critical interpretive analysis of provider training programs. *Psycho-Oncology* **14**: 861–72.

Campbell T (1998) Patient focused care: primary responsibilities of research nurses. *British Journal of Nursing* **7**(22): 1405–9.

Catania G, Poirè I, Dozin B, Bernardi M, Boni L (2008) Validating a measure to delineate the clinical trials nursing role in Italy. *Cancer Nursing* **31**(5): E11–15.

Davis M, Read S (2001) Clinical role clarification: using the Delphi method to establish similarities and differences between nurse practitioners and clinical nurse specialists. *Journal of Clinical Nursing* **10**: 33–43.

Day S (2006) The development of clinical trials. In: Machin D, Day S, Green S,(eds) *Textbook of Clinical Trials*, 2nd edn. Chichester, UK: John Wiley & Sons, pp. 3–11.

De Veer A, Francke A, Poortvliet EP (2008) Nurses involvement in end-of-life decisions. *Cancer Nursing* **31**(3): 222–8.

Flynn KE, Weinfurt KP, Seils DM, et al. (2008) Decisional conflict among patients who accept or decline participation in phase I oncology studies. *Journal of Empirical Research on Human Research Ethics* **3**(3): 69–77.

Iranmanesh S, Axelsson K, Sävenstedt S, Häggström T (2009) A caring relationship with people who have cancer. *Journal of Advanced Nursing* **65**(6): 1300–8.

Jones RB, Pearson J, Cawsey AJ, et al. (2006) Effect of different forms of information produced for cancer patients on their use of the information, social support, and anxiety: randomised trial. *BMJ* **332**(7547): 942–8.

Malone J, Fontenla M, Bick D, Seers K (2008) Protocol-based care: impact on roles and service delivery. *Journal of Evaluation in Clinical Practice* **14**: 867–73.

Manning M (2004) The advanced practice nurse in gastroenterology serving as patient educator. *Gastroenterology Nursing* **27**(5): 220–5.

Martens ML (2009) A comparison of stress factors in home and inpatient hospice nurses. *Journal of Hospice and Palliative Nursing* **11**(3): 144–53.

McNeil SD, Fernandez CV (2006) Informing research participants of research results: analysis of Canadian university based research ethics board policies. *Journal of Medical Ethics* **32**: 49–54.

Meropol NJ, Weinfurt KP, Burnett CB, et al. (2003) Perceptions of patients and physicians regarding phase I cancer clinical trials: implications for physician-patient communication. *Journal of Clinical Oncology* **21**(13): 2589–96.

Parker PA, Aaron J, Baile WF (2008) Breast cancer: unique communication challenges and strategies to address them. *Breast Journal* **15**(1): 69–75.

Raven A (1997) *Consider it Pure Joy...*, 3rd edn. Cambridge: Cambridge Healthcare Research Ltd.

Srivastava N, Tucker JS, Draper ES, Milner M (2008) A literature review of principles, policies and practice in extended nursing roles relating to UK intensive care settings. *Journal of Clinical Nursing* **17**: 2671–80.

Stead M, Eadie D, Gordon D, Angus K (2005) Hello, hello – it's English I speak!: a qualitative exploration of a patient's understanding of the science of clinical trials. *Journal of Medical Ethics* **31**: 664–9.

Stryker JE, Wray RJ, Emmons KM, Winer E, Demetri G (2005) Understanding the decisions of cancer clinical trial participants to enter research studies: factors associated with informed consent, patient satisfaction and decisional regret. *Patient Education and Counseling* **63**: 104–9.

Wagner D, Bear M (2008) Patient satisfaction with nursing care: a concept analysis within a nursing framework. *Journal of Advanced Nursing* **65**(3): 692–701.

Weinfurt KP, Castel LD, Li Y, et al. (2003) The correlation between patient characteristics and expectations of benefit from phase I clinical trials. *Cancer* **98**: 166–75.

Williams A, McGee P, Bates L (2001) An examination of senior nursing roles: challenges for the NHS. *Journal of Clinical Nursing* **10**: 195–203.

Chapter 10

Emotional work of caring in cancer nursing

Anne McQueen

The reader will appreciate that there are many types of cancer – all individual in their development, treatment and management. The specific management, the treatment options, the stage of the patient's cancer journey and the particular patient scenario will determine the specifics of their care and their relationship with professional carers. For the purpose of this chapter the concepts of caring, emotional work and the nurse–patient relationship herein will be situated in a general frame of nurses caring for patients with cancer, rather than with a specific type of cancer or individuals following a particular therapeutic approach. An over-riding factor in cancer care is not just care of the patient but care of the patient within their family context; interaction, communication and supportive work with the family is therefore inclusive in patient care and will be discussed as part of the nurse's work. This chapter will explore the concepts of caring and emotional work of nurses and proceed to illustrate the significance of these concepts in cancer care.

Caring

Concepts of care and caring are common in everyday contexts as well as in professional contexts. In social life we are familiar with maternal and paternal care for children; care for friends and for fellow human beings, and care for animals. In addition there is also a sense of care for our property: for our home and other prized possessions. In this respect Heidegger, as early as 1962, makes a useful distinction between two types of care: care for others (solicitude) and care for things (concern). The care of interest here is that of solicitude, and particularly in the context of nursing. Many authors have recognised that caring is fundamental to humanity (Clifford 1995; Brykczynska 1997; Brechin et al. 1998) and much has been written on caring in the context of nursing.

A great deal of the important work on caring and its significance in nursing dates from the 1980s. The authors of that time explored the concept, attempted to clarify its nature or meaning, they put forward their perspective and raised the profile of caring, emphasising its value in nursing. This literature is relevant here; it is invaluable in our understanding and application of caring today and it has provided a good foundation for further research.

Perspectives on Cancer Care.   Edited by Josephine (Tonks) N. Fawcett and Anne McQueen
© 2011 Blackwell Publishing Ltd

Caring is considered to be fundamental to nursing. Leininger (1984), for example, believes that caring is a central or focal issue; indeed, it is considered to be the essence of nursing. Earlier Watson (1979) also proposed that caring was at the heart of nursing. Many others have also considered caring to be at the core of nursing (Benner & Wrubel 1989; Kurtz & Wang 1991; Morrison 1992; Smith 1992; Abu Said 1993). While caring is not unique *to* nursing it may be unique *in* nursing (Roach 1992: 47). In other words, it can be argued that the physical and emotional work of caring that is part of nursing is special to nursing and can be distinguished from the caring employed by other professional groups.

Larson and Ferketich (1993) describe care as the intentional actions that convey physical care and emotional concern and promote a sense of security in another. However, some authors such as Kitson (1987) and Fealy (1995) differentiate between lay and professional caring. Lay caring can be driven by love for a member of the family, whereas professional caring is determined by a professional ethic, a professional sense of responsibility. Clearly it has an ethical dimension, partly based on human ethic (i.e. respect for persons) and partly on a professional ethic, as in a professional code of behaviour. Fealy (1995) therefore assigns a moral dimension to professional caring, indicating that caring in nursing is considered against theories of social morality and the professional imperatives that guide actions. Professional caring is suggested as a distinct type of caring, dependent on special knowledge and skills, and also on how these are used in caring situations. Fealy (1995) also acknowledges two sides to the coin of caring: the overt behaviours and the concomitant emotions. Caring *for* is concerned with doing, helping activities, and caring *about* involves feelings and emotions (concerns, anxieties, sympathy, empathy, etc.).

Swanwick and Barlow (1994) extend the concept of caring to include physical, emotional, cognitive and intuitive aspects. They therefore acknowledge the special knowledge, thought processes and judgements as well as the instinctive and perceptive qualities that come to the fore in caring. Caring is not bound by rules but is a flexible, amorphous process. Both Swanwick and Barlow (1994) and Radwin et al. (2005: 166) believe that caring is 'showing compassion, concern and kindness'.

In spite of the abundance of literature on caring and its place in nursing, it is difficult to formulate a clear, all-embracing definition of caring. Perhaps part of the problem is its subjective nature and what is caring in one situation may be interpreted as intrusiveness in another. Caring undoubtedly incorporates actions, interactions and feelings with cognitive and emotional components, and is intended to have a beneficial outcome. The input of each of these components can vary according to how people individually perceive or interpret the meaning of caring. There is clearly a need to understand the values and practices relevant to the circumstances and the culture of the person being cared for.

Unlike the overt technical work of nursing, much of caring is invisible, goes unnoticed or is taken for granted. Care is not specified or quantified. The *invisibility* of care work and lack of its documentation results in it being overlooked as part of the nurse's work, with its associated skills as well as its stresses and the fatigue it may cause. It is argued here that caring is fundamental and pervades all nursing work (feeling, thinking and doing), and the extent to which the nurse feels and thinks about caring for a patient has an important influence on the quality of nursing care experienced by the patient. The low status of care work, traditionally linked with *women's work*, belittles this important aspect of nurses' work. It is, therefore, important to identify the benefit of 'caring' for patient outcomes.

A caring relationship

Fundamental to the nature and quality of care is the relationship between the carer and the person receiving care. Over the last three decades there has been a move away from the authoritative, paternalistic attitude which characterised the relationship between health-care professionals and patients. The elite position of professionals and the power accorded to them associated with their special knowledge and skills have been challenged. Information relating to health and wellbeing, and facts relating to diseases and treatments, including cancers, are easily accessible to the public through popular magazines, books, the Internet, radio and television. Furthermore, individuals are encouraged to take responsibility for their health, to follow advice about diet and exercise, to take advantage of screening facilities and to make informed choices about care and treatment. The patient's relationship with professionals has, more generally, moved towards one of partnership; the patient and the professional working together and jointly deciding on the best course of action for the particular patient.

Government policies and healthcare initiatives demonstrate a commitment to patient participation and encourage the public to express their views for strategic planning of cancer services (Scottish Executive 2004; Scottish Government 2008). Public meetings and 'open days' are arranged to allow professionals, academics and the general public to contribute their views to policy makers and to hear about innovations in research in cancer and other diseases. If patients are to participate in discussion and debate they require access to up-to-date information. Likewise, if they are to 'become active partners when they require professional intervention, relevant information, advice, guidance and counselling are required at an individual level' (McQueen 2000: 726).

Nurses are in a unique position in the healthcare structure in that they are the personnel closest to the patients. The work of nurses can involve intimate physical contact as well as an emotional connection, and in a hospital context, their care of patients continues over the 24-hour day and night. Nurses are therefore pivotal figures and their relationship with patients is fundamental to the wellbeing of patients. The type of relationship formed will differ in different situations with different patients and is related to their healthcare needs (Morse 1991). Good interpersonal skills are required to develop a rapport that will be of therapeutic value to the patient and will enable meaningful communication with relatives. The development and maintenance of an appropriate therapeutic relationship requires work on the part of the nurse and is fundamental to a successful partnership (McQueen 2000).

Partnerships form when individuals or parties work together with a shared interest and, in this instance, implies two people coming together on a joint venture. This need not be a relationship where the participants are of equal status or contribute equally, as has been suggested by Fealy (1995), but rather one involving open negotiation, and agreed decisions being made about the contribution of each partner. Nurses bring to this their professional expertise, while patients contribute knowledge and skills based on their particular life experiences and feelings. Offering choices to patients respects their individuality and personal preferences within their particular life context. Their choices require to be honoured when patents have been provided with all the relevant information and evidence upon which to base their decisions. Having acknowledged this, making choices can be burdensome for some patients, and it is also recognised that not all patients wish to be involved in decisions relating to their treatment or care. Here they choose to delegate to the professional, whom they believe is acting in their best interests (Waterworth & Luker 1990; Cahill, 1998).

Forming valued, therapeutic relationships requires trust, closeness and mutual commitment (Muetzel 1988; Christensen 1993; Dowling 2006). Trust is fundamental to the intimacy involved, particularly in cancer care, in a nurse–patient relationship and in the physical, psychosocial and emotional aspects of nurses' work. This is illustrated in the intimate contact nurses have with patients when they assist with personal hygiene, assess and dress wounds, and administer medications and treatments. Also, intimate or personal information relating to one's psychosocial experiences and emotional reactions is shared and discussed with nurses as part of the holistic approach to care (Mok & Chiu 2004). The value of a close nurse–patient relationship is expressed by Mok and Chiu when they say that these nurses:

> show understanding of patients' suffering, are aware of their unvoiced needs, provide comfort without actually being asked, and are reliable, proficient, competent and dedicated in their care . . . Such relationships not only improve patients' physical and emotional state, but also facilitate their adjustment to their illness, ease pain and can ultimately lead to a good death experience.
>
> Mok and Chiu (2004:475)

An appropriate therapeutic relationship may develop spontaneously between nurse and patient, or some factors may inhibit a mutually satisfying relationship. Morse (1991) and Ramos (1992) describe some discordant relationships where the commitment of the two individuals appears to be at different levels of involvement. This fails to meet the needs of either partner and is unproductive. While it is recognised that 'both nurse and patient clearly contribute to the type of relationship, it is the nurse's role to encourage the development of one that is therapeutic. This calls on personal qualities, social skills and emotional work' (McQueen 2000: 727). Emotional work is not only involved in forming relationships with patients but also in the work of nursing more generally.

Emotional work

It has been shown above that the relationship nurses have with their patients, as they perform the technical skills and compassionate care of nursing, can involve both physical and emotional involvement. Close, intimate, physical work is not without thought and personal feelings for the nurse; perhaps embarrassment, distaste or shock. Nurses also face many disconcerting situations with their patients when patients' treatments result in distress or when they are informed of 'bad news' such as a very poor prognosis. Supporting patients in pain and distress also stimulates emotion in nurses as they empathise and attempt to provide compassionate care. Thus there are many situations that can give rise to emotional feelings when caring for sick individuals. However, not all emotions experienced by nurses are negative; they also share in feelings of joy when patients have 'good news' or recover, and they can experience feelings of satisfaction when they believe that they have contributed to the patient's comfort or wellbeing (McQueen 1997).

While emotional feelings associated with experiences may be spontaneous, it is not always appropriate to express these emotions. Conversely, sometimes emotional displays that are appropriate in a particular situation do not occur spontaneously. In these circumstances the management of feelings, appropriate for social situations, requires emotional work. Arlie Hochschild (1983) used the term 'emotional *labour*', emphasising the hard work or effort involved *and* the fact that managing one's emotions, within the context of one's job, is part of the job for which one is paid. She writes:

> This labor requires one to induce or suppress feelings in order to sustain an outward countenance that produces the proper state of mind in others – in this case, the sense of being cared for in a convivial and safe place.
>
> Hochschild (1983:7)

In nursing, emotional work is called for in the formation and maintenance of a relationship with patients, in supporting and educating patients and in association with the physical work, including that described by Lawler (1991) as 'dirty work'. This might include, for example, dressing a noxious smelling, fulminating wound, cleaning an incontinent patient, or performing the final act of care when someone dies. Thus emotional work parallels many other aspects of the nurse's work. Feelings are managed with the aim of portraying a positive caring manner, to encourage patients to feel valued and secure, such that they feel able to express their individuality and exert control over their care as they wish.

Management of feelings

Hochschild (1983) describes processes of surface and deep acting, as emotional work in the management of feelings. In surface acting, the individual behaves in a manner that conveys to the other that she seems to understand and appreciate the other person's situation. Facial expressions, such as tightening of the lips or furrowing of the brow, and behaviour such as a light touch on the arm can convey feelings for the other person and indicate concern and support. The surface actor works at displaying an understanding and concern, and this can be immediately effective at providing some comfort for the other person, but any feelings for the other person's situation are quite brief and at a superficial level. Deep acting, however, is more profound and can be achieved by either directly forcing the required emotion or indirectly by using one's imagination to produce the desired emotion. To illustrate this, a nurse, listening to a patient explain how he finds the fatigue associated with his cancer therapy so frustrating and debilitating, may use surface acting to demonstrate empathy and understanding. This can be achieved by her facial expression, movement of her head and perhaps a light touch of her hand on the patient's arm, in addition to any comforting words she may say; but the feelings she may have about the patient's experience require little effort and are quite short-lived. Deep acting might be experienced when the nurse intentionally thinks about the experience of intense fatigue, exhaustion, the frustration of not being able to carry out everyday activities, the limitations and restrictions this imposes, and tries to understand this from the patient's position. In other words, she has worked on her feelings by engaging in cognitive work. In situations where a nurse finds it difficult to empathise with a patient (perhaps because of different social or cultural values) more effort may be required to *create and demonstrate* the desired emotion and achieve the 'feelings of care' that will enhance the behavioural care possible. Thus emotions are worked on; some may be suppressed while others are pushed forward and are developed, so that the deep actor actually experiences the feeling being displayed.

In the course of their work nurses interact with many patients, each with their own particular health concerns and personal worries. Moving from one patient to another then demands that nurses continually mange their emotions so that they are appropriate for the particular interaction and interpersonal communication with individual patients. By way of illustration, a nurse may have been comforting a patient who has been informed that she has cancer, and on leaving this patient she moves to another patient who shares her delight in knowing that she is pregnant after several attempts at in-vitro fertilisation. Having been deeply involved with the previous patient it may be difficult to really appreciate the joy of the next one, but the correct display, with surface acting, is called for. Clearly this demonstrates how nurses require to be able to control their emotions and present the image that is appropriate to engage with their patients. This involves mental energy, and over time can be tiring and draining. While one can feel emotionally exhausted there may also be a feeling of satisfaction in knowing that one has behaved in a way that has been of benefit to the patients.

While caring relationships may be achieved without undue effort and can be a source of satisfaction, the emotional work involved in forming and maintaining therapeutic relationships may be considerable and can be a cause of mental exhaustion. In some situations deep relationships can develop almost spontaneously, in accordance with the nurse's 'true' or 'natural' feelings for a patient. However, close and intense relationships where nurses empathise deeply with their patients can add to the stress of nursing. Conversely, there may be times when nurses feel unable to engage with their patients; the situation may be too demanding. Surface action may be employed but attempting to maintain this over time, when there is a difference between the feeling and the action, results in emotive dissonance: an unpleasant experience and the cause of strain. It is important to achieve a balance between engagement and detachment in a professional, therapeutic relationship, or burnout may result (Blomberg & Sahlberg-Blom 2007).

In Hochschild's (1983) research with flight attendants, she found that it was possible for them to learn to manage their emotions by systematic training, that competence was achieved with increasing experience and that the more experienced personnel were more proficient at deep acting. These workers were more adept at separating their 'personal' and 'work' selves and this protected against burnout. This emphasises the importance of including the concept of emotional work in the nursing curriculum and assisting nurses with the use of surface and deep acting as well as the employment of appropriate defence strategies to protect their mental wellbeing (Lawler 1991; Smith 1992; Freshwater and Stickley 2004).

While emotional work focuses on the management of emotions in interpersonal situations, it seems to be an obvious advantage, if not an imperative, to be able to successfully assess and appreciate the emotions of others, if one is to respond in a way that fosters in others the desired feeling. The ability to perceive, understand and analyse emotions in a rational way is now recognised as one of many types of intelligence.

Emotional intelligence

Historically, intelligence has been associated with performance in IQ tests, but work over recent decades indicates that this is only one of many types of intelligence. Mayer (2001) describes the work on cognition and emotion from 1900 in five stages:

> (1) from 1900 to 1969, during which the psychological study of intelligence and emotions were relatively separate; (2) from 1970 to 1989, when psychologists focused on how emotions and thought influenced each other; (3) from 1990 to 1993, which marked the emergence of EI as a topic of study; (4) from 1994 to 1997, when the concept was popularized, and (5) the present era of clarifying research.
>
> Mayer (2001:4)

Work in social intelligences, first proposed by Thorndyke (1920), was a precursor to understanding emotional intelligence. In 1993 Gardner wrote about seven major types of intelligence that could be further categorised according to specific abilities. However, his perspective on social intelligence, as discrete from academic abilities, did not accept the concept of emotional intelligence. Gardner (1993) described two types of personal intelligence: interpersonal and intrapersonal. Interpersonal intelligence is demonstrated in the ability to understand other people and successfully cooperate with them. Intrapersonal intelligence is reflected in the ability to form an accurate understanding of one's self and to use this successfully in life; it requires self-awareness and acknowledgement of one's feelings, and the use of these in social encounters. Gardner (1993) recognised these abilities but he did not consider these to be allied with the concept of intelligence. However, in the early 1990s Mayer and Salovey presented a synthesis and analysis of the many strands of research reported from the previous decades; based on a review of work in the fields of emotions, aesthetics, intelligence, artificial intelligence, clinical psychology and brain research, they concluded that the mental work associated with the interpretation and understanding of emotions did constitute a type of intelligence (Mayer & Salovey 1993). Furthermore, they employed an empirical test to measure this construct. A definition of emotional intelligence put forward by Mayer et al. in 1990 is:

> A type of emotional information processing that includes accurate appraisal of emotions in oneself and others, appropriate expression of emotion, and adaptive regulation of emotion in such a way as to enhance living.
>
> Mayer et al. (1990:773)

At around the same time the concept of emotional intelligence was quickly picked up by journalists and became popular, with Golman's first publication on the subject in 1995.

The scientific understanding of the concept at this time was extended and blended with other skills and attributes including motivation, wellbeing and successful engagement in relationships and became a 'trendy', modern message for success but without the scientific rigour (Mayer 2001). Claims were made that emotional intelligence was, or could be, more important than IQ and that it was necessary for success in life. The popular interpretation of emotional intelligence actually blurs the boundaries between psychological traits and emotional intelligence itself. Mayer (2001) claims that most of what has been popularised is more akin to personality traits than emotional intelligence per se, but he concedes that this is not without value.

By 1999 a refined and expanded definition was presented, recognising emotional intelligence as an intellectual ability and acknowledging the capacity to manage emotions:

> Emotional intelligence refers to an ability to recognize the meanings of emotions and their relationships and to reason and problem-solve on the basis of them. Emotional intelligence is involved in the capacity to perceive emotions, assimilate emotion-related feelings, understand the information of these emotions and manage them.
>
> Mayer et al. (1999:267)

Scientific research continues in the field of emotional intelligence, and new measures are being developed, including performance tests and self-report questionnaires (Ciarrochi et al. 2001). Research is complex, with understandings of the concept bearing both popular and scientific features. In attempting to measure emotional intelligence as an 'intelligence' one must be clear that such tests are not measuring other personality traits or characteristics. Ciarrochi et al. (2001: 26) claims that emotional intelligence 'can be assessed reliably, that it is distinct from traditional intelligence and other related concepts'.

It is clear from the abilities identified above and the definitions put forward that emotional intelligence has a place in the context of nursing, where interactions with others are of therapeutic value. It is fitting therefore to give some attention to this in preparing nurses and to consider its relevance to emotional work. While scientific work continues to address emotional intelligence in general, research and scholarly publications specific to nursing have also emerged (Freshwater & Stickley 2004; McQueen 2004; Rego et al. 2010).

The following extract from Freshwater and Stickley (2004) shows an acknowledgment of both the technical skills and emotional work of nursing:

> Whilst the rational mind may adequately attend to the necessary technical aspects of nursing procedures, it is not the place of the rational mind to intuitively sense the needs and emotions of the person at the receiving end of care.
>
> Freshwater and Stickley (2004:93)

Furthermore, they contend that:

> An education that ignores the value and development of the emotions is one that denies the very heart of the art of nursing practice.
>
> Freshwater and Stickley (2004:93)

Other writers also indicate that emotional intelligence is an asset in care (Evans & Allen 2002). Freshwater and Stickley) 2004: 94) contend that 'it [emotional intelligence] is also fundamental to the act of caring'. Indeed, Cadman and Brewer (2001) go further, suggesting that an assessment of emotional intelligence be made prior to recruiting students to a nursing programme. Emotional intelligence has also been shown to be of value in leadership (Stichler 2006) and in teamwork (Druskat & Wolff 2001), both relevant in nursing. McQueen (2004) also suggests that emotional management calls upon emotional intelligence, in achieving successful interactions with patients, their relatives and with colleagues.

Rego et al. (2010) illustrate the complex relationship of emotional intelligence and caring when they relate emotional intelligence with caring behaviours. A total of 120 nurses and 360 patients were included in their study, which involved nurses self-reporting on specified aspects of their emotional intelligence and patients reporting on their caring behaviours. Variance, correlation and regression analyses were employed in an attempt to ascertain how the nurses' emotional intelligence explains their caring behaviours. The findings stress the importance of several dimensions of emotional intelligence, but not all dimensions of emotional intelligence result in more caring behaviours. The caring outcome was shown to depend on the particular combination of the nurse's emotional intelligence profile. While this study has its limitations, this rather complex research has advanced the work on emotional intelligence in nursing, and has shown direction for future work in this field.

Clearly, dealing with one's emotions and those of others is part of nursing, and this is particularly important in cancer care. Emotions require to be managed, in order to engage therapeutically with patients, to gain job satisfaction and to maintain a balance between intimacy and professional distance, to the benefit of both nurse and patient over time. The patient's healthcare needs and their circumstances will influence the most appropriate type of engagement, as will the nurse's ability and willingness to attain a mutually satisfying relationship. Patients with cancer meet nurses at various stages on their cancer journey and inevitably their relationships with nurses will vary with different staff and at different times as their healthcare needs change. The final section of this chapter will address nursing relationships in caring for cancer patients.

Caring in cancer nursing

Caring for patients with cancer is challenging and complex. The work for nurses can be very satisfying and rewarding; it demands specialised knowledge, technical skills, an empathetic approach (compassion) and a commitment to care. It is physically and emotionally demanding, both of which can drain the nurse and lead to feelings of exhaustion. Aside from coping with the technical and physical demands of caring for an individual with cancer and the needs of their family, a cancer diagnosis brings with it many questions, concerns and problems for individuals with respect to their health, self-image and future life. Part of nurses' work is to address these issues and this demands both professional skills and a personal input from the nurse as an individual *caring* for another human being.

While issues relevant to the care of individuals with cancer are presented here, it is important to stress that care will be individualised according to the person's specific needs and their particular situation. Many factors will influence this such as the diagnosis, the stage of disease and treatment, the person's age, their social and cultural background and their supportive network. Nurses are involved with patients faced with the initial diagnosis, through various stages of treatment, individuals enduring a recurrence, patients having palliative care and those who are dying with cancer. Throughout the patients' journeys, nurses work together with other professionals in the interdisciplinary team to address the holistic care of patients. While the specific therapy and care will address the particular patient scenario, there are underlying qualities in caring that transcend the spectrum of cancer nursing.

Cancer nursing incorporates the following aspects (Grunday 2006):

- Assisting patients and their families to adjust to and cope with a cancer diagnosis;
- Administering treatments within their competence;
- Managing side effects and problems associated with cancer and its treatments;
- Controlling and managing symptoms;
- Providing physical, psychological and social support to patients and their families;
- Providing advice and information to patients, their relatives and other health professionals;
- Evaluating nursing care and managing care delivery;
- Engaging in research to enhance quality of care;
- Showing leadership in cancer care.

Other chapters in this book specifically address the nursing care of patients with a particular type of cancer. This chapter complements this by focusing on the emotional aspects of caring for cancer patients.

While some research has suggested that patients rate competence and clinical expertise more highly than effective communication skills of the nurse (von Essen & Sjoden 1991; Widmark-Petersson et al. 1996; 2000), I would argue that this is not surprising. If a nurse is not competent to carry out safe, good-quality practical nursing then good communication skills will count for little when her nursing role is evaluated. Technical competence must be a given, but importantly affective qualities complement the quality of care that can be achieved and enhances the therapeutic nature of nursing.

Grundy (2006: 748) believes that the concept of *care* has had little attention in the context of cancer nursing. She proposes that this is due to its association with women's work, the general belief that it does not require any particular knowledge or skill, and the invisibility of caring. However, she contends that caring is central to cancer nursing and it is 'vital that nurses ... identify the caring aspects of their work and the underlying knowledge which informs that care'.

As discussed earlier in this chapter, there is a need for the nurse to be able to engage with the patient to achieve a satisfying relationship for both patient and nurse. However, a balance is required between a close personal relationship with each cancer patient, facilitating an understanding of and an almost automatic or spontaneous response to their specific, individualised needs, and ensuring a professional demeanour that provides optimal care as well as an emotional defence for the nurse's psychological wellbeing (Blomberg & Sahlberg-Blom 2007).

Relationships are dynamic; they can develop and deepen over time (Morse 1991; Ramos 1992) according to each individual's attitudes and the needs and interactions that occur between them. Over the course of a cancer journey, nursing staff and patients meet at different stages of the treatment trajectory and as a result nurses and patients can 'get to know' each other and develop a professional friendship. Thus a relationship that has been mutually relatively superficial at first meeting – perhaps at a clinic appointment – can evolve over time to one with a deep emotional involvement, satisfying both patient and nurse. Such a relationship spontaneously affords optimum quality of care for the patient and personal reward for the nurse. Forming a relationship involves input from both patients and nurses. Both contribute to develop the type of relationship they are comfortable with, and the way this develops over time. The therapeutic value is appreciated when both nurse and patient are comfortable with the same intensity of the relationship and find it mutually satisfying. The formation of such emotional bonds with cancer patients is often effortless because of the frequency of interactions over a long period and the intimate nature of the interactions, either physically or emotionally.

Dixon and Sweeney (2000) address several qualities considered to be important in a therapeutic relationship. It is particularly relevant in the care of cancer patients for the nurse to use empathy, facilitate relaxation, provide reassurance, use touch, improve self-esteem, recognise the value of laughter and encourage hope. Beyond the treatment regime and the technical care, these attributes add to the quality of care and enhance the overall therapeutic effect.

In a small phenomenological study by Bertero (1999) 10 registered nurses, caring for patients with cancer, were asked to give an account of a situation where they were able to provide good care and of one where they were unable to provide good care for a patient. One major theme emerged from analysis of the caring data: i.e. 'developing and maintaining a helping-trusting interpersonal relationship' (Bertero 1999: 414), suggesting that the relationship was fundamental to the quality of care that can be achieved. Five subthemes were also demonstrated as part of caring described by the nurses: creating an interaction with the patient and next of kin; fulfilling the needs of the patient and next of kin; experiencing feelings of frustration in caring; being affected by time factors; and developing oneself and gaining insight. The author concluded that *caring* was central to the connection between the nurses and the patients, to the sense of achievement the nurses experienced and to their personal enrichment.

In a larger study by Kendall (2007), 392 nurses were asked to describe a caring situation they had experienced, together with its impact on their learning and subsequent practice. It was clear from the language used by nurses in this study that they had a profound understanding of the magnitude and intensity of cancer for patients and their relatives. Frustration and sadness were expressed in interactions with patients. Patients' suffering and the life-threatening nature of cancer impacted on nurses' emotions, affecting them personally and professionally. Furthermore, reflecting on their practice showed insight and great potential for their future practice.

While healthcare policy advocates that patients with cancer will be treated in specialist cancer centres, the pressure on such units and the prevalence and nature of cancer in society means that a number of patients with cancer will have some of their treatment in non-specialist units or at home. As a consequence, not all nurses working with cancer patients will be expert in this specialism (Mohan et al. 2005); their expertise will lie in other fields appropriate to the main area of their work.

A qualitative study by Mohan et al. (2005) suggests that both cancer patients and the nurses caring for them in non-specialist units are at a disadvantage. The emotional nature of care was a major theme identified by the nurses, together with lack of knowledge of cancer treatment and lack of time. The nurses here found that the environment was not conducive to appropriate care and they found it difficult to deal with patients not accepting their cancer diagnosis. While the nurses in this situation were motivated to provide good patient care, they felt hindered by the environment and their lack of knowledge and training specific to cancer care. While oncology is recognised as a specialty, it must be appreciated that nurses outside such specialised units also meet patients with cancer and could benefit from some knowledge and skills appropriate to the care of patients in such settings. It is hoped that this book will be of value to nurses working in this context.

It also needs to be remembered that many patients with cancer are not in a hospital setting and are living with cancer at home. Cancer plans from the Department of Health (2000) and the Scottish Government (2008) show official commitment to the needs of cancer patients across the wider community, and healthcare policies have recognised the important involvement of district nurses, health visitors, practice nurses and school nurses to the care of cancer patients (Lane et al. 2002). However, more resources are always welcomed to make these services more widely available, to enhance an integrated service across primary, secondary and tertiary sectors.

The prevalence of cancer and its presentation in many forms result in its wide distribution across society: in general and specialist hospitals, in hospices and in the community. While it is indisputable that cancer nursing requires specialist and advanced practitioners who are '*exemplar* nurses' (Brykczynska 2002: 20), it is also true that nurses working in all areas of healthcare require adequate knowledge to provide safe and effective care for patients with cancer (Boal et al. 2000; Ward & Wood 2000). It is therefore advocated that education, to meet the needs of these nurses, is planned in association with developing cancer services and is addressed in both pre-registration and post-registration programmes, as appropriate (Grundy 2006).

Working with individuals with cancer and supporting their relatives undoubtedly can be challenging physically and emotionally for nurses, whether they work in non-specialist wards, oncology units, palliative care or a hospice setting. Caring for patients in the many contexts of cancer nursing places a heavy burden on nurses. Many factors contribute to this including, for example, the need for competence and extreme vigilance in administering special treatments, repeated exposure to pain, suffering and distress, recurring deaths, addressing existential questions from patients and their families and facing ethical dilemmas associated with their work (Sabo 2008). Lambert and Lambert (2008) also acknowledge other work-related stresses experienced by nurses more generally, relating, for example, to increasing demands of the job, lack of resources, powerlessness and lack of support. Role conflict and role ambiguity have also been implicated as sources of stress (Muncer et al. 2001). Compassion fatigue and burnout are concepts that have been applied to the resulting distress experienced by nurses who have been overwhelmed by the stresses of their work.

Payne (2001), investigating aspects of hospice nurses' work, found that high levels of emotional exhaustion, extreme depersonalisation of patients and low personal accomplishment correlated with burnout. More specifically, she found that coping with death and dying, dealing with staff conflicts and accepting responsibility contributed to nurses' experience of emotional exhaustion; staff conflicts and inadequate preparation for their job led to feelings of depersonalisation; and inadequate preparation, lack of positive appraisal and having fewer professional qualifications contributed to feelings of lower personal accomplishment.

Stress can be defined as the perception we have about a mismatch between the demands made on us and our coping ability. It therefore follows that logical coping mechanisms might include:

- alteration to the demand;
- changes to perception of demand;
- changes to perception of coping;
- enhancing coping ability.

These mechanisms can be incorporated in different coping strategies, attacking stress directly or indirectly. Lambert et al. (2004; 2007) and Chang et al. (2007) found that the most commonly used coping strategies were problem solving, self-control and seeking social support, and that these were stable across different cultures. Social support may be addressed by talking to colleagues. In this respect, Hopkinson (2002) reports that the nursing handover can provide a supportive medium for nurses, giving them an opportunity to discuss their thoughts and feelings relating to their care of dying patients. This is in addition to gaining information upon which to base their future nursing actions.

Conclusion

In conclusion, caring is fundamental to the quality of nursing provided to patients. Caring consists of actions or behaviour and corresponding thoughts and emotions; together they enhance the quality of care possible. Clearly nurses require professional knowledge and competency in clinical skills, but in addition good nursing care draws on emotional intelligence to perform the physical and emotional work of caring for others in a professional capacity. Cognitive abilities and rational judgments work synergistically with emotional intelligence to enhance the intellectual outcome. Emotional work is essentially part of nursing; nurses work on their emotions to present a caring manner, to enhance their caring behaviour, to achieve congruence between actions and feelings, and to protect their own psychological well-being.

Working with cancer patients through their cancer journey can be a demanding and stressful job. Nurses need to keep up to date with current knowledge and maintain competency in many clinical skills. In addition, skills in communication, counselling and emotion management are also called for. There are high emotional demands on nurses as they empathise with cancer patients, experiencing much physical, mental and social suffering, and as they attempt to alleviate the pain and anguish experienced by patients and their families. While cancer nursing is often challenging it can also be very satisfying when it is perceived as a privilege to care for patients and to know that the care and support given has been of value to their comfort or wellbeing or to their dignity in death. The physical, psychosocial and emotional intimacy of caring for patients through their treatment trajectory and 'getting to know' them within their family unit requires emotional work to maintain a therapeutic relationship, but the bond between nurse and patient adds to the intense satisfaction nurses experience from their work as well as to the quality of patient care they can provide.

References

Abu Said H (1993) Nursing: the science and the practice. *International Journal of Nursing Studies* **30**: 287–94.

Benner P, Wrubel J (1989) The Primacy of Caring. London: Addison-Wesley.

Bertero C (1999) Caring for and about cancer patients: identifying the meaning of the phenomenon caring through narratives. *Cancer Nursing* **22**(6): 414–20.

Blomberg K, Sahlberg-Blom E (2007) Closeness and distance: a way of handling difficult situations in daily care. *Journal of Clinical Nursing* **16**(2): 244–54.

Boal E, Hodgson D, Banks-Howe J, Husband GA (2000) Cultural change in cancer education and training. *European Journal of Cancer Care* **9**(1): 30–5.

Brechin A, Walmsley J, Katz J, Peace S (1998) *Care Matters: Concepts Practice and Research in Health and Social Care*. London: Sage.

Brykczynska G (ed.) (1997) A brief overview of the epistemology of caring. In: *Caring: The Compassion and Wisdom of Nursing*. London: Arnold, pp. 1–9.

Brykczynska G (2002) The critical essence of advanced practice. In: Clarke D, Flanagan J, Kendrick K (eds) *Advancing Nursing Practice and Palliative Care*. Basingstoke, UK: Palgrave Macmillan, pp. 20–42.

Cadman C, Brewer J (2001) Emotional intelligence: a vital prerequisite for recruitment in nursing. *Journal of Nursing Management* **9**(6): 321–4.

Cahill J (1998) Patient participation: a review of the literature. *Journal of Clinical Nursing* **7**(2): 119–28.

Chang E, Bidewell J, Huntington A, Daly J, Johnson A, Wilson H, Lambert VA, Lambert CE (2007) A survey of role stress, coping and health in Australian and New Zealand hospital nurses. *International Journal of Nursing Studies* **44**(8): 1354–62.

Christensen J (1993) *Nursing Partnership: A Model for Nursing Practice*. Edinburgh: Churchill Livingstone.

Ciarrochi J, Chan A, Caputi P, Roberts R (2001) Measuring emotional intelligence. In: Ciarrochi J, Forgas JP, Mayer JD (eds) *Emotional Intelligence in Everyday Life: A Scientific Inquiry*. Philadelphia: Psychology Press, pp. 25–45.

Clifford C (1995) Caring: fitting the concept to nursing practice. *Journal of Clinical Nursing* **4**(1): 37–41.

Department of Health (2000) *The NHS Cancer Plan: A plan for investment, a plan for reform*. London: DH.

Dixon M, Sweeney K (2000) *The Human Effect in Medicine: Theory, Research and Practice*. Abingdon, UK: Radcliffe Medical Press.

Doweling M (2006) The sociology of intimacy in the nurse–patient relationship. *Nursing Standard* **20**(23): 48–54.

Druskat VU, Wolff SB (2001) Building the emotional intelligence of groups. *Harvard Business Review* **79**(3): 80–90.

Evans D, Allen H (2002) Emotional intelligence: its role in training. *Nursing Times* **98**(27): 41–2.

Fealy GM (1995) Professional caring: the moral dimension. *Journal of Advanced Nursing* **22**: 1135–40.

Freshwater D, Stickley TJ (2004) The heart of the art: emotional intelligence in nursing education. *Nursing Inquiry* **11**(2): 91–8.

Gardner H (1993) *Frames of Mind.* New York: Basic Books.

Golman D (1995) *Emotional Intelligence.* New York: Bantam Books.

Grundy M (2006) Cancer care and cancer nursing. In: Kearney N, Richardson A (eds) *Nursing Patients with Cancer: Principles and Practice.* Edinburgh: Elsevier, pp. 741–70.

Heidegger M (1962) *Being and Time.* Trans. Macquarrie J, Robinson E. New York: Harper & Row.

Hochschild AR (1983) *The Managed Heart: Commercialisation of Human Feeling.* Berkeley, CA: University of California Press.

Hopkinson JB (2002) The hidden benefit: the supportive function of the nursing handover for qualified nurses caring for dying people in hospital. *Journal of Clinical Nursing* **11**: 168–75.

Kendall S (2007) Witnessing tragedy: nurses' perceptions of caring for patients with cancer. *International Journal of Nursing Practice* **13**(2): 111–20.

Kitson AL (1987) A comparative analysis of lay caring and professional (nursing) caring relationships. *International Journal of Nursing Studies* **24**(2): 155–65.

Kurtz RJ, Wang J (1991) The caring ethic, more than kindness, the core of nursing science. *Nursing Forum* **26**(1): 4–8.

Lambert VA, Lambert CE (2008) Nurses' workplace stressors and coping strategies. *Indian Journal of Palliative Care* **14**(1): 38–44.

Lambert V, Lambert C, Itano J, et al. (2004) Cross-cultural comparison of workplace stressors, ways of coping and demographic characteristics as predictors of physical and mental health among hospital nurses in Japan, Thailand, South Korea and USA (Hawaii). *International Journal of Nursing Studies* **41**(6): 671–84.

Lambert V, Lambert C, Petrini M, Li X, Zhang Y (2007) Predictors of physical and mental health in hospital nurses within the People's Republic of China. *International Nursing Review* **54**: 85–91.

Lane C, Kelly C, Clarke D (2002) Cancer networks: translating policy into practice. In: Clarke D, Flanagan J, Kendrick K (eds) *Advancing Nursing Practice in Cancer and Palliative Care.* Basingstoke, UK: Palgrave Macmillan, pp. 238–54.

Larson PJ, Ferketich SL (1993) Patients' satisfaction with nurses' caring during hospitalisation. *Western Journal of Nursing Research* **15**: 690–707.

Lawler J (1991) *Behind the Screens: Nursing, Somology and the Problem of the Body.* Melbourne: Churchill Livingstone.

Leininger MM (1984) *Care: The Essence of Nursing and Health.* Thorofare, NJ: Slack.

Mayer JD (2001) A field guide to emotional intelligence. In: Ciarrochi J, Forgas JP, Mayer JD (eds) *Emotional Intelligence in Everyday Life: A Scientific Inquiry.* Philadelphia: Psychology Press, pp. 3–24.

Mayer JD, Salovey P (1993) The intelligence of emotional intelligence. *Intelligence* **17**(4): 433–42.

Mayer JD, DiPaolo MT, Salovey P (1990) Perceiving affective content in ambiguous visual stimuli: a component of emotional intelligence. *Journal of Personality Assessment* **54**: 772–81.

Mayer JD, Caruso D, Salovey P (1999) Emotional intelligence meets traditional standards for an intelligence. *Intelligence* **27**: 267–98.

McQueen A (1997) The emotional work of caring, with a focus on gynaecological nursing. *Journal of Clinical Nursing* **6**: 233–40.

McQueen A (2000) Nurse–patient relationships and partnership in hospital care. *Journal of Clinical Nursing* **9**: 723–31.

McQueen A (2004) Emotional intelligence in nursing work. *Journal of Advanced Nursing* **47**(1): 105–8.

Mohan S, Wilkes LM, Ogunsiji O, Walker A (2005) Caring for patients with cancer in non-specialist wards: the nurse experience. *European Journal of Cancer Care* **14**(3): 256–63.

Mok E, Chiu PC (2004) Nurse–patient relationships in palliative care. *Journal of Advanced Nursing* **48**(5): 475–83.

Morrison P (1992) *Professional Caring in Practice*. Aldershot, UK; Brookfield, VT: Avebury.

Morse JM (1991) Negotiating commitment and involvement in the nurse–patient relationship. *Journal of Advanced Nursing* **16**(4): 455–68.

Muetzel P (1988) Therapeutic nursing. In: Pearson A (ed.) *Primary Nursing: Nursing in the Burford and Oxford Development Units*. London: Croom-Helm, pp. 89–116.

Muncer S, Taylor S, Green DW, McManus IC (2001) Nurses' perceptions of perceived causes of work-related stress. *Work and Stress* **15**(1): 40–52.

Payne N (2001) Occupational stressors and coping as determinants of burnout in female hospice nurses. *Journal of Advanced Nursing* **33**(3): 396–405.

Radwin LE, Farquhar SL, Knowles MN, Virchick BG (2005) Cancer patients' descriptions of their nursing care. *Journal of Advanced Nursing* **50**(2): 162–9.

Ramos MC (1992) The nurse–patient relationship: theme and variations. *Journal of Advanced Nursing* **17**(14): 496–506.

Rego A, Godinho L, McQueen A, Pina e Cunha M (2010) Emotional intelligence and caring behavior in nursing. *Service Industries Journal* **30**(9–10).

Roach MS (1992) *The Human Act of Caring: A Blueprint for the Health Professions*. Ottawa, Ontario: Canadian Hospital Association Press.

Sabo BM (2008) Adverse psychological consequences: compassion fatigue, burnout and vicarious traumatization: Are nurses who provide palliative and haematological cancer care vulnerable? *Indian Journal of Palliative Care* **14**(1): 23–9.

Scottish Executive (2004) *Cancer in Scotland: Sustaining Change*. Edinburgh: Scottish Health Department.

Scottish Government (2008) *Better Cancer Care: An Action Plan*. Edinburgh: Scottish Government.

Smith P (1992) *The Emotional Labour of Nursing*. Basingstoke, UK: Macmillan.

Stichler JF (2006) Emotional Intelligence: a critical leadership quality for nurse executive. *Association of Women's Health, Obstetric and Neonatal Nurses* **10**(5): 422–5.

Swanwick M, Barlow M (1994) How should we define the caring role? *Professional Nurse* **9**(4): 554–9.

Thorndyke E (1920) Intelligence and its uses. *Harper's Magazine* **140**: 227–35.

von Essen L, Sjoden PO (1991) Patients and staff perceptions of caring: review and replication. *Journal of Advanced Nursing* **16**(11): 1363–74.

Ward J, Wood C (2000) Education and training of healthcare staff: the barriers to its success. *European Journal of Cancer Care* **9**(1): 30–5.

Waterworth S, Luker KA (1990) Reluctant collaborators: do patients want to be involved in decisions concerning care? *Journal of Advanced Nursing* **15**(8): 971–6.

Watson J (1979) *The Philosophy and Science of Caring*. Boston, MA: Little, Brown & Co.

Widmark-Petersson V, von Essen L, Lindeman E, Sjoden PO (1996) Cancer patient and staff perceptions of caring vs clinical care. *Scandinavian Journal of Caring Sciences* **10**: 227–33.

Widmark-Petersson V, von Essen L, Sjoden PO (2000) Perceptions of caring among patients with cancer and their staff. *Cancer Nursing* **23**(1): 32–9.

Chapter 11

The management of rectal cancer and the consequences of treatment

Gillian Knowles and Rachel Haigh

Survival following rectal cancer has improved significantly over the last 20 years through earlier detection and improved treatments. Treatment can involve surgery, radiotherapy and chemotherapy, often in combination, which can result in a range of potential side effects over a period of time. For this reason there is an emerging focus on the long-term impact on health-related quality of life in patients that highlights the need for more robust assessment and intervention strategies. Following treatment, patients with rectal cancer can experience distressing symptoms such as faecal leakage and incontinence, urgency and stress urinary incontinence, impotence, dyspareunia, infertility and premature menopause. These symptoms can significantly impact on quality of life, social functioning and return to work.

This chapter discusses the challenges of managing symptoms following treatment for rectal cancer within the context of colorectal cancer management.

Incidence, risk factors and aetiology

Cancer of the large bowel (colon and rectum) is the third most commonly diagnosed cancer and the second most common cause of cancer death in the United Kingdom. It is the second most common cancer in women (after breast cancer) and the third most common cancer in men (after prostate and lung cancer) (Information Services Division 2009). Colorectal cancer is predominantly a disease associated with Western countries and the highest incidence rates are noted in Europe, North America and Australia. The lowest incidences are observed in South Central Asia and East, West, North and Middle Africa (Boyle & Langman 2000). It should be noted that migrants who move from a country with a low incidence of colorectal cancer to one with a high incidence are then at the same risk of colorectal cancer development as the host population (Johnson & Lund 2007). Since the 1950s, Japan has witnessed a dramatic increase in colorectal cancer incidence, so much so that the country now has one of the highest age-standardised incidences. It is suggested that modification to the Japanese diet (increased meat and animal fat consumption) and behavioural changes are contributory factors (Minami et al. 2006).

Perspectives on Cancer Care.   Edited by Josephine (Tonks) N. Fawcett and Anne McQueen
© 2011 Blackwell Publishing Ltd

Table 11.1 Percentage distribution of cases by site within the large bowel, England, 1997–2000

Site within large bowel	Distribution (%) of bowel cancer
Anus	2
Rectum	29
Rectosigmoid junction	7
Sigmoid colon	18
Descending colon	2
Splenic flexure	2
Transverse colon	4
Hepatic flexure	2
Ascending colon	5
Caecum	13
Appendix	1
Unspecified	15

Adapted from Cancer Research UK (2010a)

On average 36,500 people are diagnosed with colorectal cancer each year in the United Kingdom. This represents approximately 100 new cases every day, of which the majority occur in individuals aged 65 years and over. The lifetime risk of a male in the United Kingdom developing colorectal cancer is 1 in 18, and the corresponding risk for females is 1 in 20. Scotland, Northern Ireland and Ireland have slightly higher rates than the average UK rates. One-third of all bowel cancers are situated in the rectum and the remaining two-thirds are found in the colon (Office for National Statistics 2008; Information Services Division 2009). Table 11.1 illustrates the distribution of cancer within the large bowel, in England, 1997–2000.

The current identified risk factors for colorectal cancer are diet, lifestyle, age and genetic predisposition (Doyle 2007). The relationship between diet and cancer is well established (Redeker et al. 2009). However, evidence on the influence of red meat and high animal fat intake in the development of colorectal cancer is conflicting (Ryan-Harshman & Aldoori 2007). A diet which is high in fruit, vegetables and fish is recommended, to minimise the risk of developing colorectal cancer. There is emerging evidence regarding the importance of vitamin D and vitamin B6 intake in reducing the risk of colorectal cancer (Ryan-Harshman & Aldoori 2007; Davis 2008; Theodoratou et al. 2008). Maintaining a healthy bodyweight throughout adulthood is understood to lower the risk of developing cancer, including bowel cancer. In addition, there is evidence supporting the relationship between obesity and colorectal cancer (Johnson & Lund 2007). A key focus of health policy is to reduce individual cancer risk by promotion of a healthy lifestyle (Scottish Government Health Department (SGHD) 2008). The positive influence of physical activity on reducing cancer risk is understood and it is recommended that adults undertake 30 minutes of exercise or physical activity each day (Slattery et al. 1997; Rogers et al. 2008). Although there is less evidence to link smoking and alcohol intake with the development of colorectal cancer, it is recommended that measures are taken to stop smoking and individuals should adhere to weekly guideline amounts of alcohol intake. Adopting a healthy lifestyle does not mean that someone will not develop colorectal cancer; however, their chances of developing cancer and other associated health problems is lessened (Doyle 2007).

It is understood that 5–10% of all colorectal cancers are caused by a hereditary genetic predisposition (Mecklin 2008). In these individuals the lifetime risk of developing a bowel cancer is 80–100% (Rustgi 2007). Hereditary nonpolyposis colorectal cancer (HNPCC) is a heterozygous germline mutation (see Box 11.1) in the deoxyribonucleic acid (DNA) mismatch repair (MMR) genes *MSH2* and *MLH1*. It is typically characterised by an early onset of colorectal cancer (diagnosed under 50 years of age) with at least three relatives with a confirmed colorectal cancer (one of whom must be a first-degree relative of the other two) and at least two generations should be affected (Vasen et al. 1999). HNPCC carriers are at risk of developing multiple cancers including endometrial, ovarian and stomach cancer. Familial adenomatous polyposis coli (FAP) is a germline mutation in the *APC* gene. For those with FAP the lifetime risk of colorectal cancer is 100%. Without prophylactic surgery, which normally involves a panproctocolectomy, the onset of cancer is usually at about 40 years of age (Mecklin 2008). FAP is characterised by the presence of hundreds of polyps throughout the large bowel, which normally become visible during teenage years.

Box 11.1   Definition of heterozygous germline mutation

Heterozygous: Containing two alleles of the same gene, one normal and one altered. *Germline:* A group of reproductive cells (gametes). The genome of the person as contained in these cells, along with any mutations, may be passed on to offspring. *Mismatch Repair Gene (MMR):* A gene that makes mismatch repair protein. These proteins correct any mistakes a cell makes while copying its own DNA. A mutation in an MMR gene can result in altered MMR protein. When this occurs, any mistakes that take place while the cell is copying its own DNA become a permanent part of the DNA in all subsequent cells.

Source: NHS National Genetics Education and Development Centre (www.geneticseducation. nhs.uk)

People who have ulcerative colitis are at an increased risk of developing colorectal cancer in comparison to the general population. The longer one has ulcerative colitis, the greater is the risk. A diagnosis of ulcerative colitis for 10 years increases the lifetime risk of colorectal cancer by 2%; this risk increases to 18% after 30 years (Lakatos 2008). Long-term chronic inflammation of the bowel is recognised as a risk factor for developing cancer in ulcerative colitis, particularly if the whole of the large bowel is involved. The risk of colorectal cancer against a background of ulcerative colitis is reduced by participating in yearly colonoscopy surveillance, maintaining a healthy diet and taking regular exercise.

Following a successful pilot study of faecal occult blood testing (FOBT) in Scotland and England, the United Kingdom government implemented a national bowel screening programme. During a pilot study, men and women were asked to complete and return FOB tests. Those with positive results were counselled and asked to attend for a colonoscopy. Regular bowel screening has been shown to reduce the risk of dying from colorectal cancer by 16%. A total of 48% of all the cancers identified in the pilot study were Dukes stage A (Weller et al. 2006). All men and women who are registered with a general practitioner and are between the ages of 60 and 69 years are invited to participate (in Scotland the screening range is 50 to 74 years).

Presenting features, diagnosis and staging

The clinical features of colorectal cancer depend on the site of the tumour. Symptoms associated with rectal cancer can include the passage of bright-red blood mixed in stool, feeling of unsatisfactory defecation and tenesmus, a feeling of the need to evacuate the bowels, accompanied by spasms with little or no stool passed. Bowel symptoms are commonly experienced in the general population; it is therefore important to consider symptom and sign combinations that are associated with a high predictive value for colorectal cancer (see Box 11.2).

Box 11.2   Clinical features of colorectal cancer

- Rectal bleeding with a change in bowel habit to looser stools and/or increased frequency of defecation persistent for 6 weeks. (*age threshold: all ages*)
- Rectal bleeding without anal symptoms (soreness, discomfort, itching, lumps or pain). (*age threshold: all ages*)
- A definite palpable right-sided abdominal mass. (*age threshold: all ages*)
- A definite palpable rectal (not pelvic) mass. (*age threshold: over 50 years*)
- Change of bowel habit to looser stools and/or increased frequency of defecation, without rectal bleeding, persistent for six weeks. (*age threshold: over 60 years*)
- Iron deficiency anaemia without an obvious cause (Hb< 11 g/dL in men or <10 g/dL in postmenopausal women).
- Significant family history.

Source: Scottish Executive (2007)

Souhami and Tobias found that 38% of all colorectal cancers develop in the rectum (Souhami & Tobias 2005) and 85% of colorectal cancers occurred in individuals over the age of 60.

Where colorectal cancer is suspected, the whole of the large bowel should be examined. Colonoscopy is recommended for visualising the bowel and enabling biopsy. Before deciding on management and treatment, a range of staging investigations are required in order to determine the site of the tumour, extent of local spread and distant metastasis. This is vital when it comes to discussing treatment options with patients, particularly in the case where the disease is advanced and life expectancy limited. People often wish to balance the 'risk' associated with treatment with quality of life. Staging investigations will include:

- digital rectal examination;
- colonoscopy;
- biopsy for histological confirmation;
- liver function test, haemoglobin, urea and electrolytes;
- computed tomography (CT) scan of chest, abdomen and pelvis, to determine the extent of the primary tumour and metastatic spread;
- magnetic resonance imaging (MRI) in rectal cancer, to determine extrarectal involvement;
- serum carcino-embryonic antigen (CEA) (a serum marker that can be raised in colorectal cancer and can provide a useful indicator of tumour response to treatment).

A typical colorectal cancer is characterised as a polypoid mass with ulceration in the centre, involving part or the whole of the bowel circumference. The majority of colorectal cancers (90%) are adenocarcinomas arising from an adenomatous polyp in the bowel mucosa. The most common pattern of spread is via local lymphatic invasion. Blood-borne metastases are usually by the portal vein, with the liver being the most frequent site of distant spread. In low rectal cancers, local recurrence can occur, often leaving patients with distressing and difficult-to-control symptoms including, for example, pain. Thorough staging work-up is, therefore, of the greatest importance in determining optimal planning of treatment, followed by pathological examination of the resected specimen in determining prognosis and the need for further adjuvant treatment.

The Dukes system of pathological staging (Dukes 1937) is the most commonly referred to criterion and is based on examination of the operative specimen. Data recorded for staging purposes also includes the TNM system (Union Internationale Contre Le Cancer (UICC) 1999) for describing the anatomical extent of diseases based on the following three components (see also Chapter 6):

T – the extent of the primary tumour;
N – the absence or presence and extent of regional lymph node metastases;
M – the absence or presence of distant metastases.

Table 11.2 shows the TNM staging system together with equivalent stages in the Dukes classification. In additional, the residual tumour classification is used routinely to indicate the absence or presence of residual tumour after treatment, taking account of clinical and pathological findings (i.e. circumferential resection margin):

R0 – no residual tumour;
R1 – residual tumour demonstrated microscopically;
R2 – macroscopic residual tumour.

People who are diagnosed early have a much better prognosis. Table 11.3 gives the survival rates from colorectal cancer by stage and approximate frequency at diagnosis. Five-year survival rates have improved significantly in both men and women over the last 20 years. Overall, five-year survival in men increased from 35% in the early 1980s to 54.9% in 2004, and from 36% to 53.9% in women (Information Services Division 2007).

Table 11.2 The staging of colorectal cancer. © Cancer Research UK, reproduced with permission

UICC	TNM	Modified Dukes staging
Stage 0	Carcinoma in situ	A
Stage I	No nodal involvement, no distant metastasis	
	Tumour invades submucosa (T1, N0, M0)	
	Tumour invades muscularis propria (T2, N0, M0)	
Stage II	No nodal involvement, no distant metastasis	B
	Tumour invades into subserosa (T3, N0, M0)	
	Tumour invades into other organs (T4, N0, M0)	
Stage III	Nodal involvement, no distant metastasis	C
	1 to 3 regional lymph nodes involved (any T, N1, M0)	
	4 or more regional lymph nodes involved (any T, N2, M0)	
Stage IV	Distant metastasis (any T, any N, M1)	D

Source: Cancer Research UK (2010b). UICC, Union Internationale Contre Le Cancer

Much of the improvement is a result of earlier diagnosis and significant advances in treatment modalities.

Management and treatment

The management and treatment of rectal cancer requires a multidisciplinary approach involving a team including colorectal surgeons, clinical and medical oncologists, radiologists, pathologists and clinical nurse specialists (Scottish Intercollegiate Guidelines Network (SIGN) 2003; National Institute for Health and Clinical Excellence (NICE) 2004). Staging of rectal cancer is crucial as treatment pathways differ for operable localised disease, locally advanced disease and metastatic disease. The current treatments for rectal cancer include surgery, radiotherapy and chemotherapy and these modalities can be used in combination. Following completion of staging investigations, individual cases should be discussed at a multidisciplinary meeting. This forum enables evidence-based decisions to be made by a group of experts whilst adhering to national guidelines. The multidisciplinary meeting can also facilitate referral to colleagues, such as hepatobiliary surgeons, when indicated.

Table 11.3 Survival rates by stage and approximate frequency at diagnosis. © Cancer Research UK, reproduced with permission

Dukes stage	Approximate frequency (%) at diagnosis	5-year survival (%)
A	8.7	93.2
B	24.2	77.0
C	23.6	47.7
D	9.2	6.6

Source: Cancer Research UK (2010c)

Nurses have an important and privileged role in supporting patients throughout all stages of the treatment pathway; thus, an awareness of all steps of the patient journey is imperative. Every patient should have access to a clinical nurse specialist who has expert knowledge of colorectal cancer and is able to provide specialist support and advice. Ideally, the colorectal clinical nurse specialist should be available to the patient and their family from the point of diagnosis onwards (SIGN 2003; NICE 2004).

Surgery

Surgery continues to be the mainstay of treatment for patients with rectal cancer. Approximately 80% of all patients diagnosed with colorectal cancer in the United Kingdom undergo surgical intervention (NICE 2004). Total mesorectal excision is the preferred technique for mid and lower third rectal cancers. Total mesorectal excision involves dissection of the integral mesentery and can successfully reduce the risk of locally recurrent disease (MacFarlane et al. 1993). Total mesorectal excision is indicated in patients who have operable, mobile tumours, without the presence of metastatic disease and who are deemed fit for surgery. The tumour and a margin of healthy bowel proximal and distal to it should be removed. Any lymph nodes responsible for drainage in this area should also be removed. In patients with tumours less than 5 cm from the anorectal junction, it may be necessary to perform an abdominoperineal resection which involves formation of a permanent stoma or a low anterior resection. Wherever possible, anal sphincter function should be preserved. In very low rectal cancers, a temporary defunc-tioning ileostomy can reduce the risk of anastomotic leak (Den Dulk et al. 2007). Any patient for whom a stoma is a potential option should be counselled by a stoma care nurse specialist prior to any surgery. Postoperatively, those with a stoma require expert input and teaching to enable self-care and adjustment. During the postoperative period nurses have a role in the education of patients about recovery and rehabilitation issues. The average recovery period is 8 to 12 weeks, and during this time activities such as heavy lifting and driving should be restricted. Most patients feel able to return to work after approximately three months, but this is dependent on any subsequent requirement for adjuvant chemotherapy. Dietary advice (low fibre, eating little and often) and written and verbal information regarding bowel, bladder and sexual function should be given, and tailored to the individual. Patients who have isolated metastatic disease in the liver or lungs should be considered for surgical resection. Resection of hepatic metastases can result in cure, and approximately 43% of patients who undergo liver resection are long-term survivors (Shah et al. 2007). In situations where rectal cancer is deemed inoperable, palliative surgery can be performed to improve symptoms of bowel obstruction. This normally involves fashioning a stoma to maintain bowel patency. Symptoms such as rectal bleeding and discharge can be reduced by endoscopic lasering of the tumour, which is routinely repeated at regular intervals (Sherwood et al. 2006).

Radiotherapy

Radiotherapy is the use of high-energy waves or beams of ionising radiation to destroy cancer cells. The role of radiotherapy in reducing incidence of local recurrence in rectal cancer is well established (Kapiteijn et al. 2001). Short-course preoperative radiotherapy involves administering a total of five individual treatments (fractions) of radiotherapy over 5 consecutive days with surgical resection taking place during the following week. Preoperative radiotherapy can reduce the risk of local recurrence by 50% (NICE 2004). When a rectal cancer is deemed to be inoperable, a long course of combined chemoradiation can be considered preoperatively, known as 'downstaging'. This is given in an attempt to reduce the size of the tumour and render it operable. This regime involves 25–30 daily fractions of radiotherapy, given over 5–6 weeks, with a radio-sensitising dose of oral or intravenous chemotherapy given either continuously or intermittently for the duration of the radiotherapy. Following downstaging treatment, patients then undergo repeat imaging (MRI scan) and surgical review to assess operability.

Table 11.4 illustrates clinical indications for surgery, short-course preoperative radiotherapy or downstaging treatment. Short-course preoperative radiotherapy followed by surgical resection in the following week minimises the short-term consequences of pelvic radiotherapy such as diarrhoea, cystitis and inflammation. When caring for such patients, nurses should be aware of the potential short- and long-term side effects of pelvic

Table 11.4 Clinical indications for surgery, short-course preoperative radiotherapy and downstaging treatment

Intervention:	Surgery alone	SCPRT	Downstaging
Tumour characteristics	Operable tumour at >10 cm from anal verge. Clinical staging T1/T2 without gross nodal involvement	T3 tumour between 5 and 10 cm from anal verge with >2 mm clearance from mesorectal fascia by tumour or involved nodes Anteriorly positioned tumours in men between 5 and 10 cm from anal verge T1 and T2 tumours with grossly involved perirectal nodes	Fixed and inoperable tumours or tumours <2 mm from the mesorectum. Radiation alone can be given if chemotherapy is not suitable
Treatment regime	Specific surgical procedure	Five daily fractions of radiotherapy followed by surgery the next week	25–30 daily fractions of radiotherapy over 5–6 weeks with either intermittent intravenous chemotherapy or concurrent oral/intravenous chemotherapy

SCPRT, short-course preoperative radiotherapy

radiotherapy. For example, there is an increased risk of delayed healing associated with radiotherapy, and this is important in the wound care for surgical patients who have received radiotherapy preoperatively.

Radiotherapy can be given in the palliative care setting to patients with locally advanced or recurrent pelvic disease. This is often in combination with palliative chemotherapy and by so doing can help provide symptomatic relief from pain or rectal discharge and bleeding.

Chemotherapy

As discussed, chemotherapy can be given in combination with radiotherapy in the treatment of rectal cancer. Chemotherapy is also administered in the postoperative period to reduce the risk of recurrent or metastatic disease following curative resection. Chemotherapy is the use of drugs to kill cancer cells. Most chemotherapeutic agents interrupt the cell cycle and stop cell division. The most common drugs used in colorectal cancer are pyrimidine analogues, which belong to a group of drugs called antimetabolites. Antimetabolites such as fluorouracil, a fluoropyrimidine, disrupt the cell's capacity for DNA synthesis and therefore cause cell arrest and apoptosis. It is recommended that patients with the following high-risk pathological staging are considered for chemotherapy:

- nodal involvement (Dukes stage C, TNM stage N1–N2);
- TNM stage T4;
- extramural vascular invasion;
- perforated tumours.

The perceived benefit of adjuvant chemotherapy in those with nodal disease is approximately 4–13% (SIGN 2003; NICE 2004). Chemotherapy should commence within 8 weeks of the date of surgery; however, it is important that patients who receive chemotherapy are selected on an individual basis. Palliative chemotherapy has a role in slowing the disease process in those with widespread metastatic deposits, for example in the liver or lungs, but it is vitally important that with extended life comes improved quality of life (De Kort et al. 2006).

The clinical trialling of new and yet unlicensed chemotherapeutic drugs is an exciting development area. There is growing interest in the significance of monoclonal antibodies in the treatment of cancer. Monoclonal antibodies are specifically engineered drugs which attach to faults in cancer cells. Essentially these drugs mimic the production of natural antibodies and in doing so make the cancer cells easier for the immune system to identify and destroy. Some monoclonal antibodies can interrupt growth factors, which are known to be overexpressed by many cancer cells, including colorectal adenocarcinoma. This has implications for the future in terms of how patients are selected and treated using specific chemotherapeutic regimens (Vincenzi et al. 2008).

Treatment effects

Substantial progress has been made in rectal cancer treatment by means of improved surgical techniques, pathological staging and multidisciplinary management, leading to overall improvement in survival and reduction in local recurrence (ISD 2007). Survival is not, however, the sole aim of treatment, and recent literature suggests a shifting focus towards assessing the impact that treatment has on health-related quality of life (Ramsey et al. 2000; Camilleri-Brennan & Steele 2001; Rauch et al. 2004; Fisher & Daniels 2006; Moriya 2006; Vironen et al. 2006).

It is widely acknowledged that a diagnosis of cancer and the effects of treatment can significantly impact on an individual's physical and psychological wellbeing (Phipps et al. 2008). This has led to a growing interest in gathering the thoughts and views of patients to identify what the key issues are, and looking at interventions to help minimise symptoms. Issues that healthcare professionals identify as important may be different to those perceived by patients; therefore, working in partnership is essential.

With the increase in use of sphincter-saving surgery, fewer patients with rectal cancer undergo abdominoperineal resection with permanent stoma formation. Without compromising the cancer treatment outcomes, sphincter-saving surgery preserves the anus and sphincter muscles, enabling maintenance of normal bowel evacuation. Previous evidence suggested that patients requiring stoma formation experienced more problems in general in relation to both physical difficulties and body image perception. Preserving normal anal continence is perceived as being preferable, so long as adequate bowel function is ensured (Dehni 1998; Harris 2001; McNamara & Parc 2003). The introduction of total mesorectal excision in the 1980s, along with autonomic nerve identification, has contributed significantly to functional outcomes from rectal surgery. However, even with accurate anatomical knowledge, individuals differ and a range of factors can influence the possibility of nerve damage, such as the running patterns of nerves within the pelvis, narrow pelvis, obesity or if the cancer directly invades the autonomic nerves. There is still more to be learned about late effects of treatment and there is growing evidence to suggest that factors such as the type of surgery, use of preoperative radiotherapy, age and gender can have a significant impact on quality of life (Schmidt et al. 2004; Hendren et al. 2005; Marijnen et al. 2005; Schmidt et al. 2005). For example, while it is widely accepted that sphincter-saving is the operation of choice for mid and low rectal cancers, bowel function can be significantly disrupted, especially within the first few months following surgery, resulting in bowel frequency and urgency, faecal incontinence and soiling, and incomplete emptying (Lange et al. 2007). While bowel function generally improves with time, the impact cannot be underestimated (Nikoletti et al. 2008). Case study 11.1 starkly demonstrates one patient's experience of bowel distress following surgery for rectal cancer. The implications for sensitive expertise on the part of nursing staff, be it in the hospital or community setting, cannot be overstated.

Local recurrence

Local recurrence is a major problem in the treatment of rectal cancer and can result in patients experiencing significant disabling symptoms such as pain, bleeding, painful skin and perineal infections. Such symptoms are not only difficult to treat but also can impact on quality of life, day-to-day living, ability to work and recreational activities. In recent years, the introduction of preoperative radiotherapy in selected patients, along with improved surgical techniques, has resulted in a significant improvement in local control. Until recently, little was known about the longer-term effects of combined preoperative radiotherapy followed by surgery. However, in a large prospective study evaluating the impact of short-term preoperative radiotherapy on health-related quality of life, Marijnen et al. (2005) have shown that, while overall quality of life was good, sexual activity declined postoperatively for both men and women, along with a decline in bladder function in those who received preoperative radiotherapy. In men, a decline in erectile function was noted at up to two years, suggesting late radiation damage to the small vessels. No significant differences were noticed in defecation problems between those patients who received preoperative radiotherapy and those who did not. This is in contrast to other studies which have demonstrated delayed bowel function in patients receiving preoperative radiotherapy (Pollack et al. 2006; Lange et al. 2007) highlighting the need for ongoing evaluation.

While surgery is the mainstay of treatment for rectal cancer, patients presenting with locally advanced, inoperable rectal cancer are often considered for a longer course of radiotherapy, with or without chemotherapy over a 4- to 5-week period, in an attempt to downstage the tumour, rendering it amenable to surgery. Similar to the studies of short-course preoperative radiotherapy, patients can experience considerable bowel and urinary disruption, and sexual function has been noted to decline significantly, particularly in men (Allal et al. 2005). In a paper by Pietrzak et al. (2007) quality of life and anorectal and sexual function did not differ in patients receiving short-course radiotherapy as compared to those receiving chemoradiation.

In general, there is still limited evidence as to the long-term symptom clusters following preoperative radiotherapy and surgery and, in women in particular, even less is known in relation to adverse effects on sexual functioning. In addition, evidence on the importance that patients attach to any symptoms they might experience is still limited, and whether functional parameters are associated with adverse quality of life. Nonetheless what is known is the potential array of distressing symptoms that patients may experience, including the faecal leakage mentioned earlier, incontinence, urgency and stress urinary incontinence, impotence, dyspareunia, and also infertility and premature menopause in younger women receiving radiotherapy. Therefore, developing interventions to minimise symptoms and address sensitive issues should be part of any patient management plan. While rectal cancer is predominantly a disease of older people, assumptions cannot be made about the importance patients attach to these adverse side effects and the impact they may have on daily living.

Self-care and supportive interventions

Nurses play a very important role, both in terms of supporting patients throughout this potentially difficult time and also in providing interventions to minimise treatment side effects. There is increasing evidence to suggest that patients with cancer want to be more actively involved in their care and recovery (Bulsara et al. 2004). Engaging patients in their healthcare and supporting people to maintain an active life throughout illness is one of the key drivers for health policy (DH 2007; SGHD 2007; 2008). To achieve this, assessment is fundamental in order to provide supportive interventions that give people the confidence and skills to manage side effects and symptoms associated with illness and treatment.

Having a diagnosis of rectal cancer can have a significant impact on both the individual and people close to them. Reactions and ways of dealing with the consequences of treatment will vary enormously, therefore individual assessment forms the basis of tailored interventions.

Discussing sensitive issues, such as pelvic dysfunction, can be challenging for healthcare professionals, especially if they feel there are limited interventions available or feel uncomfortable discussing the topic (see Case study 11.1). However, healthcare providers often find they have to discuss sensitive issues and culturally may find discussing intimate personal issues difficult. As more becomes known about the late effects of pelvic treatment, and healthcare professionals overcome their own embarrassment, they require to introduce sensitive subjects, such as questions about sexual function, as part of the overall assessment (Hautomäki et al. 2007). Giving people the opportunity to share any concerns or problems that they may be experiencing can be therapeutic in itself, so long as the infrastructure is in place to refer on to the most appropriate person/service if need be. In addition, discussing sensitive issues should be introduced gradually and be done at the pace of the individual, when they feel ready and trust has been established with the healthcare professional.

In many areas, colorectal cancer nurses have taken on a key role in follow-up care, providing not only disease surveillance but also the opportunity for ongoing assessment and monitoring of pelvic symptoms and psychological functioning. Components of a pelvic function assessment should include an assessment of bowel, bladder and sexual function, the importance the patients attach to the symptom(s) experienced and the impact on daily living. Using bowel function as an example, Box 11.3 outlines a typical assessment structure.

Box 11.3   Assessment structure for bowel function

In a sensitive collaboration with the individual:

- Take a bowel symptom history (to include when the symptoms started, nature of the problem, frequency, consistency, evacuation difficulties, diet intake, exercise, effect on lifestyle, significance).
- Discuss the possible reasons for bowel changes following surgery, with or without radiotherapy and/or chemotherapy.
- Advise on specific interventions to control or minimise bowel symptoms.
- Provide information on dietary modification and pelvic floor exercises.
- Refer to other healthcare professionals or services as appropriate.
- Agree a symptom re-evaluation plan.

Interventions for symptoms experienced following rectal cancer treatment will be specific, depending on the nature of the problem. Where possible, evidence-based intervention protocols should be in place. For many people, different symptoms can occur concurrently and they can fluctuate. For this reason, supporting patients with information and providing them with the skills to manage symptoms and lifestyle changes is vital. Such support may need to be paced, involving the delivery of information over a period of time that allows the individual patient time to adjust and adapt.

Interventions to assist with functional problems are likely to include a combination of medications and lifestyle advice. For example, in patients experiencing frequency of loose, watery stool, which can be a common concern within the first few weeks after surgery, with or without radiotherapy, the intervention plan may include prescribing an anti-motility drug to slow down gut transit, in conjunction with a bulking agent. The supported lifestyle advice will comprise information on diet and fluid intake, recommending a reduction of fibre, fruit and vegetables at this time until the bowel settles, then reintroducing such foods. Similarly, avoiding stimulants such as caffeine and alcohol will help during this period. Conversely, for patients who are constipated, the use of stool softeners or stimulant laxatives to stimulate bowel transit will be considered along with advice on toilet positioning and a balanced fibre diet.

As discussed, distressing bowel symptoms such as faecal leakage, urgency and incomplete emptying can be a major source of anxiety for patients. Interventions include recommending regular anal sphincter and pelvic floor exercises, dietary advice, for example the use of extra fibre as stool bulking agents, and identifying dietary triggers, teaching relaxation and breathing techniques along with practical advice on barrier creams to protect the skin, and accessing 'Just can't wait cards' allowing access to public toilets.

Urinary difficulties may be caused by decreased muscle tone in the bladder neck, urethra or pelvic floor, causing stress incontinence, or from an inability to inhibit detrusor contractions, or may be due to damaged urethral sphincter muscles causing urge incontinence. Self-management interventions include advice on healthy fluid intake, healthy diet and avoiding constipation, pelvic floor exercises which are essential for bladder control, and encouraging people to keep a diary in order to assess progress. Oral anticholinergic medication may be considered in patients with ongoing urge incontinence, and serotonin inhibitors for stress incontinence. However, of course, all medications have their own side effects.

In relation to sexual function following treatment for rectal cancer, evidence-based interventions are limited. Acknowledging difficulties and being sensitive to concerns is fundamental (Hautomäki et al. 2007). In patients who do report sexual difficulties, carrying out a full pelvic assessment is essential. For example, it may be the sexual difficulties are arising as a consequence of ongoing faecal leakage, preventing the individual resuming an intimate relationship. In this case, dealing with the bowel symptoms in the first instance would be vital.

The evidence for the association between radiotherapy, and surgery, and sexual dysfunction in women following treatment for rectal cancer is also limited. This has resulted in inconsistencies in practice and education, for example, in the use of vaginal dilators in the prevention of stenosis, and general vaginal aftercare. Recognising the total dose of radiotherapy and whether the whole of the vagina or the lower third is included in the treatment field needs to be considered, to inform practice. In men who experience erectile difficulties, a period of recovery of at least six months will be necessary following surgery. If problems are ongoing, a more detailed assessment will then be required by an expert, in the field including advice on both dealing with erection difficulties and the use of available treatments (e.g. a phosphodiesterase type-5 inhibitor such as Viagra®).

Conclusion

Survival following rectal cancer has improved significantly over the last 20 years through earlier detection and improved treatments. However, as survival increases, there is a shifting focus on the long-term impact on health-related quality of life in patients, and a compelling need for more robust assessment and intervention strategies to deal with the range of potentially distressing symptoms experienced. Provision of supportive interventions that give people the confidence and skills to manage side effects and symptoms associated with illness and treatment is fundamental to recovery. Understanding more about the impact of treatment through patient experiences provides a more accurate account of the challenges people face. From this starting point we can then begin to work in partnership with patients and family members to look at ways of supporting adjustment to living beyond cancer.

Case study 11.1   A patient's experience

After the operation I was so relieved the cancer had been removed and that I didn't need any further treatment. My main concern had been on getting rid of the cancer, I didn't care about anything else. I was living in a very different world. I was told that my bowel function might be disrupted for a little while after the radiotherapy and surgery . . . that was understatement. Once I got home, my bowels were fairly sluggish at first, everything felt different at that time; I was still tired and needing to rest, my appetite was beginning to return but I was only 'picking' at food. After a few days all change, my bowels went from being sluggish to opening constantly. At worst I must have been going to the toilet at least 15–20 times a day and throughout the night. I was passing loose watery stool, my bottom was sore and excoriated and I was exhausted. This went on for a number of weeks. I had this incredible sensation of urgency – I just had to get to a toilet and on a number of occasions I was caught short so I started to wear pads. I desperately wanted to get my life back to normal, get back to work, be able to collect the children from school but I was scared, what if there wasn't a toilet available? What if I get caught short? . . . It was awful.

   My bowels eventually started to firm up a little and the frequency reduced but then I got this feeling of not being able to empty my bowels properly so I had to go back and forth to the toilet 3–4 times within a space of 15 minutes to really feel they were emptied. I guess it was trial and error in the end. I took medication and I experimented with my diet. Ironically, while we all know fruit and vegetables are very important, at first it was the worst thing to take, my bowels would go into overdrive. It was a nurse at the hospital who suggested cutting back on fibre for a short while and eating blander foods. I tried this and it worked, and after a time I started to re-introduce different foods. All in all, it's taken the best part of a year for things to really start settling down and my confidence is beginning to recover. Looking back, the operation was the easy bit. . .

References

Allal AS, Gervaz P, Gertsch P, et al. (2005) Assessment of quality of life in patients with rectal cancer treated by preoperative radiotherapy: A longitudinal prospective study. *International Journal of Radiation Oncology* **61**(4): 1129–35.

Boyle P, Langman JS (2000) ABC of colorectal cancer: epidemiology. *BMJ* **321**: 805–8.

Bulsara C, Ward A, Joske D (2004) Haematological cancer patients: achieving a sense of empowerment by use of strategies to control illness. *Journal of Clinical Nursing* **13**: 251–8.

Camilleri-Brennan J, Steele RJC (2001) Prospective analysis of quality of life and survival following mesorectal excision for rectal cancer. *British Journal of Surgery* **88**(12): 1617–22.

Cancer Research UK (2010a) www.info.cancerresearchuk.org/cancerstats/types/bowel/incidence (accessed April 2010).

Cancer Research UK (2010b) http://info.cancerresearchuk.org/cancerstats/types/bowel/survival/index.htm (accessed April 2010).

Cancer Research UK (2010c) http://info.cancerresearchuk.org/cancerstats/types/bowel/symptomsandtreatment/index.htm (accessed April 2010).

Davis CD (2008) Vitamin D and cancer: current dilemmas and future research needs. *American Journal of Clinical Nutrition* **88**(suppl): 565–9S.

Dehni N, Tiret E, Singland JD, et al. (1998) Long-term functional outcome after low anterior resection: comparison of low colorectal anastomosis and colonic J-pouch-anal anastomosis. *Disease of Colon and Rectum* **41**(7): 817–22.

De Kort SJ, Willemse PHB, Habraken JM, de Haes HCJM, Willems DL, Richel DJ (2006) Quality of life versus prolongation of life in patients treated with chemotherapy in advanced colorectal cancer: a review of randomised controlled clinical trials. *European Journal of Cancer* **42**: 835–45.

Den Dulk M, Smit M, Peeters K, et al. (2007) A multivariate analysis of limiting factors for stoma reversal in patients with rectal cancer entered into the total mesorectal excision (TME) trial: a retrospective study. *Lancet Oncology* **8**(4): 297–303.

Department of Health (2007) *Cancer Reform Strategy*. London: DH.

Doyle VC (2007) Nutrition and colorectal cancer risk: a literature review. *Gastroenterology Nursing* **30**(3): 178–82.

Dukes C (1937) The classification of cancer of the rectum. *Journal of Pathology* **63**(12): 323.

Fisher SE, Daniels IR (2006) Quality of life and sexual function following surgery for rectal cancer. *Colorectal Disease* **8**(suppl 3): 20–42.

Harris GJ, Lavery IC, Fazio VW (2001) Function of a colonic J pouch continues to improve with time. *British Journal of Surgery* **88**(12): 1623–7.

Hautomäki K, Miettnen M, Kellokumpu-Lehtinen PL, Analto P, Lehto J (2007) Opening communication with cancer patients about sexually-related issues. *Cancer Nursing* **30**(5): 399–404.

Hendren SK, O'Connor BI, Liu M, et al. (2005) Prevalence of male and female sexual dysfunction is high following surgery for rectal cancer. *Annals of Surgery* **242**(2): 212–23.

Information Services Division (ISD) National Services Scotland (2007) *Trends in Cancer Survival in Scotland 1980–2004*. Edinburgh: ISD.

Information Services Division (ISD) (2009) *Cancer in Scotland*. Edinburgh: NHS National Services Scotland.

Johnson IT, Lund EK (2007) Review article: nutrition, obesity and colorectal cancer. *Alimentary Pharmacology and Therapeutics* **26**: 161–81.

Kapiteijn E, Marijnen CAM, Nagtegaal ID, et al. (2001) Preoperative radiotherapy combined with total mesorectal excision for resectable rectal cancer. *New England Journal of Medicine* **345**(9): 638–46.

Lange MM, den Dulk M, Bossema ER, et al. (2007) Risk factor for faecal incontinence after rectal cancer treatment. *British Journal of Surgery* **94**: 1278–84.

Lakatos PL, Lakatos L (2008) Risk for colorectal cancer in ulcerative colitis: changes, causes and management strategies. *World Journal of Gastroenterology* **14**(25): 3937–47.

MacFarlane JK, Ryall RDH, Heald RJ (1993) Mesorectal excision for rectal cancer. *Lancet* **341**: 457–60.

McNamara DA, Parc R (2003) Methods and results of sphincter-preserving surgery for rectal cancer. *Cancer Control* **10**(3): 212–18.

Marijnen CAM, van de Velde CJH, Putter H. et al. (2005) Impact of short-term pre-operative radiotherapy on health related quality of life and sexual functioning in primary rectal cancer: report of a multicenter randomised trial. *Journal of Clinical Oncology* **23**(9): 1847–57.

Mecklin JP (2008) The implications of genetics in colorectal cancer. *Annals of Oncology* **19** (suppl 5): 87–90.

Minami Y, Nishino Y, Tsubono Y, Tsuji I, Hisamichi S (2006) Increase of colon and rectal cancer incidence rates in Japan: trends in incidence rates in Miyagi Prefecture, 1959–1997. *Journal of Epidemiology* **16**(6): 240–8.

Moriya Y (2006) Function preservation in rectal cancer. *International Journal of Clinical Oncology* **11**: 339–43.

National Institute for Health and Clinical Excellence (NICE) (2004) *Improving Outcomes in Colorectal Cancers: manual update*. London: NICE.

Nikoletti S, Young J, Levitt M, King M, Chidlow C, Hollingsworth S (2008) Bowel problems, self-care practices, and information needs of colorectal survivors at 6 to 24 months after sphincter-saving surgery. *Cancer Nursing* **31**(5): 389–98.

Office for National Statistics (2008) *Cancer Statistics Registrations: Registrations of Cancer Diagnosed in 2006 England*. London: ONS.

Phipps E., Braitman L.E., Stites S., Leighton J.C. (2008) Quality of life and symptom attribution in long-term colon cancer survivors. *Jounral of Evaluation in Clinical Practice* **14**, 254–258.

Pietrzak L, Bujko K, Nowacki MP, et al. (2007) Quality of life, anorectal and sexual functions after preoperative radiotherapy for rectal cancer: Report of a randomised trial. *Radiotherapy and Oncology* **84**: 217–25.

Pollack J, Holm T, Cedermark B, et al. (2006) Late adverse effects of short-course preoperative radiotherapy in rectal cancer. *British Journal of Surgery* **93**: 1519–25.

Ramsey SD, Anderson MR, Etzioni R et al. (2000) Quality of life in survivors of colorectal cancer. *Cancer* **88**(6): 1294–303.

Rauch P, Miny J, Conroy T, Neyton L, Guillemin F (2004) Quality of life among disease-free survivors of rectal cancer. *Journal of Clinical Oncology* **22**(2): 354–60.

Redeker C, Wardle J, Wilder D, Hiom S, Miles A (2009) The launch of Cancer Research UK's 'Reduce the Risk' campaign: Baseline measurements of public awareness of cancer risk factors in 2004. *European Journal of Cancer* **45**, 827–836.

Rogers CJ, Colbert LH, Greiner JW, Perkins SN, Hursting SD (2008) Physical activity and cancer prevention: pathways and targets for intervention. *Sports Medicine* **38**(4): 271–96.

Rustgi AK (2007) The genetics of hereditary colon cancer. *Genes and Development* **21**: 2525–38.

Ryan-Harshman M, Aldoori W (2007) Diet and colorectal cancer: review of the evidence. *Canadian Family Physician* **53**: 1913–20.

Schmidt CE, Bestmann B, Kuchler T, Kremer B (2004) Factors influencing sexual function in patients with rectal cancer. *International Journal of Impotence Research* **17**: 231–8.

Schmidt CE, Bestmann B, Kuchler T, Longo WE, Kremer B (2005) Ten-year historic cohort of quality of life and sexuality in patients with rectal cancer. *Diseases of the Colon and Rectum* **48**: 483–92.

Scottish Executive (2007) *Scottish Executive HDL (2007)09: Scottish Referral Guidelines for Suspected Cancer*. Edinburgh: Scottish Government.

Scottish Government Health Department (2007) *Better Health, Better Care*. Edinburgh: Scottish Government.

Scottish Government Health Department (2008) *Better Cancer Care, An Action Plan*. Edinburgh: Scottish Government.

Scottish Intercollegiate Guidelines Network (SIGN) (2003) *Management of Colorectal Cancer: a national clinical guideline*. Edinburgh: SIGN.

Shah SA, Bromberg R, Coates A, Rempel E, Simunovic M, Gallinger S (2007) Survival after liver resection for metastatic colorectal carcinoma in a large population. *Journal of the American College of Surgeons* **205**(5): 676–83.

Sherwood LA, Knowles G, Wilson RG, Potter MA (2006) Retrospective review of laser therapy for palliation of colorectal tumours. *European Journal of Oncology Nursing* **10**(1): 30–8.

Slattery ML, Edwards SL, Ma K, Friedman GD, Potter JD (1997) Physical activity and colon cancer: a public health perspective. *Annals of Epidemiology* **7**: 137–45.

Souhami R, Tobias J (2005) *Cancer and its Management*, 5th edn. Oxford: Blackwell Publishing.

Theodoratou E, Farrington SM, Tenesa A, et al. (2008) *Cancer Epidemiology, Biomarkers and Prevention* **17**(1): 171–82.

Union Internationale Contre Le Cancer (UICC) (1999) *TNM Atlas Illustrated Guide to the TNM/pTNM Classification of Malignant Tumours*, 4th edn. Berlin: Springer.

Vasen HFA, Watson P, Mecklin J, Lynch HT (1999) New clinical criteria for Hereditary Nonpolyposis Colorectal Cancer (HNPCC, Lynch Syndrome) proposed by the International Collaborative Group on HNPCC. *Gastroenterology* **116**: 1453–6.

Vincenzi B, Schiavon G, Silletta M, Scutini D, Tonini G (2008) The biological properties of cetuximab. *Critical Reviews in Oncology-Haematology* **68**(2): 93–106.

Vironen JH, Kairaluoma M, Aalto A-M, Kellokumpu IH (2006) Impact of functional results on quality of life after rectal cancer. *Diseases of the Colon & Rectum* **49**: 568–78.

Weller D, Moss S, Butler P (2006) English Pilot of Bowel Cancer Screening: An evaluation of the second round final report to the Department of Health. Edinburgh: University of Edinburgh.

Chapter 12

Sustaining hope in people with cancer: developments in palliative and end-of-life care

Margaret Colquhoun and Vicky Hill

'... It is the patients themselves who are the origin and the enduring source of that hope, not us. So whilst in choosing what to say we can and do influence their hopes we must remember that the hope is theirs, not ours. Whilst we ought to encourage people to hope for outcomes which are probable, and to help them adjust away from hopes for the extremely unlikely, at the same time we ought not to seek to control their hopes.'

Randall & Downie (2006:210)

Palliative care has been described as an approach to care that focuses on quality of life for patients and families facing the challenges associated with a life-threatening illness (World Health Organization 2002). It is a team approach, in which patients and families are key members of the team and where the focus is on total care embracing physical, psychological, social and spiritual issues, drawing on the expertise of all members of the team to achieve optimal wellbeing, comfort and support for patients and their families. While palliative care may be relevant to patients and families from an early stage in the illness journey, it may also encompass end-of-life care in the last days and hours of life. Providing palliative and end-of-life care requires us to look at the patient and family as a whole and to work with them towards relief of pain and other symptoms, while also providing psychological, social and spiritual support.

Fostering and sustaining hope are increasingly viewed as relevant at all stages of the illness journey. Hope, however, is considered to be a vital human response at times when an individual is confronted by loss, suffering, uncertainty and complex decisions (Herth 1990; Herth & Cutcliffe 2002) and when the individual's personal resources and strengths are depleted (Herth 1990). Endeavouring to sustain that hope is at the heart of palliative care nursing and multidisciplinary practice (McIntyre & Chaplin 2007) and is also, therefore, central to this chapter.

Being able to access competent and compassionate palliative and end-of-life care, where and when it is required, and on the basis of need rather than diagnosis, is a key issue

Perspectives on Cancer Care. Edited by Josephine (Tonks) N. Fawcett and Anne McQueen
© 2011 Blackwell Publishing Ltd

on the national agenda (Department of Health (DH) 2004; Audit Scotland 2008; Scottish Government 2008). As a result, a range of frameworks and models are being promoted to ensure a cohesive approach (DH 2004; National Institute for Health and Clinical Excellence (NICE) 2004; Scottish Partnership for Palliative Care 2007; Scottish Government 2008).

This chapter will briefly explore the nature of hope and then some of the models and frameworks recently developed to support health and social care practitioners in delivering high-quality palliative and end-of-life care. A fictitious case study of a gentleman with lung cancer is introduced and then revisited at various points throughout the chapter, to illustrate how these models and frameworks may be used to sustain hope in a patient with cancer, and in his family and friends.

The nature of hope

One of the surprising things emerging from research over the past two decades is that patients and families may, in certain circumstances, remain hopeful right up to the end of life (McIntyre & Chaplin 2007). A number of authors and researchers have endeavoured to define hope. It appears to be a complex and multifaceted concept (Herth 1990; Buckley & Herth 2004) which is difficult to capture in words. Hope is viewed as a key issue in ensuring quality of life (Herth 2000; Cooper & Cooper 2006) and a determining factor in coping with the losses associated with life-threatening illness (Gamlin & Kinghorn 1995; Cooper & Cooper 2006). An early, but often quoted, definition considers that hope in palliative care is 'not based on false optimism or benign reassurance, but is built instead on the belief that better days or moments can come in spite of the prognosis' (Scanlon 1989: 491).

Many definitions and discussions emphasise the dynamic nature of hope and how it may change or transform over the course of the illness journey (Vanistendael 2007). At the point of diagnosis, hope may focus on cure (Johnson 2007), and some indicate that this may continue into the palliative care phase of illness (Gamlin & Kinghorn 1995; Benzein et al. 2001). For some patients, however, the focus of hope may change as the illness progresses. In Herth's (1990) study patients in the palliative care phase of illness indicated that having achievable aims fosters hope, but that these aims may change over time. From having tangible aims in the early stages of the palliative care phase, individuals, as they became frailer, focused their aims on hope for family and friends. At the very end of life, however, the desire for 'serenity, inner peace and eternal rest' prevailed (Herth 1990: 1254). Others have suggested that the fragility of hope in palliative care means that it may change from day to day (Gamlin & Kinghorn 1995). While patterns of hoping may be sought and discussed, hope appears to remain a 'unique personal experience' (Owen 1989: 75).

It is important to recognise that it is patients, not practitioners, who are 'the origin and the enduring source' of hope (Randall & Downie 2006: 210). Seminal research demonstrates that it may be an individual's personal attributes, their spiritual beliefs and/or their ability to look back with satisfaction on life that generates a sense of hope (Herth 1990). While we cannot make the patient and family hopeful, it is suggested that health and social care practitioners can play a significant part in fostering and sustaining that hope

(Herth 1990; McIntyre & Chaplin 2007). Key strategies for sustaining hope are identified in the literature and are set out in Box 12.1.

Box 12.1   Key strategies for sustaining hope

- Maintaining the patient's physical comfort.
- Supporting meaningful relationships with family and the healthcare team.
- Ensuring that the patient and family feel valued as individuals.
- Encouraging the patient to identify and achieve important aims.
- Enabling the patient and family to retain choice and control.
- Promoting reflection on life and creating meaning and legacy.
- Providing opportunities for spiritual quest, expression and growth.
- Using light-heartedness and humour appropriately.

Sources: Herth (1990), Flemming (1997), Houldin (2000), Buckley & Herth (2004), Duggleby & Wright (2004), Johnson (2007), McIntyre & Chaplin (2007), Vanistendael (2007) and Boog & Tester (2008)

Conversely, some authors indicate factors that may hinder hope. These include poorly controlled pain and other distressing symptoms, not feeling valued as a person, and having a sense of isolation or abandonment (Herth 1990; Buckley & Herth 2004; McIntyre & Chaplin 2007). Although using hope-sustaining strategies, it might be argued, is integral to the role of nurses and other health and social care practitioners, it is important to remember the positive influence these approaches may have on the patient journey and, for families, on into bereavement (Field et al. 2007; Payne et al. 2008). These strategies will be referred to throughout the chapter. In the light of this discussion, what have models and frameworks currently promoted as best practice in palliative and end-of-life care to offer in relation to sustaining hope?

The use of models and frameworks in palliative care is addressed below and illustrated in a case study. The frameworks of care are then considered in relation to their value in facilitating and maintaining hope.

Models and frameworks

The need for palliative and end-of-life care for patients with cancer has been recognised for many years (Doyle et al. 2004). The belief that this type of care should be accessible to those with other life-threatening illness, for example, dementia or end-stage renal, cardiac or respiratory disease, emerged later and is gathering momentum (Scottish Government 2008). Specialist palliative care supports those with particularly complex physical, psychosocial or spiritual issues. Increasingly, however, generalist nurses in the community, acute hospital and care home settings are delivering palliative and end-of-life care, referring to specialist palliative care teams for advice in complex cases. The United Kingdom governments have therefore acted to try to ensure the availability of care to all those who require it, wherever they are being cared for (DH 2004; Audit Scotland 2008; Scottish Government 2008). As a result, in the United Kingdom two frameworks are being promoted to help non-specialist staff provide a good standard of palliative care, namely:

- The Gold Standards Framework (GSF);
- The Liverpool Care Pathway for the Dying Patient (LCP).

The GSF is a model intended to support the delivery of high-quality palliative and end-of-life care in the community by primary care teams (Thomas 2003; Thomas & Noble 2007). The LCP is a multidisciplinary care plan that guides practitioners to offer evidence-based care in the last days of life (Ellershaw & Wilkinson 2003; Ellershaw 2006). It is these initiatives, along with a further recently published model of palliative care (Dougan & Colquhoun 2006), that will be considered in relation to sustaining hope in patients and families. Case study 12.1 demonstrates the use of the models and frameworks to sustain hope in individual patients and families on their unique journey.

Case study 12.1　Part 1

Tom is a 60-year-old gentleman who was diagnosed with small-cell lung cancer last year. Tom is married to Edith and they are due to celebrate their ruby wedding anniversary next year. Neither Tom nor Edith has any brothers or sisters and they have no children. Edith explains that they are 'best friends', sharing an interest in the sea and sailing. They have, however, two close friends, Joe and his wife, Meg, whom they met at a sailing event almost 25 years ago. Both couples live in a small coastal town and have spent much of their time at a local boating club, where Joe and Meg keep their small dinghy. The four friends sail regularly. Both Tom and Joe have been sailing instructors at weekends, keen to pass on their love of the sport to local youngsters.

At the time of his diagnosis, Tom's disease responded well to chemotherapy and radiotherapy. Tom, however, found the treatment onerous and became very weak, fatigued and spoke of feeling that his situation was 'hopeless'. His GP diagnosed clinical depression and treated Tom's depression successfully with antidepressant medication. Once he was feeling better, Tom decided, however, that should his disease recur, he would not have further treatment, but would opt for palliative care. He retired from his job as a teller at the local bank on the grounds of ill health and to make more time for the things he wanted to do.

Two weeks ago Tom developed multiple pains and on admission to the local oncology unit was found to have metastatic disease in his liver and bones. Further chemotherapy was offered, but declined. Tom had palliative radiotherapy for the bone pain and was discharged home. Edith, Meg and Joe all visited during this period. Edith was pleased to have Tom home, particularly as she did not drive and she had to depend on Meg or Joe for transport into town.

When Tom was discharged home from hospital, the primary care team – in particular the GP and Mary, the district nurse – resumed his care, supported by Esther, the community specialist palliative care nurse. Figure 12.1 sets out Tom's support network on his illness journey.

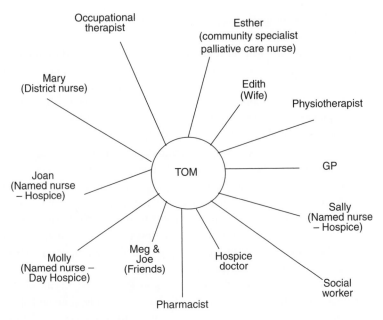

Figure 12.1 Tom's support network.

The Gold Standards Framework

The Gold Standards Framework is a programme aimed at enhancing palliative care in the community setting (Thomas 2003; King et al. 2005; Munday et al. 2007; Thomas & Noble 2007). It has been widely adopted by primary care teams across the United Kingdom, although there is 'considerable variation' in its implementation in different practices (Munday et al. 2007: 492). Central to the GSF is the development of a palliative care register to identify patients who are thought to be in the last year of life, the assessment of their needs and preferences and the setting up of a regular multidisciplinary team meeting (Thomas & Noble 2007). The purpose of this meeting is to anticipate and plan care that may be needed in response to patient and family priorities in the palliative phase and at the end of life. In a recent study, primary healthcare teams identify some of the benefits of having a palliative care register and these include increased awareness amongst general practice staff of patients' needs, fast tracking of patients for appointments or visits and ensuring effective arrangements are made for out-of-hours care (Munday et al. 2007). The framework also incorporates continuing practice-based education and audit.

As part of the GSF, the primary care team are encouraged to engage in advance care planning with patients and families in the palliative care phase of illness. Advance care planning has a variety of meanings (Horne et al. 2009), but here the term is used to describe an ongoing process of discussion between an individual and their healthcare provider, and sometimes those close to them, about future care (NHS End of Life Care Programme 2007; Conroy et al. 2009). It generally takes place 'in the context of an anticipated deterioration' in the patient's condition (NHS End of Life Care Programme 2007: 4) and is intended to alleviate patient concerns (Barnes et al. 2007). It may include discussion of the patient's understanding of illness, prognosis and their preferences for type and place of care. In relation to the complex issue of preferred place of care, it is suggested that, although approximately 50% of people with a life-threatening illness wish to die at home, less than 20% do so (DH 2004). A recent study indicates that identifying preferred place of care and planning to achieve it may lead to a significant increase in the number of patients dying at home (Wood et al. 2007), but more studies are required. Care must be taken, however, to ensure that the patient wishes and is ready to have this type of advance care conversation (Barnes et al. 2007; Conroy et al. 2009; Horne et al. 2009).

For the staff at Tom's GP practice the GSF builds upon existing high standards of care and supportive team relationships – both features that make a primary care team 'much better placed' to provide high-quality palliative care (Munday et al. 2007: 493). Mary, Tom's district nurse, and his GP have taken part in a local education project that involves shadowing their specialist palliative care counterparts at the local hospice. As a consequence of the GSF and the shadowing project, the primary care team are aware of the importance of early involvement of the community specialist palliative care team. Esther is the community specialist palliative care nurse linked to their practice, and her involvement in Tom's care was initiated at the multidisciplinary GSF meeting.

Together Esther and Mary start the process of advance care planning with Tom and, at Tom's request, involving his wife Edith. Over a number of visits Mary and Esther explore Tom and Edith's understanding of his illness and its prognosis, concerns about pain and symptom control and concerns about emotional and spiritual issues. They discuss the quality of communication and support available to Tom and Edith through Meg, Joe and other friends and neighbours. Tom is concerned that Edith is getting weary and 'hasn't a moment to herself'. Esther suggests that Tom might like to consider attending the day hospice one day a week. Mary and Esther sensitively discuss the possibility of dying and decisions that Tom and Edith might wish to make. Tom indicates that he would like to die at home with his wife and close friends at his side. Tom and Edith's wishes are documented and he is assured that he can review these at any time. Following each meeting, Esther and Mary reflect on what has been learned from this discussion and how they might continue the process of advance care planning as time goes on. They reflect upon and share the emotions that these conversations have evoked in them. The information from the advanced care planning is shared with other members of the primary care team at the next GSF meeting, and plans to enable Tom to stay at home are commenced.

Hope and the Gold Standards Framework

While more research is needed to evaluate the patient and family outcomes when using the GSF and the advance care planning process (King et al. 2005; Munday et al. 2007; Horne et al. 2009), the principles that underpin them are clearly linked with approaches for fostering hope. For Tom, being placed on the palliative care register and having his data on the out-of-hours record means that he and Edith do not always need to repeat the story of his illness journey to the GP practice receptionist, locums and the out-of-hours services. This prevents the sense of isolation and abandonment that can confront patients and their families at times of crisis, hindering hopefulness (Herth 1990; Buckley & Herth 2004). Early involvement of the district nurse, GP and community specialist palliative care nurse has enabled Mary and Esther to build a therapeutic and caring relationship with Tom and Edith. It has also ensured that pain and symptom assessment and management have been carefully addressed with the use of local palliative care guidelines (NHS Lothian 2009). The process of advance care planning is underpinned by a patient-centred approach that empowers Tom and Edith to make choices and to maintain a sense of control over events, so important for sustaining hope (Flemming 1997). The conversations with Mary and Esther have made Edith and Tom feel valued as individuals by the healthcare team. A recent study indicates that providing opportunities for patients and families to discuss their suffering and hope may also promote a trusting relationship with healthcare professionals and provide opportunities for a couple to explore and discover new strategies for coping with the palliative care phase of illness (Benzein & Saveman 2008).

During his attendance at the day hospice, Tom has shared any concerns he has with Molly, his named nurse for day care services. He has enjoyed looking out at the sea from the day hospice windows and working with the occupational therapist on his life story. Life review is considered an important means of fostering hope (Johnson 2007; Boog 2008a). The life-book that Tom and the occupational therapist are developing in partnership reflects on how Tom's life and that of Edith, Meg and Joe are all intertwined with their shared love of the sea and sailing. Tom is having two copies bound – one for Edith and one for Meg and Joe. This work has allowed Tom to share uplifting memories and create a legacy for his wife and friends, thus contributing to the sustaining of hope (Johnson 2007; Boog 2008a; Boog & Tester 2008).

Case Study 12.1   Part 2

Over a period of two months Tom is cared for by the primary care team, the community specialist palliative care nurse and the day hospice team. Tom becomes increasingly breathless and he has multiple pains that are proving difficult to control, despite careful assessment and review of his symptoms and a number of changes of medication. Esther, the community specialist palliative care nurse, suggests to the primary care team that it may be useful for Tom to go into the hospice for a brief spell to try to get his complex symptoms under control with a view to returning home again. She discusses this with Tom, who feels that he now knows the hospice well enough to consider this. It is agreed that he and Edith will go to the hospice the following morning.

On admission to the hospice, Tom and Edith are introduced to Sally and Joan, who explain their role as named nurses. During the admission assessment, Tom tells Sally and the doctor that his pain has become worse over the last few weeks and it is 'getting him down'. This feeling is obvious in his demeanour during the admission interview and, having received a comprehensive past medical history from the GP, the hospice doctor wonders briefly about depression. Tom, however, becomes more animated when he talks about the support Edith gives him and he describes her as his 'best friend'. Tom continues to speak in an animated tone when he mentions his love for the sea. He admits that he has been unable to go on boat trips due to the increased pain and feeling of breathlessness.

When Sally asks Tom about his expectations of coming into the hospice, he states that he would like his pain resolved, to feel stronger and to get back to his home. Tom explains to Sally that he knows he is 'not going to beat the cancer' and understands that he is going to die. If it is possible he would like to die at home with Edith. Over the next few days Tom's medications are reviewed and his comfort levels monitored. He spends his days chatting with Edith, Joe and Meg, over sips of espresso coffee and enjoying short walks in the garden. Tom also spends time alone in the hospice's quiet space, appreciating the peace, tranquillity and beautiful sea view. Every Monday, he enjoys reading his weekly boating magazine with a cup of his favourite espresso coffee, something he has not missed in 25 years.

Person-centred care

A recent model of palliative care (see Figure 12.2) promotes patient- and family-centred care whilst identifying how responses to loss and maintaining aspects which give pleasure can be influential in improving quality of life (Dougan & Colquhoun 2006). This model is used to consider Tom and Edith's care at the hospice.

A patient who is facing a life-threatening illness will undoubtedly experience multiple losses from many aspects of their life. Supporting adjustment to these losses is important in

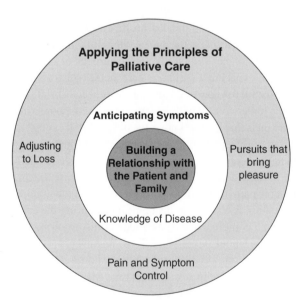

Figure 12.2 Model of palliative care.
Copyright © Elsevier 2006, reproduced with permission.

providing person-centred care (Dougan & Colquhoun 2006). Losses for Tom may include his job, the boat trips with friends and perhaps also the work with young people as a sailing instructor. Initial contact with hospice services can provide the opportunity to identify aspects affecting social and spiritual wellbeing (Prince-Paul 2008). This requires good communication skills which, it has been suggested, can be acquired from experience and reflection (Pennell & Bryan 2008). These skills are particularly important in identifying patient concerns; Heaven and Maguire (1996) state that inadequate communication can result in inadequate assessment within this area. Demonstration of sound communications skills, such as displaying empathy and using active listening, are key to this. It is suggested that understanding the patient's experience is central to building relationships (Stein-Parbury 2005). The process of understanding another person's situation can be challenging. However, the responsibility lies with the nurse to create an environment where this understanding can be facilitated (Stein-Parbury 2005). Dougan and Colquhoun (2006) use the named nurse concept to implement their model of palliative care, as this role presents an ideal opportunity for the nurse, patient and family to build a therapeutic relationship.

Teamwork is integral to palliative care and, where this involves an increase in team membership, which is often seen in palliative care, this presents challenges for effective team working and communication (Pearce & Duffy 2005). Often when caring for very ill patients, other healthcare professionals have information which is required for successful care delivery (Hall et al. 2007). In the palliative care phase of a patient's illness, there can be many health professionals involved from a variety of care settings (see Figure 12.1). Patients are often asked the same questions repeatedly by different team members (Faulkner 1998). With fatigue a common symptom (Sweeney et al. 2004), it is vital that communication is coordinated. In this case study, the named nurse role is particularly important at this point in the coordination and communication of care to the many healthcare professionals involved, especially during admission to, and discharge from, different care services. These principles are central to national and local palliative and end-of-life care policy (Scottish Government 2008).

Hope and person-centred care

Prior to admission, Tom had been experiencing increased pain and episodes of breathlessness. The doctors, pharmacist and nurses work together in assessing the effectiveness of interventions. Tom requires to be open and honest about his symptoms if physical comfort is to be achieved. The management of symptoms is considered to be hope-sustaining in itself (McIntyre & Chaplin 2007) and the process is key to building relationships. Tom's symptoms are managed over the next few days and Edith is relieved to see that he is settled. Tom has identified that friends, Joe and Meg, are very important to him. The hospice team should take opportunities to build relationships to support everyone who is involved in Tom's life. Building relationships is vital, not only in supporting Tom and Edith, but also for promoting and sustaining hope (Buckley & Herth 2004; McIntyre & Chaplin 2007).

The multidisciplinary team work together closely. The doctor and Sally, the named nurse, ensure that the admission of Tom is carried out together. Not only does this promote a team approach, it also reduces time spent on admission and conserves Tom's energy for the things that are important to him. Tom frequently speaks about his love for the sea. It is clear that this has been an important pleasure which he shares with his wife and close friends. Facilitating opportunities that can bring pleasure may support patients and families in remaining hopeful (McIntyre & Chaplin 2001). These pleasures are often small things, illustrated by Tom's enjoyment over many years of reading his weekly boating magazine with his favourite espresso coffee. As a result of his illness, Tom is no longer able to go on boat trips with his friends. However Tom, adjusting to this loss, can still enjoy looking at the sea view with his friends and reminiscing over holiday photographs and memories. This is also an example of how hope may change and transform over the illness journey (Herth 1990; Houldin 2000; Vanistendael 2007). Tom spends some time alone, reflecting on events of the past – for example friendships, hobbies – and it is suggested that this process can also inspire hope (McIntyre & Chaplin 2001; Boog 2008a).

If hope is to be sustained, it is important that any identified goals are achieved where possible and for the patient and family to retain choice and control (Flemming 1997). Tom's request to die at home is discussed at the hospice's weekly multidisciplinary team meeting a few days later. The occupational therapist, physiotherapist, social worker, pharmacist, doctors, community specialist palliative care nurse and the named nurses attend this meeting. Afterwards Joan and the doctor meet with Tom and Edith to discuss discharge. Discharge planning is started, aiming for Tom to go home on the following Wednesday. Joan, Tom's named nurse, is identified as the discharge coordinator and she will oversee the discharge process. Tom has been placed on the GSF palliative care register and the hospice doctor will ensure up-to-date information is available for access by the GP and out-of-hours services. This communication is vital in supporting Tom and Edith at home. As part of the discharge process, Tom's resuscitation status requires to be considered. The district nurse and the GP discussed this sensitively with Tom and Edith as part of the advance care planning discussion before admission to the hospice. The appropriate form indicating Tom's resuscitation status was completed and this was reviewed by the hospice doctor on admission and now prior to discharge (NHS Lothian 2007). Joan organises ambulance transport for Tom, and she informs the ambulance team that the end-of-life care plan, recently devised by the Scottish Ambulance Service, is relevant (Scottish Ambulance Service & Scottish Partnership for Palliative Care 2008). Joan also discusses the discharge with Molly, who is Tom's named nurse in the day hospice. Molly comes to see Tom and Edith and explains that he will be able to return to the day hospice following his discharge home. Edith visits Tom at the hospice every day and the named nurses, Joan and Sally, update her with information regarding the discharge. They also ascertain if Edith requires any additional support.

There are many professionals involved in discharge arrangements and this is evident in Tom's care (see Figure 12.1). Tom and Edith are encouraged to participate in the discharge planning. Creating such a partnership with patients, where democratic decision making and retaining a sense of control are maintained, is considered fundamental to fostering hope (Cutcliffe 1995).

Case study 12.1   Part 3

When Edith visits on Sunday she mentions to Joan that she thinks Tom is sleepy today. Edith explains that Tom was not feeling able to go and have his usual afternoon coffee and she has left him looking at photographs from their boating holidays over the years. Joan confirms that Tom had requested to stay in bed today. Edith decides to leave early and get some rest before Tom comes home on Wednesday. The following morning, before her visit, Edith telephones to ask how Tom is. Sally informs her that he had become frightened and very breathless overnight and has only managed a small amount of cereal before going back to sleep. When Edith visits, Tom is again very sleepy and is not interested in the magazine or coffee. Edith speaks to Sally of her concerns about taking Tom home, as she wonders if it is now too late. They agree that Sally should discuss this with the doctors and other members of the hospice team. A little later, the doctor and Sally speak with Edith. Edith says she thinks that Tom is less well and thinks he might be dying. Sally and the doctor confirm that these are their thoughts too and that it may be best for Tom to remain at the hospice, as Edith has suggested. When asked about staying at the hospice, Tom says 'that's okay – as long as I am comfortable and can see the sea sometimes – that will be fine' before drifting off to sleep.

After this conversation with Edith and Tom, Sally and the multidisciplinary team discuss how Tom has perhaps entered the last few days of his life. Sally spends time with Edith, explaining how the end-of-life care that Tom will receive will be supported by the Liverpool Care Pathway for the Dying Patient. Sally ascertains whether Edith feels she wants to be involved in Tom's care and she also tries to identify how Edith is coping now that Tom's condition has deteriorated.

Edith, Meg and Joe are supported by Joan and Sally, who inform them of any changes in Tom's condition. They stay at the hospice night and day until at 9 a.m. on Thursday morning Tom dies very peacefully with Edith and his close friends, Meg and Joe, at the bedside.

After Tom has died Sally, the named nurse, encourages Edith, Joe and Meg to sit with Tom for as long as they wish, before leading them to the hospice quiet room. While the doctor certifies the death, Sally makes tea for Edith and her friends. Over tea, Edith talks about Tom, his illness and his peaceful death and then she asks what she needs to do now. Sally, who has been actively listening to Edith, gently explains about registering Tom's death and arranging the funeral. Joe has done this recently for an elderly uncle and offers to assist Edith. Sally also speaks with Edith about the nature of bereavement and of available sources of support, should she need it. Written information on the practical and psychological issues is also given. Once Edith has sat with Tom one last time, Joe and Meg take Edith home. After they have left, Sally contacts Mary, the district nurse, and Esther, the community specialist palliative care nurse, to let them know of Tom's death. The hospice doctor contacts the GP. This allows for support in the community. A bereavement risk assessment is completed by Sally and the hospice doctor, highlighting the close relationship of Edith with Tom. At the multidisciplinary meeting the following week the hospice team have the opportunity to reflect on the care of Tom and Edith. The LCP document is audited at a later date.

Liverpool Care Pathway for the Dying Patient

The LCP is a multidisciplinary care plan that guides practitioners to offer evidence-based care in the last days of life (Ellershaw & Wilkinson 2003; Ellershaw 2006). When a patient is believed to be in their last days of life it is at this point that the pathway becomes the 'central organising tool for clinical activity' whilst incorporating clinical policies and procedures (Ellershaw & Murphy 2005: 132). It is based around a set of goals relating to physical comfort and psychological, social and spiritual care. The LCP also provides a structure for education and audit, allowing practitioners to measure outcomes of care for a particular patient and across a service.

Mirando et al. (2005) highlight the importance of achieving excellence when caring for the dying person, and that the care provided at this time should be evidence-based. Palliative care faces the challenge of transferring what is regarded as best practice principles for caring for the dying from the hospice sector into other healthcare settings (Ellershaw & Murphy 2005). The LCP was originally devised to take the hospice model of caring for the dying into non-hospice settings (Jack et al. 2003; Ellershaw & Murphy 2005; Gambles et al. 2006). More recently it has been implemented in hospice settings, as can be seen in the case study.

Recognising the dying process can be difficult (Ellershaw & Ward 2003). The LCP aids this identification by outlining criteria for starting to use the document. However, introducing the LCP does not take the place of clinical judgement, but supports decision making (Ellershaw & Murphy 2005). The document comprises three sections: initial assessment undertaken when the patient is thought to be dying, ongoing assessment and care after death. Box 12.2 summarises the goals of the LCP, which is regularly revised. An example of the current version of the LCP can be found at the website of the Marie Curie Palliative Care Institute Liverpool (2009).

Box 12.2 Summary of LCP goals

1 Initial assessment

Current medication assessed and non-essentials discontinued.
PRN subcutaneous medication written up.
Discontinue inappropriate interventions.
Ability to communicate in English assessed as adequate.
Insight into condition assessed (patient and family).
Religious and spiritual needs assessed (patient and family).
Identify how family is to be informed of patient's impending death.
Family given information about hospice facilities.
GP practice is aware of patient's condition.
Plan of care discussed with patient and family.
Family express understanding of plan of care.

2   Assessment of ongoing care

Regular assessment of: pain, agitation, respiratory tract secretions, nausea and vomiting, dyspnoea, mouth care, micturition, bowel care, medication given safely and accurately, pressure area care, psychological insight, religious and spiritual support, care of family and others.

3   Care after death

GP practice contacted about patient's death.
Procedure for last offices followed.
Procedure following a death discussed.
Family given information on hospice procedures.
Hospice policy followed for patient's valuables and belongings.
Necessary documentation and advice is given to appropriate person.
Bereavement leaflet given.

Reproduced with kind permission from the LCP Central Team UK at the Marie Curie Palliative Care Institute Liverpool

The initial assessment explores areas such as resuscitation status although, in many cases, this discussion will have taken place prior to the LCP being considered. The LCP also encourages anticipatory prescribing for key symptoms that may occur in the last hours and days of life – pain, nausea, agitation and restlessness, breathlessness and respiratory tract secretions (Glare et al. 2003). Anticipating symptoms is also a key component of the model of palliative care in Figure 12.2 (Dougan & Colquhoun 2006). Following the initial assessment, the ongoing process allows regular assessment of specific goals (see Box 12.2) to be either achieved or at variance. A variance is where, for some reason, a goal is not achieved. For example, if a patient is assessed to have pain, this would be recorded as a variance. Action would be taken, such as the administration of analgesia, and the situation reviewed.

There is a growing body of evidence showing the potential benefits and challenges of using the LCP in non-hospice settings (Jack et al. 2003; Hockley et al. 2005) and in hospice settings (Ellershaw et al. 2001; Gambles et al. 2006) (see Table 12.1). In a study by Gambles et al. (2006), for example, participants highlight many benefits of the LCP including the streamlined documentation which allows more time for practitioners to spend with patients and families. Others also argue that the LCP has an important role in hospice care to provide a structured, multidisciplinary document which evidences care given in the last days of life (Foster et al. 2003; Gambles et al. 2006). Care pathways can be used as an education and audit tool that empowers staff to monitor and improve care (Ellershaw et al. 2001; Foster et al. 2003; Mirando et al. 2005). However, the study by Gambles et al. (2006: 421) also suggests the possibility that the pathway's structured approach may negatively affect the 'art' or 'intuitiveness' integral to providing care in the dying phase, although these fears are not confirmed by the study results. However, interestingly, Kelly (2003: 39) suggests there is a risk that the dying process may become 'standardised to such a degree that reality is reduced to a flow diagram and palliative care is

Table 12.1 Potential benefits and challenges of the LCP

Potential benefits	Challenges
Reduced workload due to more appropriate referrals to services (Mellor et al. 2004)	'Another paper exercise' (Mellor et al. 2004)
Reduced documentation and time saving (Gambles et al. 2006)	Increased workload (Mellor et al. 2004)
Incorporates policies and procedures (Ellershaw & Murphy 2005)	Time needed for education (Mellor et al. 2004)
Aide-memoire (Jack et al. 2003; Gambles et al. 2006)	Lack of palliative care knowledge (Watson et al. 2006)
Continuity of care – being able to 'track care' (Ellershaw & Murphy 2005; Gambles et al. 2006)	Difficulty in 'diagnosing death' (Jones & Johnstone 2004; Watson et al. 2006)
Promotes appropriate communication (Gambles et al. 2006)	Staff/organisations not being open and receptive to change (Watson et al. 2006)
Teaching and education tool (Gambles et al. 2006)	Implementation can be resource intensive (Jones & Johnstone 2004; Mirando et al. 2005)
Research and audit tool (Gambles et al. 2006)	Challenge to change culture within an organisation (Ellershaw & Murphy 2005)

simply a series of boxes to be ticked by professional care givers'. Some of these arguments about the benefits and risks are also rehearsed in recent press coverage of the LCP (Bunyan & Smith 2009; Smith 2009). Taylor (2005), however, emphasises the importance of education to promote the LCP, not as a means of standardising care, but rather of ensuring a high standard of care. More research into the outcomes of using the LCP is required.

The final section of the LCP sets a number of goals for care after death (See Box 12.2). The LCP guides staff on key issues such as advice to relatives around legal and practical procedures following the death. Psychological aspects of care are also included, such as offering information to relatives about the impact of bereavement and facilitating grieving, by enabling the family to reflect on the death that has just taken place (Wilkinson & Mula 2003).

It is argued, therefore, that the LCP can contribute in some ways to meeting the challenges of improving care of the dying, while also encouraging future developments in practice, education and research (Ellershaw & Murphy 2005). Using the LCP may also have the potential to sustain hopefulness.

Hope and the Liverpool Care Pathway for the Dying Patient

Implementing the LCP can be daunting in that it creates a 'time frame' for the dying process (Lhussier et al. 2007). However, through the use of a pathway, staff may be able to communicate more confidently to families the uncertainties present at this time (Lhussier et al. 2007). Where the nurse has had the opportunity to build a relationship with the patient and family, interaction can be more meaningful. Effective communication is a vital thread that runs through all aspects of end-of-life care and is central to good patient care (Wilkinson & Mula 2003). The LCP not only acts as a tool to aid communication within the team, but also encourages communication with patient and family (Hockley et al. 2005; Gambles et al. 2006). As indicated earlier, sound communication and carefully built relationships are considered to engender hopefulness.

The initial assessment allows the hospice team to review Tom's condition, to ensure that non-essential treatments are discontinued and that anticipatory prescribing to promote physical comfort is in place. The doctor explains to Edith that, due to increased periods of sleepiness, Tom is not managing his oral medications and suggests that he would now benefit from receiving medications subcutaneously via a syringe driver. Using the local palliative care guidelines (NHS Lothian 2009), the doctor converts Tom's oral analgesia into a subcutaneous preparation to ensure that Tom remains comfortable. The LCP supports evidence-based practice in relation to pain and symptom control. By assessing symptoms regularly, there is a record of care given to Tom, with clear documentation of whether any symptom control intervention has been effective or not. If not, action is taken and the situation is reviewed. Edith expresses her reassurance at the level of care Tom is receiving and feels relieved that Tom is comfortable. The importance of physical comfort in sustaining hope in the patient and family has been mentioned previously (Herth 1990; Houldin 2000; Buckley & Herth 2004; McIntyre & Chaplin 2007). Tom is now unconscious and so Edith spends her day holding his hand, helping with his mouth care and recalling events of their 39 years together.

Central to the care delivered with the LCP is the spiritual dimension, which is now considered an integral aspect of practice (Speck 2003). Spirituality is described as a unique concept for each individual and may encompass a search for meaning within life experiences which enables 'transcendence and hope' (Speck 2003: 91). It may also incorporate the individual's 'hopes and aspirations' (Boog 2008b: 70). Tom and Edith do not belong to any religious or faith group. The named nurse is in a privileged position to support Tom and Edith in identifying what is important to them. She can also encourage them to retain choice and control when adjusting to the losses experienced in the dying process. In earlier stages of Tom's illness, he has adjusted to many losses, but has gained control of aspects of his life that have given him pleasure and purpose. Spiritual issues for Tom are evident in the relationships he has with Edith, Joe and Meg. These relationships are further entwined with Tom's passion for the sea. Opportunities for spiritual quest and reflection on life have been identified as hope-fostering strategies (Vanistendael 2007). Health professionals can therefore encourage an environment conducive to hope by facilitating this process.

After Tom has died the LCP goals act as a guide for Sally, the named nurse. Much of the preparation for bereavement is undertaken through the care of the patient and family before the death (Field et al. 2007; Payne et al. 2008). For example, risk factors for the bereavement period may be identified by the hospice team at an earlier stage on the illness journey. The period after death, however, is particularly important and 'constant support' of the family is needed (Wilkinson & Mula 2003: 86). The use of good communication skills such as active listening and empathy by the named nurse over tea in the quiet room facilitates Edith to share uplifting memories of Tom, which may foster hopefulness

(Herth 1990; Buckley & Herth 2004). The LCP assists the named nurse, Sally, to have confidence in discussing bereavement and sources of support with Edith. Giving written information and ensuring that the primary care team and community specialist palliative care team know of Tom's death are important issues. It means that the GP, district nurse and community specialist palliative care nurse can be in contact with Edith, preventing her from feeling isolated and abandoned after Tom's death (Wilkinson & Mula 2003). Again this may help to sustain hope. The hospice multidisciplinary team meeting provides an opportunity for staff to reflect on episodes of end-of-life care, especially in situations which have been complex and challenging. This is not only about improving care for the future, but also about providing mutual support for staff – an important factor in sustaining hopefulness in the palliative care team.

A few months later Edith, Meg and Joe come, by invitation, to the Time of Remembrance event that is held in the hospice. This event brings bereaved families and their friends together with hospice staff to remember a life. Edith, Meg and Joe join the gathering in the quiet space with the view of the sea, and think back over times shared with Tom and of the legacy left, before setting out for home. Uplifting memories and legacy are recognised as hope-sustaining (Boog & Tester 2008).

The care of Tom and Edith, Meg and Joe in the last days of Tom's life indicates therefore how the LCP may be used to support the delivery of care before and after death. Summarising the role of the LCP, Cicely Saunders, founder of the hospice movement, said:

> All the careful details of the pathway . . . are a salute to the enduring worth of an individual life. Such an ending can help those left behind to pick up the threads of memory and begin to move forward.
>
> Saunders (2003: vi)

Models, frameworks and hope

While we have argued that there is the potential for palliative and end-of-life frameworks to sustain hope, more research is required into the outcomes of these frameworks (King et al. 2005; Main et al. 2006; Munday et al. 2007; Horne et al. 2009). Moreover, models and frameworks do not in themselves ensure good practice, as suggested in the recent media debate on the LCP (Bunyan & Smith 2009; Smith 2009). If models are to be effective they require to be thoughtfully introduced in a way that is in keeping with both the philosophy of palliative care and of successful change management. Teams need to feel ownership of the initiatives (King et al. 2005). Listening to staff, involving staff in reflective practice and providing education to support the use of frameworks are essential (Murphy 2003). When used in generalist settings, such as acute hospitals and care homes, education must include not only learning about the frameworks, but also further learning about palliative care. Ongoing facilitation is vital too, as demonstrated by Hockley et al. (2008) when introducing the GSF into a number of care homes in central Scotland. Finally, models and frameworks should be introduced in a culture that empowers staff to be reflective, that enables those caring for palliative care patients to look back and critically analyse the care they have offered and be motivated to progress their palliative and end-of-life practice. The delivery of good palliative and end-of-life care is dependent not only on the knowledge and skills of the practitioner but also on their self-awareness, motivation and life experience (Dougan & Colquhoun 2006).

Conclusion

As indicated at the outset, it is patients who are 'the origin and enduring source' of hope (Randall & Downie 2006: 210) and therefore healthcare staff cannot make patients and families hopeful. Similarly, the implementation of models and frameworks does not necessarily generate hope. There are, however, strategies that nurses can use, such as ensuring the patient's physical comfort and valuing the patient and family as individuals, that may sustain hope. The careful introduction of the models and frameworks outlined in this chapter may promote these strategies and support the delivery of high-quality and hope-sustaining palliative and end-of-life care wherever the patient may be – at home in the community, in the ambulance, in the hospital, in a care home or hospice.

Acknowledgements

We wish to thank current and former members of the St Columba's Hospice multi-disciplinary team for their comments on the first draft of this chapter. We are also grateful to Professor John Ellershaw, director, and Deborah Murphy, associate director, of the Marie Curie Palliative Care Institute Liverpool and Professor Keri Thomas, national clinical lead for the Gold Standards Framework Centre, for permitting us to discuss the concept of hope in palliative care in the context of their frameworks.

References

Audit Scotland (2008) *Review of Palliative Care Services in Scotland*. Available at: http://www.audit-scotland.gov.uk/docs/health/2008/nr_080821_palliative_care.pdf.

Barnes K, Jones L, Tookman A, King M (2007) Acceptability of an advance care planning interview schedule: a focus group study. *Palliative Medicine* 21: 23–8.

Benzein EG, Saveman B-I (2008) Health-promoting conversations about hope and suffering with couples in palliative care. *International Journal of Palliative Nursing* 14(9): 439–45.

Benzein E, Norberg A, Saveman B-I (2001) The meaning of the lived experience of hope in patients with cancer in palliative home care. *Palliative Medicine* 15(2): 117–26.

Boog K (2008a) Telling tales – the importance of narrative in our lives. In: Boog KM, Tester CY (eds) *Palliative Care: A Practical Guide for the Health Professional: Finding meaning and purpose in life and death*. Edinburgh: Churchill Livingstone/Elsevier.

Boog K (2008b) Spirituality. In: Boog KM, Tester CY (eds) *Palliative Care: A Practical Guide for the Health Professional: Finding meaning and purpose in life and death*. Edinburgh: Churchill Livingstone/Elsevier.

Boog K, Tester C (2008) All that was left . . . hope. In: Boog KM, Tester CY (eds) *Palliative Care: A Practical Guide for the Health Professional: Finding meaning and purpose in life and death.* Edinburgh: Churchill Livingstone/Elsevier.

Buckley J, Herth K (2004) Fostering hope in terminally ill patients. *Nursing Standard* **19**(10): 33–41.

Bunyan N, Smith R (2009) Pensioner died after being wrongly put on 'death pathway'. *Daily Telegraph* [online] 13 October. Available at: http://www.telegraph.co.uk/news/uknews/6311473/Pensioner-died-after-being-wrongly-put-on-death-pathway.html.

Conroy S, Fade P, Fraser A, Schiff R (2009) Advance care planning: concise evidence-based guidelines. *Clinical Medicine* **9**(1): 76–9.

Cooper J, Cooper DB (2006) Hope and coping strategies. In: Cooper J (ed.) *Stepping into Palliative Care 1: Relationships and Responses*, 2nd edn. Oxford: Radcliffe Publishing.

Cutcliffe JR (1995) How do nurses inspire and instil hope in terminally ill HIV patients? *Journal of Advanced Nursing* **22**: 888–95.

Department of Health (2004) Building on the Best: End of life Care Initiative. Available at: http://www.dh.gov.uk/en/Publicationsandstatistics/Lettersandcirculars/Dearcolleagueletters/DH_4084872.

Dougan HAS, Colquhoun MM (2006) The patient receiving palliative care. In: Alexander MF, Fawcett JN, Runciman PJ (eds) *Nursing Practice Hospital and Home: The Adult*, 3rd edn. Edinburgh: Churchill Livingstone/Elsevier.

Doyle D, Hanks G, Cherny NI, Calman K (2004) Introduction. In: Doyle D, Hanks G, Cherny N, Calman K (eds) *Oxford Textbook of Palliative Medicine*, 3rd edn. Oxford: Oxford University Press.

Duggleby W, Wright K (2004) Elderly palliative care: cancer patients' descriptions of hope-fostering strategies. *International Journal of Palliative Nursing* **10**(7): 352–9.

Ellershaw JE (2006) Integrated care pathways. In: Cooper J (ed.) *Stepping into Palliative Care 1 – Relationships and Responses*, 2nd edn. Oxford: Radcliffe Publishing.

Ellershaw JE, Murphy D (2005) The Liverpool Care Pathway (LCP): influencing the UK national agenda on the care of the dying. *International Journal of Palliative Nursing* **11**(3): 132–4.

Ellershaw J, Ward C (2003) Care of the dying patient: the last hours or days of life. *BMJ* **326**: 30–4.

Ellershaw J, Wilkinson S. (eds) (2003) *Care of the Dying: A Pathway to Excellence*. Oxford: Oxford University Press.

Ellershaw J, Smith C, Overill S, Walker SE, Aldridge J (2001) Care of the dying: setting standards for symptom control in the last 48 hours of life. *Journal of Pain and Symptom Management* **21**(1): 12–17.

Faulkner A (1998) *Effective Interaction with Patients*, 2nd edn. New York: Churchill Livingstone.

Field D, Payne S, Relf M, Reid D (2007) Some issues in the provision of adult bereavement support by UK hospices. *Social Science and Medicine* **64**(2): 428–38.

Flemming K (1997) The meaning of hope to palliative care cancer patients. *International Journal of Palliative Nursing* **3**(1): 14–18.

Foster A, Rosser E, Kendall M, Barrow K (2003) Implementing the Liverpool Care Pathway for the Dying Patient (LCP) in hospital, hospice, community and nursing home. In: Ellershaw J, Wilkinson S (eds) *Care of the Dying: A Pathway to Excellence*. Oxford: Oxford University Press.

Gambles M, Stirzaker S, Jack BA, Ellershaw JE (2006) The Liverpool Care Pathway in hospices: an exploratory study of doctor and nurse perceptions. *International Journal of Palliative Nursing* **12**(9): 414–21.

Gamlin R, Kinghorn S (1995) Using hope to cope with loss and grief. *Nursing Standard* **9**(48): 33–5.

Glare P, Dickman A, Goodman M (2003) Symptom control in care of the dying. In: Ellershaw J, Wilkinson S (eds) *Care of the Dying: A Pathway to Excellence*. Oxford: Oxford University Press.

Hall P, Weaver L, Gravelle D, Thibault H (2007) Developing collaborative person-centred practice: A pilot project on a palliative care unit. *Journal of Interprofessional Care* **21**(1): 69–81.

Heaven CM, Maguire P (1996) Training hospice nurses to elicit patient concerns. *Journal of Advanced Nursing* **23**: 280–6.

Herth K (1990) Fostering hope in terminally-ill people. *Journal of Advanced Nursing* **15**(11): 1250–9.

Herth K (2000) Enhancing hope in people with a first recurrence of cancer. *Journal of Advanced Nursing* **32**(6): 1431–41.

Herth K, Cutcliffe JR (2002) The concept of hope in nursing. 3: hope and palliative care nursing. *British Journal of Nursing* **11**(14): 977–83.

Hockley J, Dewar B, Watson J (2005) Promoting end-of-life care in nursing homes using an 'integrated care pathway' for the last days of life. *Journal of Research in Nursing* **10**(2): 135–52.

Hockley J, Watson J, Murray SM (2008) *The Midlothian 'Gold Standards Framework in Care Homes' Project*. Edinburgh: University of Edinburgh.

Horne G, Seymour J, Payne S (2009) Advance care planning: evidence and implications for practice. *End of Life Care* **3**(1): 58–64.

Houldin AD (2000) *Patients with Cancer: Understanding the Psychological Pain*. Philadelphia: Lippincott.

Jack BA, Gambles M, Murphy D, Ellershaw JE (2003) Nurses' perceptions of the Liverpool Care Pathway for the dying patient in the acute hospital setting. *International Journal of Palliative Nursing* **9**(9): 375–81.

Johnson S (2007) Hope in terminal illness: an evolutionary concept analysis. *International Journal of Palliative Nursing* **13**(9): 451–9.

Jones A, Johnstone R (2004) Reflection on implementing a care pathway for the last days of life in nursing homes in North Wales. *International Journal of Palliative Nursing* **10**(10): 507–9.

Kelly D (2003) A commentary on 'An integrated care pathway for the last two days of life'. *International Journal of Palliative Nursing* **9**(1): 39.

King N, Thomas K, Martin N, Bell D, Farrell S (2005) 'Now nobody falls through the net': Practitioners' perspectives on the Gold Standards Framework for community palliative care. *Palliative Medicine* **19**: 619–27.

Lhussier M, Carr SM, Wilcockson J (2007) The evaluation of an end-of-life integrated care pathway. *International Journal of Palliative Nursing* **13**(2): 74–81.

Marie Curie Palliative Care Institute Liverpool (2009) Example of the Liverpool Care Pathway for the Dying Patient (LCP). Available at: www.mcpcil.org.uk.

McIntyre R, Chaplin C (2001) Hope: the heart of palliative care. In: Kinghorn S, Gamlin R (eds) *Palliative Nursing: Bringing Comfort and Hope*. Edinburgh: Baillière Tindall.

McIntyre R, Chaplin J (2007) Facilitating hope in palliative care. In: Kinghorn S, Gaines S (eds) *Palliative Nursing: Improving End-of-life Care*, 2nd edn. Edinburgh: Churchill Livingstone/ Elsevier.

Main J, Whittle C, Treml J, Woolley J, Main A (2006) The development of an Integrated Care Pathway for all patients with advanced life-limiting illness – the Supportive Care Pathway. *Journal of Nursing Management* **14**: 521–8.

Mellor F, Foley T, Connolly M, Mercer V, Spanswick M (2004) Role of a clinical facilitator in introducing an integrated care pathway for the care of the dying. *International Journal of Palliative Nursing* **10**(10): 497–501.

Mirando S, Davies PD, Lipp A (2005) Introducing an integrated pathway for the last days of life. *Palliative Medicine* **19**(1): 33–9.

Munday D, Mahmood K, Dale J, King N (2007) Facilitating good process in primary palliative care: does the Gold Standards Framework enable quality performance? *Family Practice* **24**: 486–94.

Murphy D (2003) The education strategy to implement the Liverpool Care Pathway for the Dying Patient. In: Ellershaw J, Wilkinson S (eds) *Care of the Dying: A Pathway to Excellence*. Oxford: Oxford University Press.

National Institute for Health and Clinical Excellence (NICE) (2004) *Improving Supportive and Palliative Care for Adults with Cancer: the Manual.* Available at: http://www.nice.org.uk/nicemedia/pdf/csgspmanual.pdf.

NHS End of Life Care Programme (2007) *Advance Care Planning: A Guide for Health and Social Care Staff.* Available at: http://www.endoflifecareforadults.nhs.uk/eolc/files/F2023-EoLC-ACP_guide_for_staff-Aug2008.pdf.

NHS Lothian (2007) Do Not Attempt Resuscitation (DNAR) Policy. Available at: http://www.nhslothian.scot.nhs.uk/ourservices/palliative/documents/nhslothian_DNAR_policy_1207.pdf.

NHS Lothian (2009) Lothian Palliative Care Guidelines. Available at: http://www.palliativecareguidelines.scot.nhs.uk/

Owen DC (1989) Nurses' perspectives on the meaning of hope in patients with cancer: a qualitative study. *Oncology Nursing Forum* **16**(1): 75–9.

Payne S, Lloyd-Williams M, Kennedy V (2008) Bereavement care and hope. In: Lloyd-Williams M (ed.) *Psychosocial Issues in Palliative Care*, 2nd edn. Oxford: Oxford University Press.

Pearce CM, Duffy A (2005) Holistic care. In: Lugton J, McIntyre R (eds) *Palliative Care: The Nursing Role*, 2nd edn. Edinburgh: Churchill Livingstone/Elsevier.

Pennell M, Bryan L (2008) Key tips in communication skills when giving information. *End of Life Care* **2**(2): 27.

Prince-Paul M (2008) Relationships among communicative acts, social well-being, and spiritual well-being on the quality of life at the end-of-life in patients with cancer enrolled in hospice. *Journal of Palliative Medicine* **11**(1): 20–5.

Randall F, Downie RS (2006) *The Philosophy of Palliative Care: Critique & Reconstruction.* Oxford: Oxford University Press.

Saunders C (2003) Foreword. In: Ellershaw J, Wilkinson S (eds) *Care of the Dying: A Pathway to Excellence.* Oxford: Oxford University Press.

Scanlon C (1989) Creating a vision of hope: the challenge of palliative care. *Oncology Nursing Forum* **16**(4): 491–6.

Scottish Ambulance Service and Scottish Partnership for Palliative Care (2008) *End of Life Care Plan.* Available at: http://www.palliativecarescotland.org.uk/assets/files/publications/SAS_-_EOLCP_08-08.pdf.

Scottish Government (2008) *Living and Dying Well: A national action plan for palliative and end-of-life care in Scotland.* Edinburgh: NHS Scotland.

Scottish Partnership for Palliative Care (2007) *Palliative and end-of-life care in Scotland: the case for a cohesive approach.* Available at: http://www.palliativecarescotland.org.uk/assets/files/publications/Palliative_and_End_of_Life_Care_in_Scotland.pdf.

Smith R (2009) More training needed following concerns about death pathway: cancer tsar. *Daily Telegraph* [online] 17 October. Available at: http://www.telegraph.co.uk/health/healthnews/6345372/More-training-needed-following-concerns-about-death-pathway-cancer-tsar.html.

Speck P (2003) Spiritual/religious issues in care of the dying. In: Ellershaw J, Wilkinson S (eds) *Care of the Dying: A Pathway to Excellence.* Oxford: Oxford University Press.

Stein-Parbury J (2005) *Patient and Person: Interpersonal Skills in Nursing*, 3nd edn. Sydney, Australia: Churchill Livingstone/Elsevier.

Sweeney C, Neuenschwander H, Bruera E (2004) Fatigue and asthenia. In: Doyle D, Hanks G, Cherny N, Calman K (eds) *Oxford Textbook of Palliative Medicine*, 3rd edn. Oxford: Oxford University Press.

Taylor A (2005) Improving practice with the Liverpool Care Pathway. *Nursing Times* **101**(35): 36–7.

Thomas K (2003) *Caring for the Dying at Home: Companions on the journey.* Abingdon, UK: Radcliffe Medical Press.

Thomas K, Noble B (2007) Improving the delivery of palliative care in general practice: an evaluation of the first phase of the Gold Standards Framework. *Palliative Medicine* **21**: 49–53.

Vanistendael S (2007) Resilience and spirituality. In: Monroe B, Oliviere D (eds) *Resilience in Palliative Care: Achievement in Adversity*. Oxford: Oxford University Press.

Watson J, Hockley J, Dewar B (2006) Barriers to implementing an integrated care pathway for the last days of life in nursing homes. *International Journal of Palliative Nursing* **12**(5): 234–40.

Wilkinson S, Mula C (2003) Communication in the care of the dying. In: Ellershaw J, Wilkinson S (eds) *Care of the Dying: A Pathway to Excellence*. Oxford: Oxford University Press.

Wood J, Storey L, Clark D (2007) Preferred place of care: an analysis of the 'first 100' patient assessments. *Palliative Medicine* **21**: 449–50.

World Health Organization (2002) *National Cancer Control Programmes: Policies and managerial guidelines*, 2nd edn. Geneva: WHO. Available at: http://www.who.int/cancer/media/en/408.pdf.

Conclusion

Tonks N. Fawcett and Anne McQueen

This book has provided a compilation of perspectives across the range of cancer care. It has not addressed the whole range of aspects relevant to the care of individuals with cancer, nor has this been the intention. The aim has been to provide readers with a selection of highly relevant topics in cancer care, chosen to enhance their knowledge and understanding. The authors have demonstrated their particular expertise and passion in their area of cancer care and it is hoped that this will encourage readers to use and apply this in their practice.

While each chapter has a particular focus and is presented in a different style according to the author's position and perspective, the collected work brings together important features relevant to cancer care. The different perspectives illustrate the diverse nature of cancer care, including issues directly relevant to patients, nurses and doctors. The science and art of therapy and care are brought together in discussing treatments and care issues for patients and their families. The sensitivity necessary in caring for individuals with cancer is highlighted throughout the text.

The importance of ongoing research in medical and nursing care and the application of worthy science are paramount in advancing the quality of patient care. Progress in science and technology has facilitated improved diagnostic and therapeutic techniques, extended knowledge of genetics and enabled the development of more effective treatment options. This, combined with the increasing understanding of the psychosocial implications of a cancer diagnosis for the patient and the family and the emotional work of professional and lay carers, has added immensely to the quality of cancer care. While this book presents a limited view within the field of cancer care it has, through the text, illustrated the value of research in practice, the significance of advances in science, such as genetics, and the important contribution of work on the emotional aspects of caring.

Index